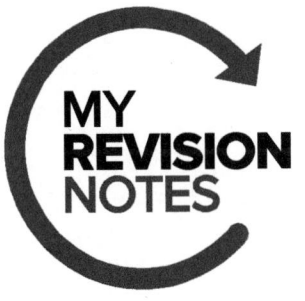

T-LEVELS
THE NEXT LEVEL QUALIFICATION

HEALTH

Liz Blamire
Stephen Hoare

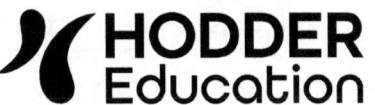

'T-LEVELS' is a registered trade mark of the Department for Education.

'T Level' is a registered trade mark of the Institute for Apprenticeships and Technical Education. The T Level Technical Qualification is a qualification approved and managed by the Institute for Apprenticeships and Technical Education.

Photo credits

p.16 © Dglimages/stock.adobe.com; **p.20** *l* © Martin Lee/stock.adobe.com; *r* © Andrey Popov/stock.adobe.com; **p.21** © AB Forces News Collection/Alamy Stock Photo; **p.30** Image taken on 13/01/2022 from www.instituteforapprenticeships.org – this information is subject to change and this URL should be used to access the most up to date information; **p.31** © Peenat/stock.adobe.com; **p.37** © Mykola Kovalchynsky/stock.adobe.com; **p.39** Contains public sector information published by the Health and Safety Executive and licensed under the Open Government Licence v3.0; **p.43** © Stocksolutions/stock.adobe.com; **p.44** © Gary L Hider/stock.adobe.com; **p.67** © Javidestock/stock.adobe.com; **p.69** © **Tyler Olson/stock.adobe.com**; **p.70** *l* © Sherry Young/stock.adobe.com; *r* © Anamejia18/stock.adobe.com; **p.80** © Monkey Business/stock.adobe.com; **p.85** © Lumos sp/stock.adobe.com; **p.86** © Tatsiana/stock.adobe.com; **p.87** © Zinkevych/stock.adobe.com; **p.95** © Tetiana/stock.adobe.com; **p.98** © Vector Archive/stock.adobe.com; **p.101** Crown Copyright/OHID in association with the Welsh government, Food Standards Scotland and the Food Standards Agency in Northern Ireland; **p.107** *l* © Jbrown/stock.adobe.com; *r* © Peakstock/stock.adobe.com; **p.108** © Rawpixel.com/stock.adobe.com; **p.112** Contains public sector information licensed under the Open Government Licence v3.0; **p.116** © Romaset/stock.adobe.com; **p.133** *b* © Aldona/stock.adobe.com; **p.136** © VectorMine/stock.adobe.com; **p.143** © GUNILLA ELAM/SCIENCE PHOTO LIBRARY; **p.158** © Olga/stock.adobe.com; **p.159** *t* © VectorMine/stock.adobe.com; *b,r* © STEVE GSCHMEISSNER/SCIENCE PHOTO LIBRARY; **p.173** *r* © Sakurra/stock.adobe.com; **p.177** © Vecton/stock.adobe.com; **p.183** © Designua/stock.adobe.com; **p.191** © Macrovector/stock.adobe.com; **p.193** © Olando/stock.adobe.com

Acknowledgements

p.13 © Institute for Apprenticeships and Technical Education 2024. This information is licensed under the Open Government Licence v3.0. To view this licence visit https://www.nationalarchives.gov.uk/doc/open-government-licence/; **p.113** © World Health Organization 2021. Licence: CC BY-NC-SA 3.0 IGO.

Although every effort has been made to ensure that website addresses are correct at time of going to press, Hodder Education cannot be held responsible for the content of any website mentioned in this book. It is sometimes possible to find a relocated web page by typing in the address of the home page for a website in the URL window of your browser.

Hachette UK's policy is to use papers that are natural, renewable and recyclable products and made from wood grown in well-managed forests and other controlled sources. The logging and manufacturing processes are expected to conform to the environmental regulations of the country of origin.

To order, please visit www.hoddereducation.com or contact Customer Service at education@hachette.co.uk / +44 (0)1235 827827.

ISBN: 978 1 3983 7894 0

© Liz Blamire and Stephen Hoare, 2024

First published in 2024 by
Hodder Education,
An Hachette UK Company
Carmelite House
50 Victoria Embankment
London EC4Y 0DZ

www.hoddereducation.co.uk

Impression number	10 9 8 7 6 5 4 3 2
Year	2028 2027 2026 2025 2024

All rights reserved. Apart from any use permitted under UK copyright law, no part of this publication may be reproduced or transmitted in any form or by any means, electronic or mechanical, including photocopying and recording, or held within any information storage and retrieval system, without permission in writing from the publisher or under licence from the Copyright Licensing Agency Limited. Further details of such licences (for reprographic reproduction) may be obtained from the Copyright Licensing Agency Limited, www.cla.co.uk

Cover photo © Drazen - stock.adobe.com

Illustrations by Aptara Inc. Barking Dog Art and Integra Software Services Pvt. Ltd

Typeset by Aptara Inc.

Printed and bound by CPI Group (UK) Ltd, Croydon, CR0 4YY

A catalogue record for this title is available from the British Library.

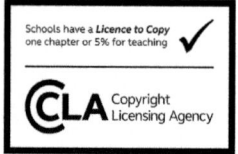

Get the most from this book

Everyone has to decide their own revision strategy, but it is essential to review your work, learn it and test your understanding. These Revision Notes will help you to do that in a planned way, topic by topic. Use this book as the cornerstone of your revision and don't hesitate to write in it – personalise your notes and check your progress by ticking off each section as you revise.

Tick to track your progress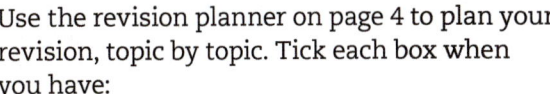

Use the revision planner on page 4 to plan your revision, topic by topic. Tick each box when you have:
+ revised and understood a topic
+ tested yourself
+ practised the exam questions and gone online to check your answers and complete the quick quizzes.

You can also keep track of your revision by ticking off each topic heading in the book. You may find it helpful to add your own notes as you work through each topic.

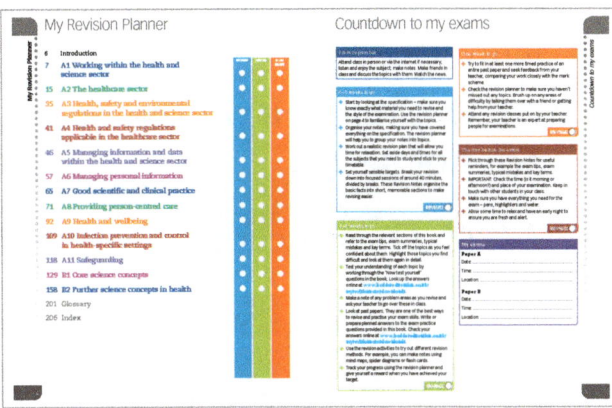

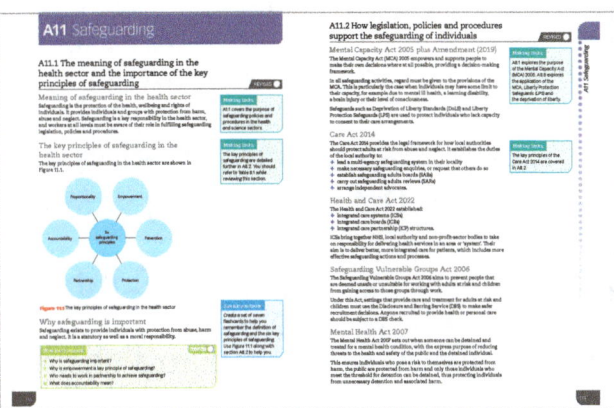

Features to help you succeed

Exam tips
Expert tips are given throughout the book to help you polish your exam technique and maximise your chances in the exam.

Typical mistake
The authors identify the typical mistakes candidates make and explain how you can avoid them.

Now test yourself
These short, knowledge-based questions provide the first step in testing your learning. Answers are provided online at www.hoddereducation.co.uk/myrevisionnotesdownloads

Definitions and key words
Clear, concise definitions of essential key terms are provided where they first appear.

Key words from the specification are highlighted in bold throughout the book.

Making links
This feature identifies connections between topics and tells you how revising these will aid your exam answers.

Revision activities
These activities will help you to understand each topic in an interactive way.

Exam practice
Exam-style practice questions are provided for each topic. Use them to consolidate your revision and practise your exam skills.

Online
Go online to check your answers to the questions and try out the extra quick quizzes at www.hoddereducation.co.uk/myrevisionnotesdownloads

My Revision Notes: Health T Level

My Revision Planner

- 6 Introduction
- 7 **A1 Working within the health and science sector**
- 15 **A2 The healthcare sector**
- 35 **A3 Health, safety and environmental regulations in the health and science sector**
- 41 **A4 Health and safety regulations applicable in the healthcare sector**
- 46 **A5 Managing information and data within the health and science sector**
- 57 **A6 Managing personal information**
- 65 **A7 Good scientific and clinical practice**
- 71 **A8 Providing person-centred care**
- 92 **A9 Health and wellbeing**
- 109 **A10 Infection prevention and control in health-specific settings**
- 118 **A11 Safeguarding**
- 129 **B1 Core science concepts**
- 158 **B2 Further science concepts in health**
- 201 Glossary
- 206 Index

Check your understanding and progress at www.hoddereducation.co.uk/myrevisionnotes

Countdown to my exams

From September

Attend class in person or via the internet if necessary; listen and enjoy the subject; make notes. Make friends in class and discuss the topics with them. Watch the news.

6–8 weeks to go

+ Start by looking at the specification – make sure you know exactly what material you need to revise and the style of the examination. Use the revision planner on page 4 to familiarise yourself with the topics.
+ Organise your notes, making sure you have covered everything on the specification. The revision planner will help you to group your notes into topics.
+ Work out a realistic revision plan that will allow you time for relaxation. Set aside days and times for all the subjects that you need to study and stick to your timetable.
+ Set yourself sensible targets. Break your revision down into focused sessions of around 40 minutes, divided by breaks. These Revision Notes organise the basic facts into short, memorable sections to make revising easier.

REVISED ◯

2–6 weeks to go

+ Read through the relevant sections of this book and refer to the exam tips, exam summaries, typical mistakes and key terms. Tick off the topics as you feel confident about them. Highlight those topics you find difficult and look at them again in detail.
+ Test your understanding of each topic by working through the 'Now test yourself' questions in the book. Look up the answers online at www.hoddereducation.co.uk/myrevisionnotesdownloads.
+ Make a note of any problem areas as you revise and ask your teacher to go over these in class.
+ Look at past papers. They are one of the best ways to revise and practise your exam skills. Write or prepare planned answers to the exam practice questions provided in this book. Check your answers online at www.hoddereducation.co.uk/myrevisionnotesdownloads.
+ Use the revision activities to try out different revision methods. For example, you can make notes using mind maps, spider diagrams or flash cards.
+ Track your progress using the revision planner and give yourself a reward when you have achieved your target.

REVISED ◯

One week to go

+ Try to fit in at least one more timed practice of an entire past paper and seek feedback from your teacher, comparing your work closely with the mark scheme.
+ Check the revision planner to make sure you haven't missed out any topics. Brush up on any areas of difficulty by talking them over with a friend or getting help from your teacher.
+ Attend any revision classes put on by your teacher. Remember, your teacher is an expert at preparing people for examinations.

REVISED ◯

The day before the exam

+ Flick through these Revision Notes for useful reminders, for example the exam tips, exam summaries, typical mistakes and key terms.
+ IMPORTANT: Check the time (is it morning or afternoon?) and place of your examination. Keep in touch with other students in your class.
+ Make sure you have everything you need for the exam – pens, highlighters and water.
+ Allow some time to relax and have an early night to ensure you are fresh and alert.

REVISED ◯

My exams

Paper A

Date: ....

Time: ....

Location: ....

Paper B

Date: ....

Time: ....

Location: ....

My Revision Notes: Health T Level

Introduction

The T Level exam papers

REVISED

In the first year of your T Level Health qualification, you will take two exams and complete an employer set project (ESP). This book focuses on the two exams, which assess the two core elements that you will learn in year one.

There are two papers – Paper A and Paper B – that cover the core elements between them.

	Paper A	Paper B
Weighting	34%	36%
Time allowed	2 hours 30 minutes	2 hours 30 minutes
Maximum marks	116	118
Section A	A1 – Working in the health and science sector A2 – The healthcare sector A7 – Good scientific and clinical practice	Body Systems 1: Cardiovascular system, respiratory system, nervous system and musculoskeletal system
Section B	A5 – Managing information and data within the health and science sector A6 – Managing personal information	Body Systems 2: Digestive system, renal system, integumentary system, reproductive system and endocrine system
Section C	A3 – Health, safety and environmental regulations in the health and science sector A4 – Health and safety regulations applicable in the healthcare sector A10 – Infection prevention and control in health-specific settings	Body Systems 3: Synoptic section that can assess any of the B1 and B2 content in combination. Core science concepts (B1) and cancer (B2.30 and B2.31) can be assessed in any section.
Section D	A8 – Providing person-centred care A9 – Health and wellbeing A11 – Safeguarding	

The remaining 30% of your grade is allocated to the ESP.

Question types

There are three types of question in papers A and B:
+ multiple-choice
+ short answer
+ extended response.

You need to be familiar with each type of question. Extended-response questions are usually worth more marks than multiple-choice and short-answer questions.

It is always a good idea to read through the whole exam paper before you start. This gives you a chance to calm your nerves and prepare yourself.

Take note of the types of questions on the paper and the marks allocated for each, as this will help you to know how much time to spend on each question. You need to make sure you leave yourself sufficient time for the extended response questions, which attract more marks.

Look carefully at the command words at the beginning of each short-answer and extended-response question, as these give you the instructions for answering the question. A list of the command words used in T Levels can be found on the NCFE website: www.ncfe.org.uk/qualification-search/qualification-detail/t-level-technical-qualification-in-health-level-3-delivered-by-ncfe-1644

Check your understanding and progress at www.hoddereducation.co.uk/myrevisionnotes

A1 Working within the health and science sector

A1.1 The purpose of organisational policies and procedures in the health and science sector

REVISED

Equality, diversity and inclusion policy

Equality, diversity and inclusion policies exist to ensure fair and equitable treatment of individuals and to prevent prejudice and discrimination. These are legal requirements for public-sector bodies such as the NHS.

An organisation's equality, diversity and inclusion policy sets out what it will do to comply with legislation. It helps to ensure equality in how people are treated and makes sure that an organisation does not practise discrimination. Following these procedures is beneficial for several reasons:
+ social inclusion is promoted
+ individuals are respected, celebrated and valued
+ the cycle of disadvantage is tackled.

Legislation governing equality, diversity and inclusion includes the Equality Act 2010 and, to some extent, the Human Rights Act 1998. Policies and procedures will reflect this legislation. Under the Equality Act 2010, it is illegal to discriminate against people based on certain protected characteristics:
+ age
+ disability
+ gender reassignment
+ marriage and civil partnership
+ pregnancy and maternity
+ race
+ religion or belief
+ sex
+ sexual orientation.

Discrimination may be direct or indirect and occurs when people are treated unfairly due to protected characteristics.

Policies and procedures are supported by the Human Rights Act 1998. This ensures that people are treated with dignity and respect and protects the freedoms and rights of people as individuals and as members of groups.

Safeguarding policy

Safeguarding policies provide guidelines on what an organisation must do to protect the health, wellbeing and human rights of individuals. These policies establish how individuals should be protected from harm, such as abuse and neglect. This includes service users, as well as staff and visitors, with particular responsibility for children, young people and more vulnerable adults.

Safeguarding policies should outline clearly the roles of different agencies involved in safeguarding, for example the role of:
+ local authority adult and children's social care services
+ GPs
+ hospitals
+ education settings
+ Ofsted
+ the Care Quality Commission (CQC).

> **Equality** Ensuring every individual has equal opportunities in life.
>
> **Policy** A document that sets out what an organisation will do, usually based on laws or regulations.
>
> **Legislation** A law or set of laws passed by Parliament.
>
> **Procedure** Instructions for how to follow an organisational policy.
>
> **Cycle of disadvantage** The concept that people who grow up in poverty are more likely to suffer from health problems, social isolation, housing instability and unemployment and are less likely to reach their full potential in life. This disadvantage, in turn, is transmitted to the next generation.
>
> **Safeguarding** The protection of the health, wellbeing and rights of individuals.

Typical mistake

Equality means ensuring everyone has equal opportunities and is treated the same. However, sometimes equity is required – when a person has different needs to reach an equal outcome. This could be providing sign language interpreters for people who are deaf or installing accessible toilets for people who use wheelchairs and other people with disabilities. Do not confuse equality with equity.

Making links

A11 looks at safeguarding in detail. For more on the roles of Ofsted and the CQC, see A8.3.

My Revision Notes: Health T Level

Employment contracts

All employees have an employment contract with their employer, to make clear the expectations the employer has of the employees and what they can expect in return.

There are four main elements of each employment contract, known as its terms (see Table 1.1).

Table 1.1 Employment contract terms

Terms	Examples
Employment conditions	Notice periods; salary/wages; dress code (if applicable)
Rights (guaranteed by the employer)	At least meeting the National Minimum Wage; holiday leave and pay; protection against unlawful discrimination
Responsibilities (of the employee)	To obey lawful and reasonable orders; to take reasonable care for health and safety
Duties	Tasks that are undertaken in a particular role, for example to assist service users with activities of daily living; also includes contributing to health and safety standards as per the Health and Safety at Work etc. Act 1974.

> **Exam tip**
> Although your exam paper is split into sections, the questions will draw upon knowledge from across the elements of the specification. For example, safeguarding is a fundamental concept and could be relevant to numerous questions.

Performance reviews

A performance review is a regular process carried out between manager and employee. The objectives of performance reviews are to:
+ evaluate employee performance against standards and expectations
+ provide feedback to the employee on how to improve
+ give the employee an opportunity to raise concerns
+ ensure there is continuing professional development (CPD), for instance by identifying further training needs.

Disciplinary policy

A disciplinary policy states how problems with employee performance or conduct will be dealt with by an organisation.

Disciplinary policies:
+ set out and maintain the expected standards of work and conduct
+ establish the procedures and sequence for disciplinary action when these standards are not met
+ ensure all employees are treated consistently and fairly.

For example, if an employee consistently failed to follow the correct handwashing procedure, the disciplinary policy would outline how their manager should deal with this. Should the employee continue to fail to comply, the disciplinary policy would outline next steps, such as supervised practice, final warning or termination of employment.

Grievance policy

A grievance policy provides a way for employees to formally raise concerns (grievances) at work. Grievance policies:
+ provide the opportunity for employees to raise a grievance confidentially
+ establish the procedure for employees to follow when raising a grievance, including how to appeal if they do not agree with any conclusions or decisions made.

> **Continuing professional development (CPD)** A process of continual learning and development to keep skills and knowledge up to date so that employees can work safely and effectively.
>
> **Grievance** A concern, problem or complaint someone may have at work.

For example, an employee makes a request for flexible working arrangements, as they are entitled to under law, but their manager refuses to review the request. The grievance policy outlines who the employee raises their grievance with, how to do this and the procedure their employer must follow in reviewing and making their decision on the grievance.

> **Revision activity**
>
> Make a concept map of the protected characteristics of the Equality Act 2010 and list examples for each of policies and procedures that can ensure discrimination does not occur.

> **Typical mistake**
>
> It is easy to confuse disciplinary, grievance and complaints policies. Remember: Employers can discipline their staff. Employees can raise grievances about their workplace. Service users can complain about their care.

> **Now test yourself** TESTED
>
> 1 Name **two** laws that underpin equality, diversity and inclusion.
> 2 What is the purpose of a safeguarding policy?
> 3 Name **three** things normally covered in an employment contract.
> 4 Why is a performance review important for employees?
> 5 What is the difference between a disciplinary and a grievance policy?

A1.2 The importance of adhering to quality standards, quality management and audit processes within the health and science sector

REVISED

Quality standards and quality management are sets of good practice, methods, systems or requirements to ensure consistent and safe products, processes and services.

Both can apply to internal working practices, such as purchasing and using equipment that is proven to be safe, as well as to the provision of care, such as following evidence-based practice when treating a patient.

Audit processes can help with continuous improvement and form part of objective, independent reviews, for example enquiries into failed safeguarding.

Various organisations at local, national and international level have responsibility for establishing quality standards and quality management.

The importance of adhering to quality standards, quality management and audit processes is shown in Figure 1.1.

> **Audit** An on-site verification activity, which checks compliance with an agreed standard.

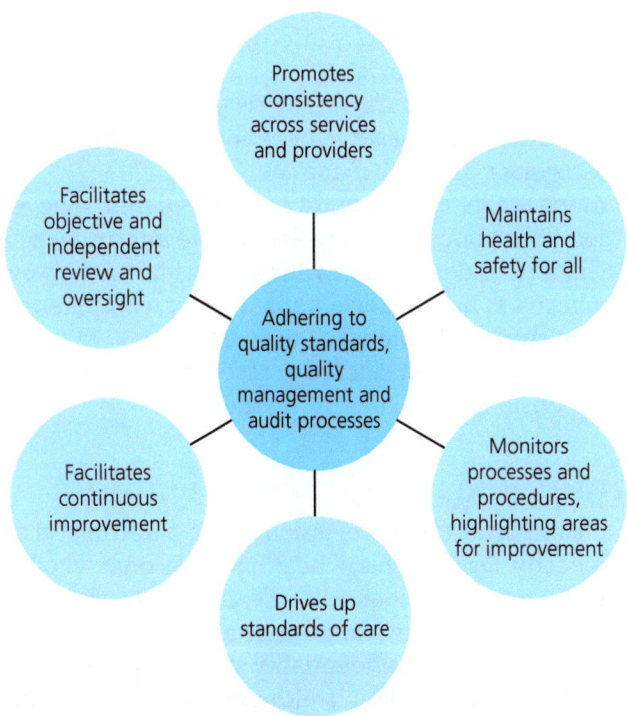

Figure 1.1 Reasons why it is important to adhere to quality standards, quality management and audit processes within the health and science sector

My Revision Notes: Health T Level

> **Now test yourself** TESTED
>
> 1 Give **two** reasons why it is important to follow quality standards, quality management and audit processes.
> 2 Describe what is meant by the term *audit*.

> **Typical mistake**
>
> Students sometimes forget that quality standards, quality management and audit processes are not just important for the safety of service users. Every quality standard, health and safety and safeguarding process also serves to protect the health, safety and wellbeing of individual staff members and their colleagues, as well as visitors to the setting.

> **Exam tip**
>
> It is useful to know some specific real-life examples of quality standards, quality management and audit processes used in the health and science sector. Then you can provide evidence of your knowledge and understanding in your answers.

A1.3 The key principles of ethical practice in the health and science sector

REVISED

Ethical practice describes ways of working that apply ethical values and decision-making. It is required in the everyday work of health professionals.

Ethical principles can also be used to enable difficult decisions to be made or dilemmas to be solved.

Autonomy and informed consent

- Within the health sector, personal autonomy describes the right of competent adults to make decisions about their care.
- This is directly linked to informed consent.
- To make an autonomous decision about proposed care or treatment, an individual must be fully informed about that care or treatment and must voluntarily agree to it.
- When an individual's capacity is under question, the Mental Capacity Act 2005 offers a framework for acting in the person's best interests when decisions need to be made.
- Young adults aged 16 and 17 are considered to have the capacity to make decisions about their care and to give informed consent.
- Children under the age of 16 can consent to their own treatment if they are believed to have sufficient intelligence, competence and understanding of what they are being asked to agree to.
- If a child is not considered to meet these conditions, an adult with parental responsibility can consent for them.

Truthfulness and confidentiality

- It is important that professionals are truthful and share information honestly. For example, a health professional who has taken a blood sample to test for an infectious disease must be truthful when discussing the results with the individual concerned.
- The principle of confidentiality states when and how information is to be shared. For example, a health professional only shares the result of the test with the individual concerned. This information can only be shared with others with the individual's consent.
- A responsibility to be truthful arises from the duty of candour, which is a requirement to be open and honest. This includes making individuals aware when mistakes are made in their care or treatment, apologising for these mistakes and, when possible, putting things right.

> **Ethical values** Moral principles that guide behaviour and conduct.
>
> **Autonomy** A person's ability to act in their own interests.
>
> **Competent** Having the necessary knowledge, skill or ability to do something.
>
> **Capacity** The ability to decide for yourself what is in your own best interest.

> **Making links**
>
> A8.1 covers more about mental capacity and discusses the Mental Capacity Act 2005 plus Amendment (2019) in detail.

> **Making links**
>
> The Data Protection Act 2018 and General Data Protection Regulations 2018 are two pieces of legislation that govern information handling, including principles and practice of confidentiality. They are covered in A5.6.
>
> The duty of candour is covered more fully in A6.9.

Beneficence

- **Beneficence** requires professionals to act in ways that benefit others, for example by choosing or promoting the best medical treatment for an individual.
- It does not override an individual's autonomy.
- What is best must be considered from the perspective of the individual and their values and choices.
- What is best for one individual is not necessarily best for another.

Nonmaleficence

- **Nonmaleficence** is the principle of not causing harm to others.
- This requires that professionals do not cause harm through an action, such as reusing disposable equipment, or an omission, such as failing to complete a scheduled check-up on a patient.

Justice

- Justice requires that any action taken by a health professional is compatible with the law, compatible with an individual's rights and is both fair and balanced.
- An example would be providing care and treatment to all individuals that require it, regardless of their protected characteristics under the Equality Act 2010, and ensuring individuals are not subject to inhuman treatment as prohibited by the Human Rights Act 1998.

> **Beneficence** The act of doing or producing something good.
>
> **Nonmaleficence** Not to do or allow harm to others.

> **Making links**
>
> The ethical principle of beneficence links strongly to person-centred care and the Care Act 2014 (see A8.2).

> **Exam tip**
>
> It is not enough just to know the meanings of terms such as nonmaleficence. You will need to be able to apply your knowledge of ethical terms to scenario-based questions. To prepare yourself for this, ensure you can give examples of each ethical principle in a healthcare context.

> **Now test yourself** TESTED
>
> 1. Why are the principles of autonomy and beneficence important to individuals?
> 2. What does the term *informed consent* describe?
> 3. How is nonmaleficence different to beneficence?
> 4. Which pieces of legislation are important to the principle of justice?

> **Revision activity**
>
> Draw a table and list each of the key principles of ethical practice. Write your own definition of each one and then find an example of this ethical principle being used in a healthcare setting.

A1.4 The purpose of following professional codes of conduct

REVISED

A code of **conduct** is a set of rules surrounding behaviour, attitudes, standards, values and principles which professionals must agree to follow.

Professionals, service users and the public can refer to a code of conduct and immediately see:
- the **mission**, values, principles and standards to which everyone working within the organisation must adhere
- the expected professional behaviours and attitudes of everyone working in the organisation
- the rules and responsibilities within the organisation.

A code of conduct also promotes confidence and trust in an organisation and those working within it.

> **Conduct** The way in which a person behaves, especially in a particular place or situation, such as at work.
>
> **Mission** An organisation's mission defines why it exists and what it intends to do (its purpose).

A code of conduct may be written by a professional body such as the Nursing and Midwifery Council (NMC), an organisation such as Skills for Health, or an employer.

Examples of what might be covered in a professional code of conduct include:
+ accountability
+ upholding privacy, dignity and rights
+ working safely and in collaboration with others
+ using open and honest communication
+ respecting confidentiality
+ improving the quality of the service provided
+ promoting equality, diversity and inclusion.

> **Accountability** To accept that you are responsible for your own actions.

Revision activity

Use the internet to find the *Code of Conduct for Healthcare Support Workers and Adult Social Care Workers in England*. Draw a spider diagram to illustrate how each of the seven points of the code of conduct support:
+ healthcare assistants
+ service users.

Typical mistake

When working in health and social care settings, workers are not just accountable to their employer and any relevant professional bodies, they are also accountable to the public. Health and social care workers are obliged to consider and work in the best interests of everyone.

Now test yourself — TESTED

1. Explain what the term *conduct* means in relation to a future job role you are interested in.
2. List **two** professional bodies for health professionals that have a code of conduct.
3. What is the purpose of following a professional code of conduct?

A1.5 The difference between technical, higher technical and professional occupations in health, healthcare science and science

REVISED

Table 1.2 outlines the difference between technical, higher technical and professional occupations in health with examples.

Table 1.2 The difference between technical, higher technical and professional occupations in health

	Occupational level		
	Technical occupations	**Higher technical occupations**	**Professional occupations**
Entry route, skills and qualifications required	Skilled occupations that a college leaver or an apprentice would be entering, typically requiring qualifications at levels 2/3	Require more knowledge and skills acquired through experience in the workplace or further technical education, and typically require qualifications at levels 4/5	There is a clear career progression from higher technical occupations, through university degrees, as well as occupations where a degree apprenticeship exists (level 6)
Type of role	Health assistant	Health practitioner	Health professional
Brief description of role	Provide direct patient contact and care, undertaking routine, well-defined clinical duties	Provide direct patient contact and high-quality care with in-depth knowledge of the factors influencing health and ill health using specialist expertise	Provide direct patient contact along with high-quality diagnosis and care, working independently and with other health professionals

Check your understanding and progress at www.hoddereducation.co.uk/myrevisionnotes

Examples	<ul><li>Ambulance support worker</li><li>Community health and wellbeing worker</li><li>Dental nurse</li><li>Healthcare support worker</li></ul>	<ul><li>Associate ambulance practitioner</li><li>Healthcare assistant practitioner</li><li>Hearing-aid dispenser</li><li>Nursing associate</li><li>Oral health practitioner</li></ul>	<ul><li>Diagnostic radiographer</li><li>Doctor</li><li>Midwife</li><li>Nurse</li><li>Occupational therapist</li><li>Psychological wellbeing practitioner</li></ul>

Table 1.3 Examples of healthcare science and science occupations

	Occupational level		
	Technical occupations	**Higher technical occupations**	**Professional occupations**
Examples	Healthcare science:<ul><li>Dental laboratory assistant</li><li>Pharmacy technician</li></ul>Science:<ul><li>Food technologist</li><li>Laboratory technician</li></ul>	Healthcare science:<ul><li>Clinical Dental technician</li><li>Dental Technician</li></ul>Science:<ul><li>Embalmer</li><li>Laboratory manager</li></ul>	Healthcare science:<ul><li>Dispensing Optician</li><li>Pharmacist</li></ul>Science:<ul><li>Biochemist</li><li>Laboratory Scientist</li><li>Physicist</li></ul>

Source: Adapted from the IfATE occupational maps, www.instituteforapprenticeships.org/media/1868/health-pdf.pdf

> **Exam tip**
>
> The questions in your exam contain contextual information. Some will specify a particular healthcare role. It is important to pay attention to this information because knowing the extent of the role (what the individual can and cannot do) will influence the content of your answer.

> **Revision activity**
>
> Healthcare scientists are a large group of workers in healthcare and have numerous roles at technical, higher technical and professional levels. Open the website: https://occupational-maps.instituteforapprenticeships.org/maps/route/health-science
>
> Scroll down to Healthcare Science. Make a table that lists two roles at each occupational level. Follow the layout of Table 1.2.

> **Now test yourself** TESTED
>
> 1 Write **two** sentences to describe the difference between technical, higher technical and professional occupations.
> 2 List **three** occupations at each occupational level that you are interested in.

> **Typical mistake**
>
> Remember, a medical doctor is the only professional that can always diagnose a medical condition and prescribe medication. Some other healthcare professions can do this, but only after undertaking additional training and/or qualifications. Ensure you are familiar with the extent of common roles and responsibilities for healthcare workers.

A1.6 Opportunities to support progression within the health and science sector

REVISED

There are several ways to progress your career. Figure 1.2 shows ways to support career progression within the health and science sector. Each way presents an opportunity to develop knowledge, skills and abilities, and to move up or gain entry to learning, training or a job, at one of the occupational levels described in A1.5.

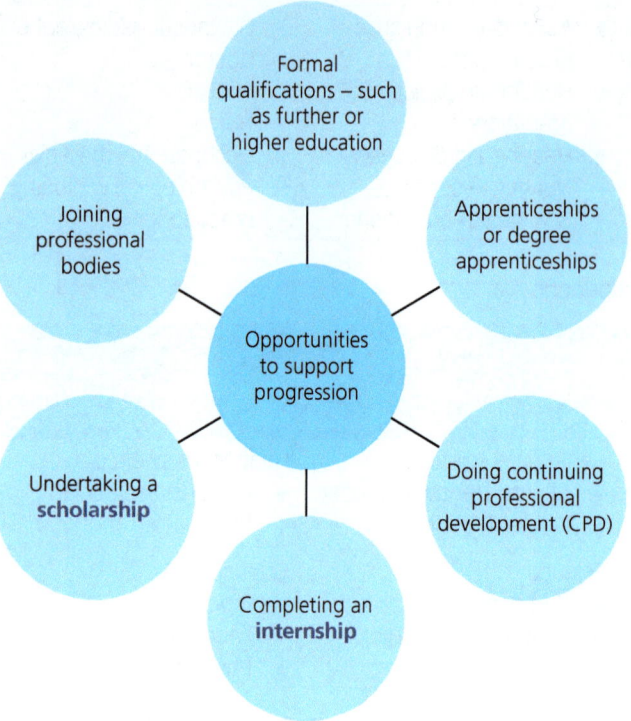

Internship The process of working within an organisation, sometimes without pay, to learn and gain experience.

Scholarship A grant or payment made to support a period of learning.

Figure 1.2 Ways to support career progression within the health and science sector

Now test yourself
TESTED

1 Write **one** sentence to describe how undertaking a course of further education can support the progression of your career.
2 Write your own definition of *continuing professional development (CPD)*.

Exam practice

1 Jig is in hospital. His religious beliefs require him to eat a vegetarian diet.
   State **one** policy which a hospital must have in order to protect and promote Jig's rights. [1]
2 Becca is on an induction programme for her job as a healthcare support worker. She is learning about the hospital's equality, diversity and inclusion policy.
   Explain **one** benefit of equality of opportunity. [2]
3 State **one** reason why an employer must have a grievance policy. [1]
4 Megan is in labour with her first child. She has a complex medical history.
   Explain why adhering to quality standards is important in a large hospital where service users like Megan are cared for. [3]
5 Darius is 15 years old and has a serious medical condition. His doctor needs to gain consent to carry out a difficult surgical procedure to improve Darius' quality of life. Discuss how the doctor might obtain consent in this situation. [6]
6 Jenna is attending her first day of work as a mental health support worker. As part of her induction, she is being asked to read and agree to a code of conduct prepared by her employer.
   a Identify **one** aspect of a professional code of conduct. [1]
   b Explain the purpose of following this aspect of the code of conduct, considering how it supports Jenna and the service users she will work with. [2]
7 Dominic has completed his Level 3 T Level in Health.
   a Identify **one** occupation he can now undertake. [1]
   b State the occupational level of this occupation. [1]
8 Jamal is on his summer break, having completed his T Level in Health. Jamal is interested in progressing towards a career in the ambulance service.
   Briefly explain **one** way that Jamal could exploit an opportunity for progression within the health and science sector. [2]

Check your understanding and progress at www.hoddereducation.co.uk/myrevisionnotes

A2 The healthcare sector

A2.1 The diversity of employers and organisations within the healthcare sector

REVISED

The NHS

The NHS is the largest employer in the UK healthcare sector. It is publicly funded (through taxation and government money). Key decisions regarding funding and policy are directed by the government.

Most NHS services remain free at the point of use for UK citizens, for example visiting the GP and receiving emergency and routine care at the hospital.

Private healthcare

Private suppliers charge a fee for their healthcare services and aim to make a profit from this. The profits benefit the owners and shareholders of the organisation.

Examples of large private healthcare providers in the UK include HCA Healthcare UK, Nuffield Health and Spire Healthcare.

Private/non-profit organisations

Healthcare is also provided by third-sector, or non-profit, organisations (such as charities). Their primary aim is to contribute positively to society and therefore any money remaining after costs are covered is put back into the organisation to improve service provision.

Figure 2.1 shows some examples of non-profit healthcare providers.

Social care services

Social care describes support services, personal care and practical assistance for children, young people and adults that require additional help with daily living.

Local authorities have responsibility for children's, young people's and adults' social care, although they may commission private or non-profit organisations to provide the relevant services.

Other examples of social care include housing services and youth and community services.

> **Making links**
>
> A2.5 covers the origins and development of the healthcare sector.
>
> A2.6 covers the potential impact of future developments in the healthcare sector.

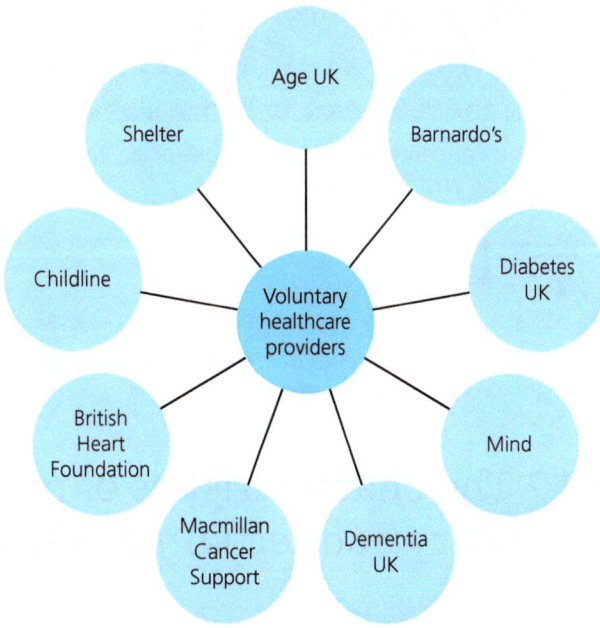

Figure 2.1 Examples of non-profit healthcare providers

> **Typical mistake**
>
> Social care is not just for the elderly! All types of people may require social care at different points in their lives. For example, someone may be temporarily disabled after surgery and require social care for a short time.

Diverse working environments

Healthcare and social care are provided in the setting that best meets the needs of the service user. Therefore, working environments are diverse and include:
+ hospitals
+ GP surgeries
+ community settings, such as family/children's centres or schools
+ residential settings, such as elderly care homes
+ the homes of service users
+ prisons and youth offender institutions
+ local authority departments, such as the housing office.

> **Exam tip**
>
> Many of your exam questions will have a scenario featuring a wide variety of settings where care can be delivered. Ensure you are familiar with all the settings mentioned in this part of the specification, as well as those that appear later, for example hospices, in A8.12.

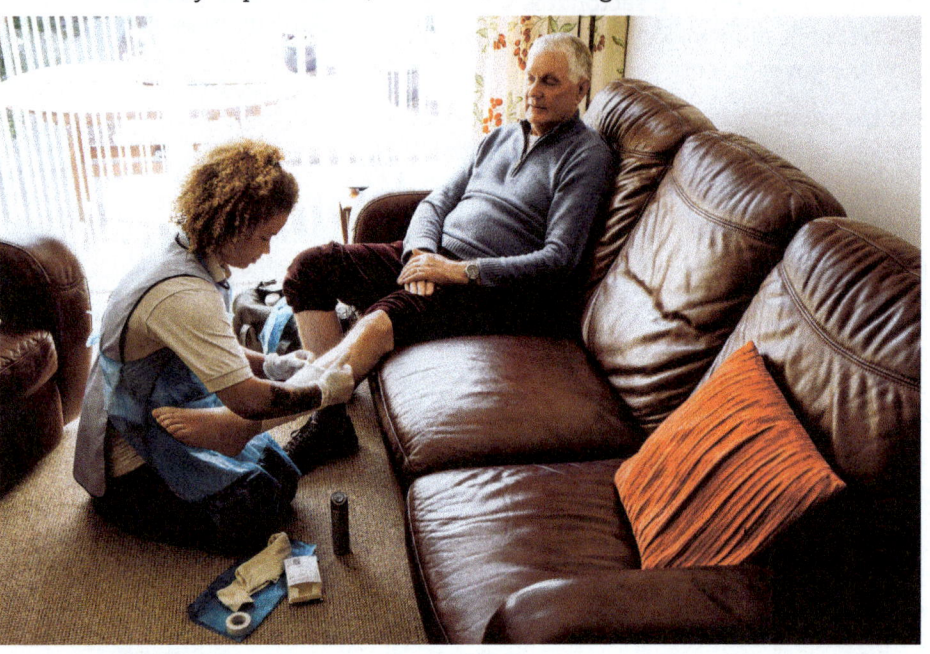

Figure 2.2 For some healthcare professionals, the homes of service users are their main working environment.

> **Now test yourself** TESTED
>
> 1. What are the **three** types of healthcare employers?
> 2. List **three** environments where healthcare or social workers may carry out their job.

A2.2 The characteristics of primary, secondary and tertiary healthcare tiers

REVISED

Primary care

Primary care is often the first point of contact that service users have with healthcare. It can be accessed directly, either by 'walking in' or making an appointment. Think of primary care as the 'front door' of the NHS.

Examples of primary care services include:
+ general practice (GP services)
+ walk-in centres
+ accident and emergency (A&E)
+ NHS 111 telephone service
+ dental care
+ opticians
+ specialist community public health services, such as health visitors and school nurses.

Primary care services may meet acute, chronic or preventative care needs. They provide general care, with the option to make referrals to secondary, specialised care services.

Public participation is encouraged at primary care levels. This means that patient groups are established to provide feedback for the improvement of services.

Secondary care

Individuals requiring specialised healthcare are referred to secondary care by primary health professionals such as GPs or dentists.

Secondary healthcare is usually:
+ centred in hospitals; individuals referred there receive planned care designed to meet their specific needs
+ organised by specialism, for example cardiology clinics, wards, nurses and consultants provide care for patients with heart conditions.

An individual requiring care and treatment over several days will usually be admitted as an inpatient.

Outpatient services, such as clinics and day surgery, do not require overnight stays.

Primary healthcare professionals, schools and other agencies can also refer to social care services, for example when there is a safeguarding concern or when someone requires additional assistance with personal care or the activities of daily living.

Tertiary care

Tertiary care can be provided in hospital or community settings but also in the service user's own home.

Tertiary care is generally used to provide:
+ highly specialised care over extended periods for complex or long-term conditions
+ respite care for families.

Examples of tertiary care include:
+ hospice care and end-of-life care
+ burns units
+ transplant services
+ secure mental health units.

> **Typical mistake**
>
> It can be easy to confuse secondary and tertiary care. Secondary care is specialised to meet a specific need, usually in isolation. Tertiary care is for individuals with more complex and ongoing needs, needing multiple specialists.

> **Revision activity**
>
> Create a table to illustrate the different secondary care specialisms found in most NHS hospitals. Remember to include a description of the specialist area. Challenge yourself to learn the spellings!

> **Now test yourself** 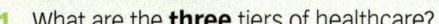 TESTED
>
> 1 What are the **three** tiers of healthcare?
> 2 Give an example of **one** service in each healthcare tier.
> 3 Summarise the role of each healthcare tier.

Acute health conditions These are sudden in onset and usually short term. For example, if you fall and break your arm, you go to A&E.

Chronic health conditions These are persistent or long-lasting conditions, requiring ongoing care and management. For example, having high blood pressure and visiting the GP for six-monthly checks and a prescription.

Preventative healthcare Describes practices that aim to prevent or detect issues with health before they become problematic, for example vaccinations.

Referral The action of sending someone for further review, consultation or action, such as a GP referring a patient with a skin condition that is not responding to treatment to a dermatologist.

Respite care Planned or emergency temporary care of an individual (usually with complex needs) to provide their usual carers, often family, with a short break.

Hospice care Care given to individuals with a terminal illness with the aim of improving quality of life and wellbeing, either in a residential care home setting or the service user's own home.

A2.3 The diverse range of personal factors that would dictate the services accessed by an individual including barriers to service access

REVISED

Range of personal factors

A unique range of factors dictates which health service(s) an individual accesses. Table 2.1 lists examples of personal factors.

Table 2.1 A range of personal factors for why an individual would access healthcare services

Personal factor	Reason	Example of service
Pre-existing health conditions	To prevent deterioration, conditions require monitoring, regular reviewing and management (including self-management) of treatment, as well as health education information and advice.	A multidisciplinary diabetes clinic for individuals with type 1 and type 2 diabetes, staffed by specialist endocrine doctors or diabetologists, diabetes specialist nurses and dieticians
Physical disabilities	Services support the maintenance of good physical condition, mobility and independence.	Physiotherapy, occupational therapy and medical care as necessary (from a GP or specialist doctor)
Mental health conditions	Services monitor and regularly review the condition and its management/treatment.	A community mental health team, staffed by mental health nurses, mental health support workers and psychiatrists (specialist mental health doctors that can prescribe treatment)
Learning difficulties	Services support the maintenance of good health and wellbeing, dignity and independence.	Annual health checks with the GP and learning disability nurse, as well as access to community learning disability services
Age group	At different ages and life stages, individuals have different needs. Health screening is linked to the age when risks for certain conditions increase.	The provision of regular breast screening for all women once they reach their 50th birthday. Vaccination programmes may be targeted at certain life stages as risk increases, for example HPV vaccinations for adolescents as they develop towards sexual maturity.
Gender	Individuals may require services linked to their biological sex/sex assigned at birth, and/or their gender, which is a way to describe a person's innate sense of their own gender, whether male, female, or non-binary, which may not correspond to the sex registered at birth.	Biological females/individuals assigned female at birth require access to screening for cervical cancer once they reach 25 years of age and may require maternity services if they become pregnant. Individuals experiencing gender dysphoria can be referred to a gender dysphoria clinic by their GP to be assessed by a specialist team.
Social care needs	Individuals may require social care for a variety of factors, such as requiring support to complete activities of daily living.	Personal hygiene and grooming, nutrition and hydration, or to maintain service users' independence, for example help with managing finances and travel to shops and appointments.

Pre-existing health conditions Any long-term health conditions that a service user has, is aware of and is being treated for.

Multidisciplinary An approach where health professionals from a range of specialties (disciplines) work together to achieve the best outcomes for service users.

Health screening A way of identifying whether apparently healthy people have an increased risk of a particular condition. Part of preventative healthcare.

Vaccination A treatment given via injection, administered orally (by mouth) or sprayed into the nose. The vaccine triggers the body's immune system to create antibodies against the target disease. Part of preventative healthcare.

Gender dysphoria Deep sense of distress that may occur when an individual's biological sex does not match their gender identity.

> **Exam tip**
>
> Remember that many individuals in the healthcare sector have multiple needs. For example, an individual with a physical disability may require treatment from a doctor for a health condition and assistance from a social care service to meet their daily needs. Ensure you read the scenarios on the exam paper carefully so you do not miss anything.

Barriers to accessing healthcare services

Service users may experience barriers to accessing healthcare services. These are shown in Table 2.2.

Table 2.2 Examples of barriers to accessing healthcare services

Barrier	Example
Socioeconomic	Influenced by an individual's role in society or financial status, for example being unable to afford to park your car in the hospital car park during a medical appointment
Psychological	Linked to the way that individuals think, for example the fear of being judged for having a particular health condition such as a sexually transmitted infection
Physical	Factors linked to the physical world/built environment or a person's physical condition, for example steps but no ramp into a hospital being a barrier for a wheelchair user
Cultural and language	Linked to a person's culture and language/the predominant culture and language, for example being unable to accept personal care from a person of the opposite sex due to religious requirements
Geographical	Determined by the location of an individual or a service, for example secondary care and specialist services are not usually local to most people

> **Exam tip**
>
> If a question asks you to explain barriers to accessing healthcare services, ensure you cover who is affected, how they are affected and why they are affected by the barrier.

> **Now test yourself**
>
> 1 List **three** personal factors that dictate what service an individual may need to access.
> 2 What type of services may individuals with pre-existing conditions need to access?
> 3 List the **five** types of barriers to accessing healthcare services. Give an example for each barrier.
>
> TESTED

A2.4 How the use of different developments in technology supports the healthcare sector

 REVISED

Health applications

Apps are software designed to carry out specific tasks and are available for use on personal computers or devices such as mobile phones and tablets. Some apps that support healthcare are listed in Table 2.3.

Table 2.3 Examples of health apps and their benefits

App	Benefit
NHS App	This provides advice and support to enable service users to make healthy choices; it can also be used to order repeat prescriptions, book appointments and get health advice.
My Diabetes My Way	This provides the means for service users to manage their condition independently (for example eLearning courses on diabetes management).
FreeStyle (blood glucose monitoring system)	This supports the management and monitoring of an individual's ongoing condition by healthcare professionals. For example, diabetic users can share blood glucose data with health professionals using the apps that are provided with their monitor.
Evergreen Life	This allows service users to book and change appointments and health teams to manage these.

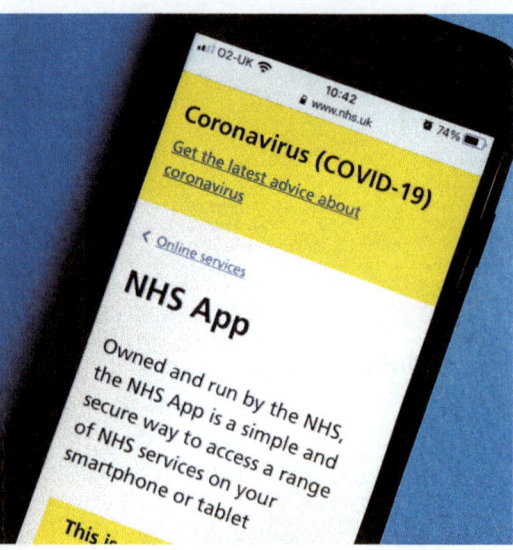

Figure 2.3 The NHS App provides several functions, including access to your health record, vaccination record and the NHS health A–Z

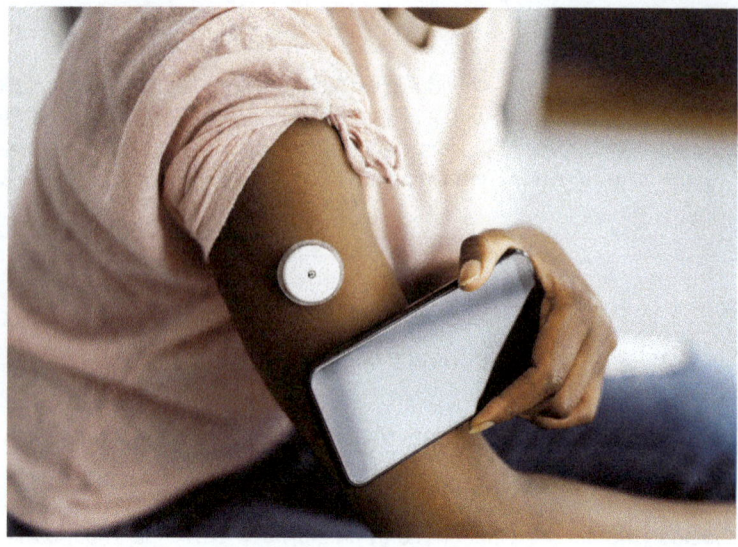

Figure 2.4 Smartphone apps can be used to record and share data collected from continuous blood glucose monitoring systems; these give service users greater control over their own condition and provide vital information to healthcare professionals to manage these conditions remotely

Assistive computer technology

Assistive computer technology is being continuously developed for healthcare to provide innovative ways to treat and manage conditions.

There are two main benefits of using assistive computer technology:
+ It supports the health team to treat or manage conditions more efficiently.
+ It provides solutions that may not have been previously available in order to support conditions.

Table 2.4 provides examples of assistive computer technology and explains how they can be used in healthcare.

Table 2.4 Examples of assistive computer technology and their uses in healthcare

Technology	Use
CAD/CAM/3D printing	This technology can be used to design and produce **prosthetics** that are custom built to the requirements of individual service users, cheaply and quickly. It is possible to 3D print models of organs and surgical instruments. In future, 3D printing of tissues and organs may be approved for human use.
Health implants	Devices (for example internal pacemakers or defibrillators) can be placed inside the body for medical purposes to support the health team so that medical conditions can be managed and treated more efficiently.
Robotic surgery	Using robotics for surgery offers several advantages: + It can make complex, delicate procedures possible. + It is minimally invasive (it limits the size of the surgical opening, promoting faster healing and reducing the risk of infection). + It can be used remotely, enabling skilled surgeons to operate on service users in different geographical locations (**telesurgery**).

Prosthetics An artificial body part, such as an arm, a foot or a tooth, used to replace a part that is missing, either from birth or due to accident or surgery.

Telesurgery Technology that uses robotics and wireless networking to enable surgeons to operate on patients who are not in their immediate geographical location.

> **Making links**
>
> A2.6 covers the potential impacts of future developments in the healthcare sector in relation to care provision.

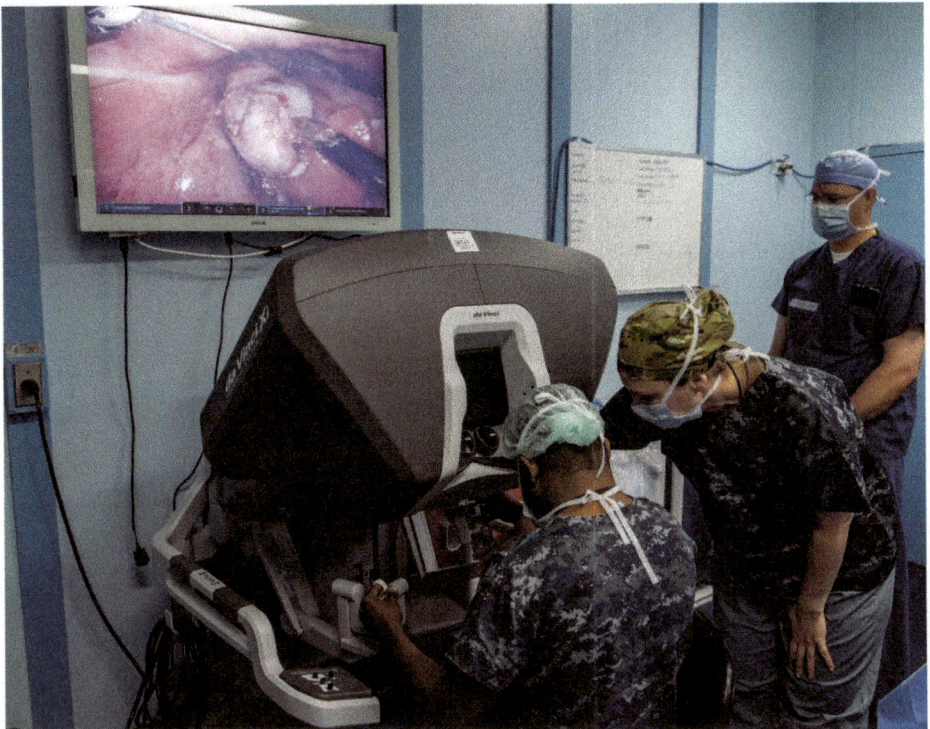

Figure 2.5 During telesurgery, the surgeon controls the surgical robot from a console

Artificial intelligence technologies

Artificial intelligence (AI) technologies are those intended to perform tasks such as decision-making, speech recognition and visual perception.

In radiology, computers are used to identify complex patterns emerging in images (such as MRI scans) and then classify those images according to the identified patterns based on complex algorithms.

This enables radiologists to make faster decisions or even replaces radiologist decisions with AI-made decisions. This means that machines can be used to make diagnoses.

Other uses of AI can support health professionals:
+ It gathers large sets of data to be used and shared beyond the usual geographical boundaries.
+ It keeps health professionals informed of trends in conditions and responses by providing data from a wide range of individuals.

> **Typical mistake**
>
> Radiology and radiography are not the same. Radiology is a branch of medicine, so radiologists are medical doctors. They are experts in reading and interpreting scans for the purpose of diagnosing illness and disease. Radiography describes the process of performing scans and other imaging techniques to obtain images. Therefore, a radiographer is an expert clinical technician who performs imaging tests.

> **Now test yourself** TESTED
>
> 1 List the benefits of health apps.
> 2 What is a health implant? Describe **one** example.
> 3 What is meant by the term *artificial intelligence*?

A2.5 The origins of the healthcare sector and how this has developed into the current healthcare sector

Origins of the healthcare sector in the UK

In the early 1900s, there was a lot of debate and discussion about the health of the population in the UK. This led to the founding of the government-provided National Health Service (NHS) on 5 July 1948.

The NHS Act 1946, introduced by Health Minister Aneurin Bevan, was the law on which the NHS was founded.

The Act stated that the purpose of the NHS was to improve physical and mental health, through prevention, diagnosis and treatment of illness. The NHS was the first completely free, universal (open to all) healthcare service in the world.

How the healthcare sector has developed since 1945

The NHS

The NHS has undergone many changes, updates and reorganisations. It needs to develop so that it continues to meet the needs of the population and remains financially viable.

The NHS is currently funded through general taxation and the National Insurance (NI) scheme.

As the UK's population has increased, its needs have become more complex. Advancements in medical care and treatment are expensive.

As expenditure has now exceeded demand, some NHS services are no longer free. For example, prescription charges were first introduced in 1952, with exemptions for certain members of the population.

Community care and multi-agency working

Since 1945, there has been an increased emphasis on community care, enabling people to live and be cared for within their own local communities and to maintain independence and live in their own homes as much as possible.

Currently, there is more focus on multi-agency working, to ensure the holistic needs of individuals are met and that gaps in care do not arise.

Private-sector healthcare and charities

In parallel to the NHS, healthcare services have been developed by private healthcare companies (paid for through medical insurance or individual payments). This sector is continuing to expand.

Healthcare services provided by charities, such as Marie Curie hospices, have also developed to support health and wellbeing.

> **Exam tip**
>
> Look out for questions that indicate a number of required elements in your answer, for example 'give one' or 'outline two'. If you do not give the required number, you will miss out on marks.

> **Revision activity**
>
> Create a basic timeline to illustrate the origins and development of the healthcare sector in the UK.

> **Now test yourself**
>
> 1. What date was the NHS founded?
> 2. What is the main way that the NHS is funded?
> 3. Give **two** reasons why the NHS is no longer completely free.
> 4. What **two** parts of the healthcare sector have developed alongside the NHS?

A2.6 The potential impacts of future developments in the healthcare sector in relation to care provision

REVISED

The healthcare sector will need to continue developing to meet demands. Table 2.5 lists some developments and their potential impacts on healthcare provision.

Table 2.5 The potential impacts of future developments in the healthcare sector

Development	Potential impact on healthcare provision
Artificial intelligence (AI)	Improved diagnostic procedures – AI speeds up diagnosis and can reveal new diagnostic methods
	Improved triaging – speedier decisions, based on larger amounts of data than humans can easily process
Technological infrastructure	Provides remote access for professionals – no need to see patients face to face
	Enables greater collaboration between experts and services – no need to meet face to face
Regenerative medicine	Could provide new treatments and therapies – for example, it could restore function to damaged organs or tissues or even grow whole new organs
Biomarkers	Expanding the use of biomarkers and discovering new biomarkers could: + assist earlier diagnosis of early onset cardiovascular disease + increase discovery, testing and success rates of new drug therapies + accelerate availability of other novel treatments.
Remote care	Provides the opportunity for remote services, such as online clinics, virtual consultations, mobile clinics and screening
	Enables individuals with reduced mobility or chronic pain conditions to access care more easily
	Cost-efficient model of care that reduces long-term funding required for services
Patient self-management	Wearable devices for monitoring physiological functions such as blood pressure or existing conditions such as diabetes
Funding of services	Stretched funding as more people access the services
Private healthcare provision	Can provide a greater number of services to a greater number of people with shorter waiting times
Changes in patient/ service user demographics	Changes in life expectancy, an increase in complex care needs and rates of obesity will drive demand for services and increase funding requirements
	Changes will also drive the need for innovation in treatments and service provision

Triage Deciding the urgency of a medical case based on signs and symptoms presented.

Regenerative medicine Multidisciplinary science that aims to replace or regenerate human cells, tissues or organs to restore or establish normal functioning.

Biomarkers A broad category of medical signs that can be measured accurately. They can indicate a normal biological process, a pathogenic process (one caused by disease) or a response to medication. Biomarkers range from blood pressure measurements to blood cholesterol tests to chemical reactions at the cellular level.

Physiological Relating to the functioning of the human body or body system.

Typical mistake

It can be easier to focus on negative impacts in healthcare. Remember that for every challenge in the healthcare sector, such as increasing rates of obesity, there are both potentially negative impacts (stretched funding) as well as positive impacts (the drive to innovate and seek new treatments or ways to deliver care).

Revision activity

Make a list of some of the demands on healthcare services. For each demand, provide an example of a future development that could alleviate it.

Now test yourself

1. Which individuals may benefit from remote care?
2. What is a biomarker and how is it used?
3. What are some of the possible impacts on the health sector of the use of regenerative medicine?

TESTED

My Revision Notes: Health T Level

A2.7 The importance of adhering to national, organisational and departmental policies in the healthcare sector including the possible consequences of not following policy

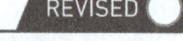

Importance of adhering to national, organisational and departmental policies

A policy ensures that in specific situations, all staff act in the same way. As policy is underpinned by legislation and evidence of best practice, this means that:

+ high-quality, standardised care is provided for all patients and service users
+ the safety of all service users is maintained
+ errors are prevented
+ there is consistency of practice
+ health and wellbeing are promoted for service users
+ the safety and wellbeing of practitioners are ensured.

> **Making links**
> A1.1 outlines the purpose of organisational policies and covers safeguarding, disciplinary and grievance policies.

> **Making links**
> A2.9 covers evidence-based practice.

Possible consequences of not following policy

The consequences of not following policy can range from the individual level up to the organisational level. They are listed in Table 2.6 with examples.

Table 2.6 Consequences of not following policy

Consequence	Example
Health and safety risks	Failing to follow a policy on the safe and secure storage of chemical cleaning agents could expose service users to risk.
Harm to self and others	Chemical cleaning agents that have not been stored safely and securely could lead to chemical burns.
Termination of employment	Employment contracts require employees to follow organisational policy; not doing so could lead to dismissal.
Negative media coverage	A news story could be published about a service user experiencing chemical burns from unsafe and insecure storage of chemical cleaning agents.
Implications for inspection/grading	If during an inspection the Care Quality Commission (CQC) finds that an organisation has failed to follow a policy on the safe and secure storage of chemical cleaning agents and is in breach of a regulation, it can issue a requirement notice.
Deregistration for registered practitioners	If a registered healthcare practitioner fails to follow policy and harm occurs, they may be subject to a striking-off order.
Potential criminal prosecution or civil legal action against an employer or individual	Legal action could be pursued in respect of harm caused through failing to store chemical cleaning agents safely and securely.

> **Deregistration** The act of removing a professional from an official register (of practice).
>
> **Criminal prosecution** Criminal law relates to offences and breaches that have an impact on the whole of society. If an action goes against UK law, this is a criminal offence and criminal legal action is taken.
>
> **Civil legal action** Used for non-criminal offences, such as breach of contract, personal injury or negligence. Civil law is concerned with the rights and property of individual people or organisations.

> **Revision activity**
>
> Fill an A4 page with everything you can think of relating to policies in the healthcare sector and why it is important to follow them. Then turn your page over and fill it with consequences of not following policies. Don't forget to illustrate your points with examples.

> **Now test yourself** — TESTED
>
> 1 Write **one** sentence to outline the purpose of having policies in a healthcare organisation.
> 2 Give **two** reasons why it is important to follow policy in the healthcare sector.
> 3 Explain **three** consequences of not following policy in the healthcare sector.

A2.8 The different ways in which the sectors are funded

REVISED

Each of the sectors that provide healthcare services are funded in different ways. These are shown in Table 2.7.

Table 2.7 Ways in which health sectors are funded

Health sector	How it is funded
Public	+ Income tax + National Insurance (NI) + Patient contributions (for example prescription charges)
Private	+ Insurance premiums (may be paid by individuals or employers as part of the benefits package of a job) + One-off payments direct to the provider
Voluntary/charity	+ Donations + Fundraising + Grant funding

It is important to know that rates of taxation vary over time, because of changing government economic policy and in response to requirements for increased funding of public services.

Similarly, governments can decide to increase or reduce the amount of funding received by health and social care services.

> **Now test yourself** — TESTED
>
> 1 How does the government fund public health services?
> 2 How do individuals pay for private healthcare?
> 3 What methods can be used to fund services provided by the voluntary/charity sector?

A2.9 The meaning of evidence-based practice, its application and how it benefits and improves the healthcare sector

REVISED

Meaning of evidence-based practice

Evidence-based practice is the use of rigorously conducted research and data collection to inform working practice and decision-making.

It may also include leading or taking part in scientific or mathematical research into best practice.

The application of evidence-based practice

Understanding when evidence-based practice is applicable to a specific situation and using it to inform working practices requires several skills. These include the ability to:
+ combine research findings with clinical expertise and professional judgement
+ assess findings from research, such as the validity of any information and data presented, to make judgements about the accuracy and rigour of that research
+ draw conclusions from research and know when they can be applied to improve practice or introduce innovations
+ monitor and review the impact of any changes or innovations made, such as deciding whether working practices informed by evidence are successful.

How evidence-based practice benefits and improves the healthcare sector

Research is an essential part of continuous learning and improvement in the healthcare sector. Table 2.8 lists who benefits from evidence-based practice.

Table 2.8 Who benefits from evidence-based practice

Who benefits	Benefits and improvements
The population	+ Facilitates improvements in person-centred care + Improves outcomes for individuals + Improves safety + Promotes equity in provision + Informs health-promotion requirements
The healthcare sector	+ Encourages quality provision + Improves cost effectiveness + Improves capability and competency of the workforce
The healthcare practitioner	+ Job satisfaction + Empowerment + Continuous professional development

> **Research validity** The extent to which the concept being studied is accurately measured. This requires the design and methods of the study to be well chosen.

> **Typical mistake**
> While *conducting* research may not be a part of most people's everyday work in the healthcare sector, evidence informs all activities carried out. For example, handwashing, manual handling, pressure-area care and cleaning hard surfaces with chemicals are all working practices that are informed by evidence drawn from research. Therefore, everyone working in healthcare occupations is an evidence-based practitioner.

> **Now test yourself**
> 1. Write your own definition of evidence-based practice.
> 2. Summarise what is meant by validity in research.
> 3. Identify **two** groups who benefit from evidence-based practice and for each, state **two** benefits.
>
> TESTED

A2.10 The different types of organisational structures within the healthcare sector and the resulting job roles

REVISED

Flat structure and tiered hierarchical structure

The structure of an organisation can be flat or hierarchical.

Flat structure
+ Has fewer layers of management
+ Employees have more responsibility
+ More open communication and improved co-ordination
+ Confusion can result if employees do not have a person to report to
+ Hard to maintain for larger organisations
+ Example: teams working within a hospital, small organisations (for example a specialist service provided by a charity)

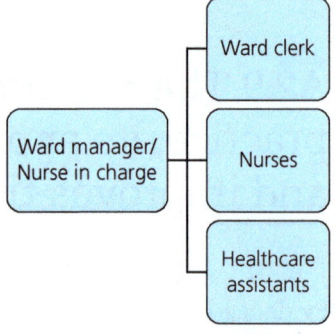

Figure 2.6 An example of the flat structure of a ward in an NHS hospital

Tiered hierarchical structure
+ Features numerous layers of management, cascading down from the top
+ Employees have a specialty and can see a clear career path
+ Innovation/change can be slowed down due to levels of bureaucracy
+ Example: an NHS hospital

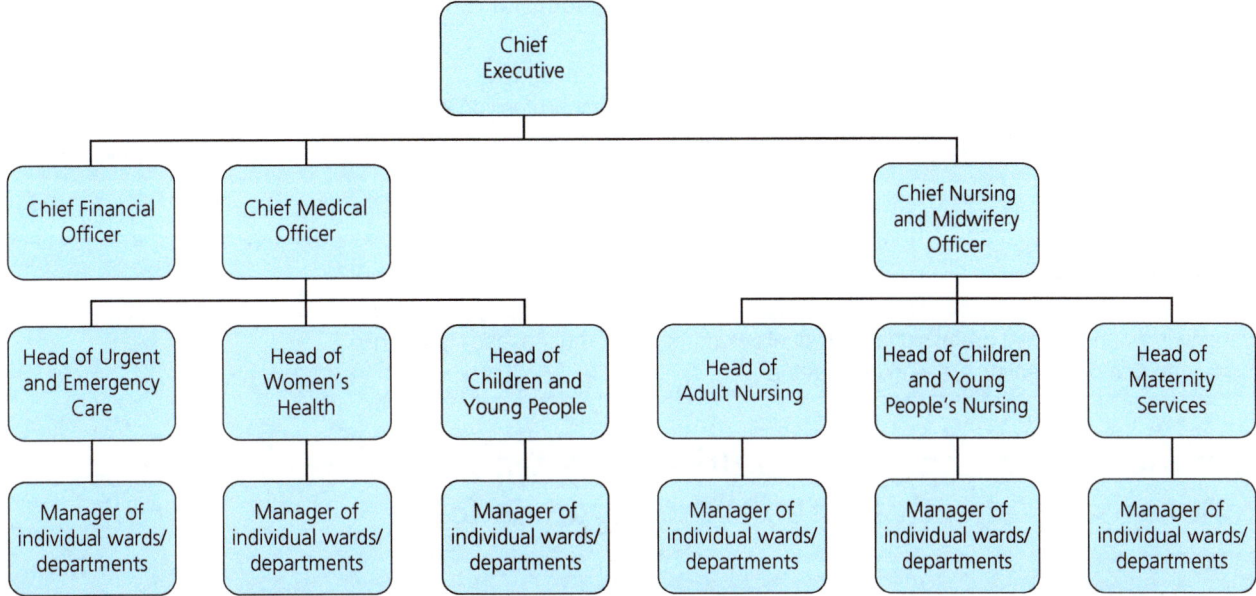

Figure 2.7 Example of a tiered hierarchical structure in an NHS hospital

Job roles
Types of job roles in flat and tiered hierarchical organisational structures are shown in Table 2.9.

Table 2.9 The job roles in flat and tiered hierarchical organisational structures

Role	Description
Management	Many management roles in the healthcare sector are carried out by clinicians.
	The more senior the role, the less likely the manager is to be actively practising their clinical role.
	Some very senior management roles, such as Chief Financial Officer, would be undertaken by a professional in that area (for example finance).
Caring	This includes: doctors and other medically trained individuals (such as physician's associates); allied health professionals (such as radiologists); nurses and midwives; healthcare assistants and other roles that provide hands-on care but are not professionally registered.
Ancillary	This includes: domestic staff (cleaning and food preparation roles); porters; site management.

External agencies
In the healthcare sector, common functions fulfilled by external agencies include domestic cleaning, catering and security.

Agencies may also be used to cover shortages of professional staff, for example doctors, midwives and nurses. These roles may be part of a long-term contract between the healthcare organisation and the agency.

External agency roles may be integrated within the service delivery and managed within the organisational structure, or non-integrated and managed entirely by the external agency.

Teams working within healthcare organisations

Multidisciplinary team working is a common feature of the healthcare sector. A multidisciplinary team may consist of those with caring and management roles, as is the case for a team managing bed and workload allocation. For example, when planning the discharge of a vulnerable patient from hospital, the NHS, adult social care and a private residential nursing home may work together.

> **Multidisciplinary team** A team made up of people from different professional fields (disciplines) or with different job functions coming together to achieve a common goal for an individual.

> **Typical mistake**
>
> The terms *multidisciplinary* and *multi-agency* are not interchangeable. Multidisciplinary working is when different professional individuals work together; multi-agency is when more than one organisation are working together.

How multidisciplinary and multi-agency teams work together effectively as part of organisational structures

Multidisciplinary and multi-agency team working enhances respect and builds rapport (bonds) between colleagues and organisations to create a positive working culture.

Each member of the team is required to take ownership of their own role and responsibilities.

Key features of good team working include:
+ giving and receiving constructive feedback
+ sharing best practice
+ contributing to discussions to support problem-solving
+ actively listening to colleagues' contributions and sharing relevant information
+ collaborating to support the continuity of care, particularly between the healthcare and social care sectors.

> **Exam tip**
>
> Remember, some questions carry marks for the quality of your written communication. You can gain marks through appropriate use of technical language, so ensure you can use key terms such as *multidisciplinary* and *multi-agency* with precision and confidence.

> **Now test yourself** TESTED
>
> 1 List the characteristics of a tiered hierarchical organisational structure.
> 2 What are **three** types of role found in healthcare organisations?
> 3 Write a definition of multidisciplinary team working.
> 4 Write a definition of multi-agency working.
> 5 What are the benefits of team working?
> 6 How can a professional working in a team maximise their contributions to that team?

Check your understanding and progress at www.hoddereducation.co.uk/myrevisionnotes

A2.11 The importance of job descriptions and person specifications and how this defines roles and responsibilities

REVISED

When applying for or starting a new job, the job description and person specification should be consulted.

Job description

Table 2.10 What a job description should include

What a job description should include	Meaning
Scope of the role	The number of different tasks required in a job and the frequency of those tasks
Purpose of the role	How the role fulfils one or more of the functions of the organisation
Responsibilities	The tasks and duties expected to be completed
Reporting lines	Who is in charge of the work done and who tells the employee what work needs to be done
Accountabilities	How the fulfilment of the job will be measured

Person specification

Person specifications define:
+ experience required
+ essential and desirable skills
+ attributes required
+ qualifications required
+ mandatory training and continuing professional development required, including reflective practice
+ registration requirements where appropriate, for example if the person must be a registered nurse.

Together, the job description and person specification ensure the employee knows what is expected of them and the employer recruits the person with the right qualifications, skills and attributes for the job.

> **Reflective practice**
> Thinking about situations and actions in a structured way and drawing points of learning from them.

Typical mistake

Do not confuse the job description and the person specification. While they are both required to understand what is expected of the job, the job description sets out roles and responsibilities that the employer expects the applicant to fulfil while working, whereas the person specification sets out the experience, skills and attributes that the applicant must already have.

Now test yourself

TESTED

1. What is the purpose of a job description?
2. What is the purpose of a person specification?
3. List the features of a typical job description.
4. List the features of a typical person specification.

A2.12 The career pathway opportunities for employment and progression within the healthcare sector

REVISED

The IfATE maps the availability and progression of careers in the health pathway. The 'healthcare assistant' role represents a 'technical occupation'. This is the first level of occupation.

Healthcare assistant roles are those where direct patient contact and caring occur, and tasks undertaken are routine, well-defined clinical duties.

Figure 2.8 shows the health pathway from healthcare assistant to health professional.

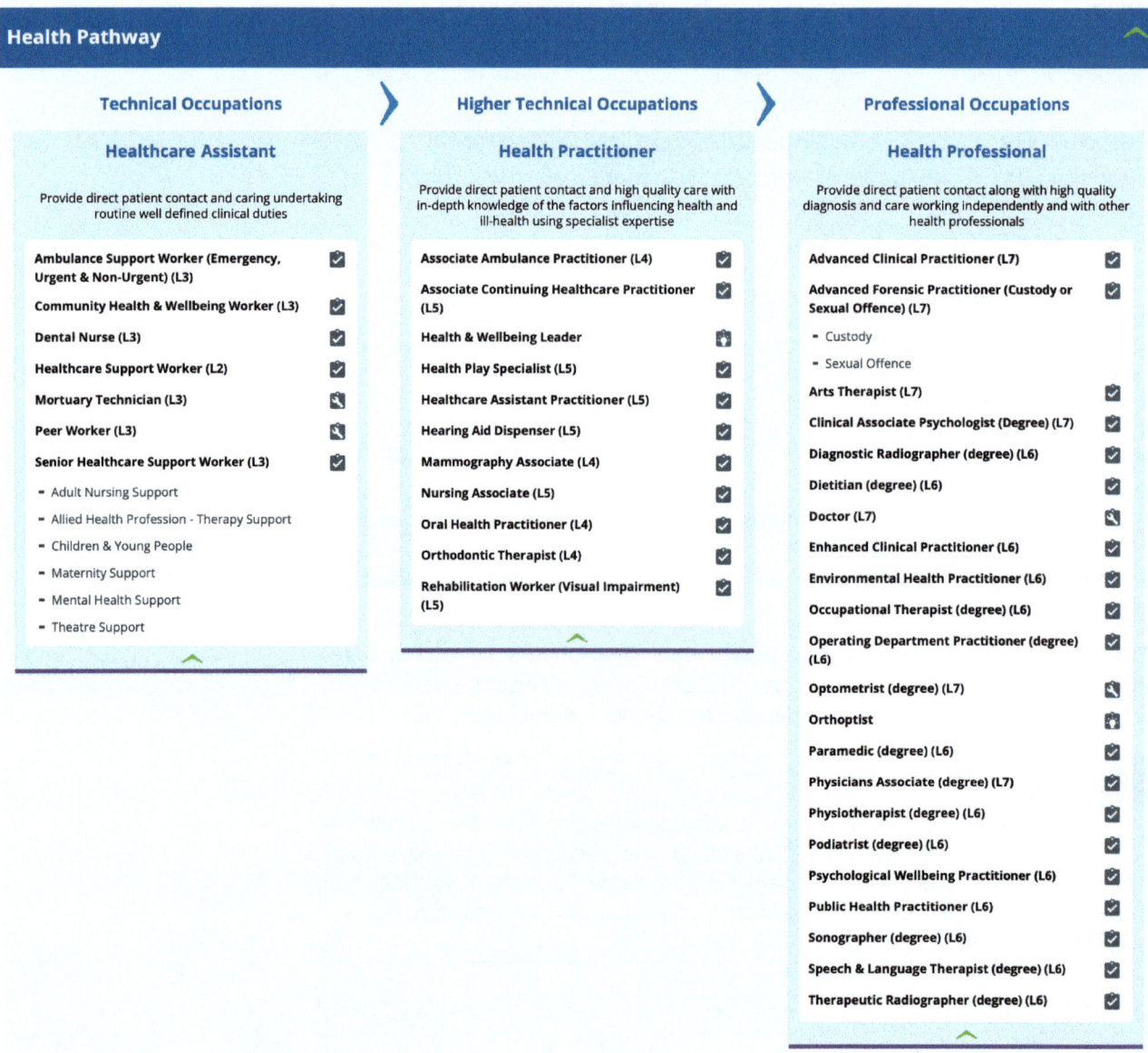

Figure 2.8 The health pathway from healthcare assistant to health professional

Source: Image taken on 13/01/2022 from www.instituteforapprenticeships.org – this information is subject to change and this URL should be used to access the most up-to-date information

> **Now test yourself** TESTED
>
> 1 Name **three** roles of a healthcare assistant.
> 2 Name **three** roles of a senior healthcare support worker.
> 3 What are the differences between healthcare support workers and senior healthcare support workers?

Check your understanding and progress at www.hoddereducation.co.uk/myrevisionnotes

A2.13 The potential impact of external factors on the activities of the healthcare sector

REVISED

External factors

There are certain external factors that may have an impact on the activities of the healthcare sector, shown in Figure 2.9.

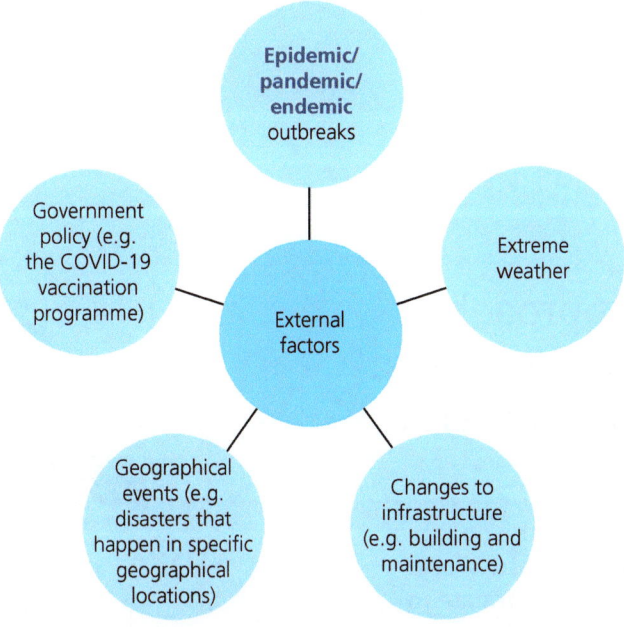

Figure 2.9 External factors that may have an impact on the activities of the healthcare sector

Epidemic The widespread occurrence of a disease in a community at a particular time.

Pandemic A disease outbreak that is prevalent across a whole country or geographical area.

Endemic A disease or condition regularly found in certain populations or local areas.

Supply chain The network of all the individuals, organisations and processes involved in the creation, sale and receipt of a product.

Impacts of external factors

The impacts of external factors on the activities of the healthcare sector may include:
+ service overload (e.g. too many people requiring treatment)
+ insufficient staff resources
+ inaccessible services
+ damage to facilities
+ additional resource requirements (e.g. equipment and materials)
+ effect on the supply chain (e.g. costs and delivery capacity)
+ contingency plan implementation requirements (e.g. a disaster recovery plan).

Exam tip

You can use examples from recent events to demonstrate your knowledge of the impact of external factors. A good example is the COVID-19 global pandemic that caused a service overload on the NHS. The NHS struggled to cover the additional staffing requirements and additional resource requirements such as for personal protective equipment (PPE) and ventilation equipment.

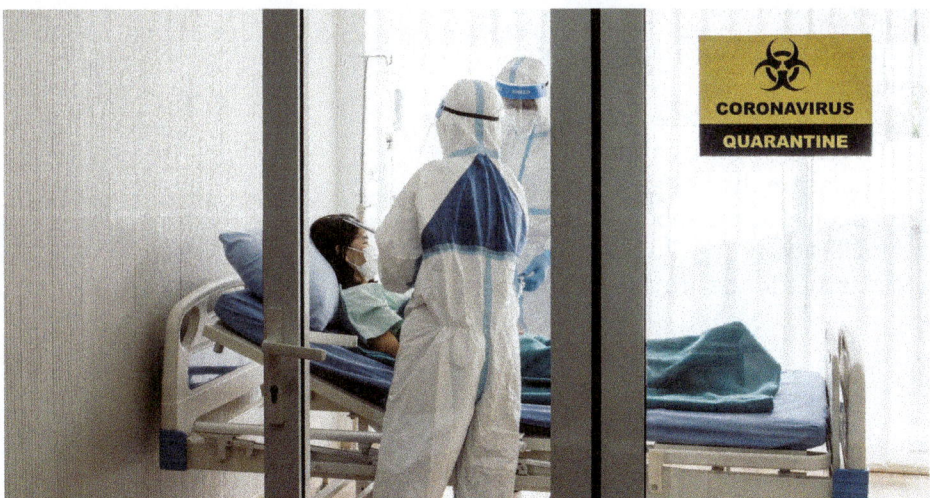

Figure 2.10 At the peak of the COVID-19 pandemic, there was extreme demand on healthcare services in terms of beds, staff and resources such as PPE

My Revision Notes: Health T Level

> **Revision activity**
>
> Create a table of external factors that may have an impact on the activities of the healthcare sector. For each factor, list at least two relevant examples. Then for each example, list all the possible impacts.

> **Now test yourself** TESTED
>
> 1 Give **two** external factors that can affect the activities of the healthcare sector.
> 2 Give **two** impacts on healthcare activities of the two factors chosen as your answer to question 1.
> 3 How might extreme weather affect the activities of the healthcare sector?
> 4 What impacts on the activities of the healthcare sector may arise when large amounts of building work are undertaken at a hospital?

A2.14 The role of public health approaches and how this benefits regional and national population health through prevention and improvement initiatives

REVISED

Public health is about protecting, promoting and improving the health of entire populations of people and communities. For example, the World Health Organization (WHO) was established in 1948 with a mandate to promote worldwide health.

Public health activities are often government-led, and in the UK, the government departments responsible for public health are the:
+ UK Health Security Agency (UKHSA)
+ Office for Health Improvement and Disparities (OHID)
+ Department of Health and Social Care (DHSC).

> **Typical mistake**
>
> The UK Health Security Agency and the Office for Health Improvement and Disparities *replaced* Public Health England (PHE) in April 2021. Therefore, you should not refer to PHE in your answers.

The role of public health approaches

Key approaches in public health include:
+ determining health issues by collecting information regarding their extent, whom they impact and their effects
+ determining why a particular health issue might occur and factors that may contribute to it or increase the risk of it occurring
+ determining what could help to decrease the risk and providing interventions to a wide range of people, in a number of different health-related environments and locations
+ determining the impact of social issues for health and wellbeing.

The benefits of public health approaches to regional and national health

Public health approaches have numerous benefits, which are shown in Figure 2.11.

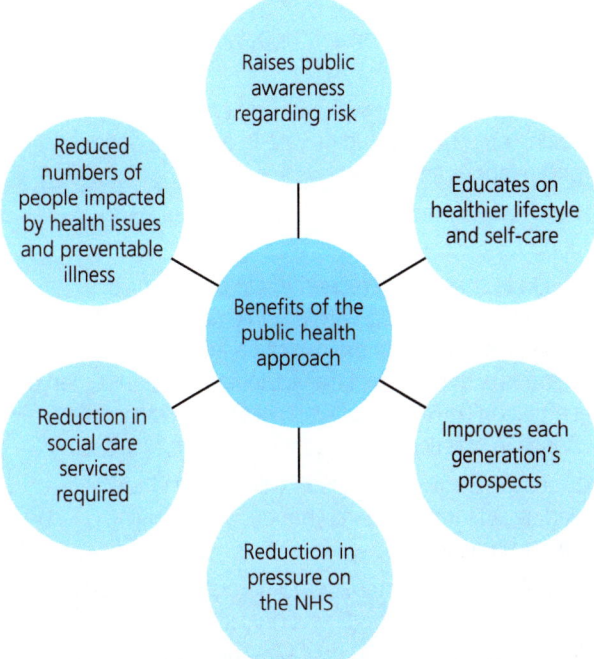

Figure 2.11 The benefits of the public health approach

Revision activity

Create a table or diagram to demonstrate as many links as you can between the different public health approaches and their benefits.

Typical mistake

Students sometimes use the terms *public health*, *health education* and *health promotion* interchangeably. Public health is about protecting, promoting and improving the health of entire populations of people and communities. Approaches used within this include health education (individuals learning about how to take action to improve health) and health promotion (raising awareness about how health can be supported by individuals, families, organisations and society).

Now test yourself

1. What is 'public health'?
2. Which government agency is responsible for public health in the UK?
3. What does WHO stand for?
4. List the **four** public health approaches.
5. Identify **two** benefits of public health approaches.

Exam practice

1. Gracie is a health visitor and she is going to conduct a routine 9–12-month health and development review on a child.
   a. Identify the most likely employer of Gracie. [1]
   b. State **three** settings where Gracie may carry out this review. [3]

2. a. Describe the healthcare service provided by **one** named non-profit organisation. [1]
   b. State **two** examples of healthcare workers that work in the homes of service users. [2]

3. Jin works as a healthcare assistant on a cardiology ward.
   a. Identify the healthcare tier that Jin works in. [1]
   b. Describe **one** characteristic of that tier. [1]

4. Zendaya lives in a small village and has just celebrated her 50th birthday. She has multiple sclerosis, a condition that causes problems with her vision, arm and leg movements, and balance.
   a. Identify **two** services that Zendaya might want to access. [2]
   b. Explain **three** barriers that Zendaya might experience when trying to access these services. [6]

5. Jeanetta has had type 1 diabetes for 15 years. She finds it difficult to manage her condition while busy at university. She has heard about a medical implant for people with type 1 diabetes.
   Discuss the benefit of a continuous blood glucose monitoring system and smartphone app for individuals like Jeanetta. [3]

6. Faizal is 82 years old. He has type 2 diabetes, which has caused a deterioration in his eyesight. He is also showing signs of dementia. Faizal lives alone in a small house.
   Explain why the healthcare sector now uses integrated care systems to provide joined-up working between health and social care services for individuals like Faizal. [3]

7. Kit Yee is a health economist. She is looking at cost-effective ways that healthcare services can be developed to meet the needs of older people with co-morbidities.
   a. Identify **two** future developments for Kit Yee to research. [2]
   b. Explain briefly the impact that each development will have. [4]

8. Dawood is a healthcare assistant in a large hospital. His line manager has asked him to read the health and safety policy for the acute admissions unit where he works.
   Discuss why it is important for Dawood to read the policy as requested. [6]

9. Valentina is pregnant with her first child. She is looking at both NHS and private healthcare options for the labour and birth.
   Discuss how these **two** healthcare sectors are funded. [6]

10. Nelson is conducting research into pain-control options for individuals with chronic pain conditions. He wants to compare the use of pharmacological methods with the use of transcutaneous electrical nerve stimulation (TENS) to see if he should recommend a change in practice in his healthcare setting.
    Discuss the skills that Nelson will require when reading scientific research papers and applying them to practice. [6]

11. Describe the characteristics of an organisation or a team that has a flat organisational structure. [2]

12. The person specification for an adult nurse job states that all nurses are expected to meet registration requirements and to regularly undertake reflective practice. Briefly explain these **two** features of the person specification. [4]

13. Mushtaq has just started his first job as a healthcare support worker in a hospital setting.
    Identify **three** senior healthcare support worker specialisms Mushtaq could work towards. [3]

14. An outbreak of the infectious disease mpox has occurred in a large city.
    Explain **two** ways in which an outbreak of an infectious disease could have an impact on the healthcare sector. [4]

15. During the COVID-19 pandemic, the UK government ran multiple public health campaigns, based on a variety of public health approaches. One of the key messages was:
    Wear a face covering. Wash your hands. Stay two metres apart.
    a. Identify the **two** public health approaches underpinning this message. [2]
    b. Explain the linked benefits of these public health approaches in the context of COVID-19. [4]

Check your understanding and progress at www.hoddereducation.co.uk/myrevisionnotes

A3 Health, safety and environmental regulations in the health and science sector

A3.1 The purpose of key legislation and regulations in the health and science sector

There are many key pieces of legislation and regulations in the health and science sector. Table 3.1 lists some of them.

Table 3.1 Key legislation and regulations in the health and science sector

Legislation	Purpose	Examples
Health and Safety at Work etc. Act 1974	Defines employers' responsibilities to protect the health, safety and welfare at work of employees and members of the public defines employees' duties to protect themselves and each other	+ Employers must have a health and safety policy which sets out how health and safety will be managed. + Health and safety is the responsibility of everyone, therefore everyone must report hazards and take reasonable steps with their own safety and that of those around them.
Management of Health and Safety at Work Regulations 1999	Aim to reduce the number and severity of accidents in the workplace through assessment and management of risk	+ Employers must risk assess working conditions and processes. + Employers must introduce safety measures to control any identified risks. + Employers must provide clear information and training on health and safety.
Control of Substances Hazardous to Health (COSHH) Regulations 2002 (amended 2021)	Define employers' responsibilities to control substances hazardous to health by reducing or preventing employees' exposure to them.	+ Chemicals must be stored safely. + Hazardous substances (including blood and contaminated sharps) must be disposed of safely.
Personal Protective Equipment at Work (Amendment) Regulations 2022	Define employers' responsibilities to provide appropriate personal protective equipment (PPE) to reduce harm to employees, visitors and clients; this can include safety helmets, masks, goggles and gloves	+ Where risk cannot be eliminated, PPE must be provided by the employer. + PPE must take into account any protected characteristics, for example pregnancy. + Employees must know where PPE is located and how to use it. + Employees must take responsibility for using PPE.

> **Exam tip**
> When an exam question asks about legislation, ensure you name relevant legislation accurately and provide the date. In discuss and evaluate questions, choose the most relevant legislation and link it directly to your discussion or evaluation points. For example, you might demonstrate the importance of a particular procedure by explaining how it fulfils legal requirements.

A3 Health, safety and environmental regulations in the health and science sector

Legislation	Purpose	Examples
Reporting of Injuries, Diseases and Dangerous Occurrences Regulations (RIDDOR) 2013	Define employers' duties to report serious workplace accidents, occupational diseases and specified dangerous occurrences ('near misses')	The list of serious workplace accidents includes any that cause death, significant fractures or burns, loss of limb or sight.
Environmental Protection Act (EPA) 1990	Makes provision for the improved control of pollution to the air, water and land by regulating the management of waste and the control of emissions	Organisations have a duty to keep any land they own or control free of litter.
Special Waste Regulations 1996 (Scotland only) Note: In England and Wales, these regulations are revoked by the Hazardous Waste Regulations 2005 (see below)	Outline measures relating to: the regulation and control of the transit, import and export of waste (including recyclable materials); the prevention, reduction and elimination of pollution caused by waste; and the requirement for an assessment of the impact on the environment of projects likely to have significant effects on the environment	The regulations specify whether waste is hazardous or not and how to dispose of it safely.
Hazardous Waste (England and Wales) Regulations 2005	Control the storage, transport and disposal of hazardous waste (waste stream) to ensure it is appropriately managed and any risks are minimised	+ Coloured waste bags must be used according to waste type, to eliminate contamination and control risk. + Specialist removal and disposal companies (waste carriers) must be used to eliminate risks.
Waste Electrical and Electronic Equipment (WEEE) Regulations 2013	Aim to reduce the amount of electrical and electronic equipment incinerated or sent to landfill sites, with the onus placed on all businesses to store and transport electrical waste correctly	Batteries and electronic equipment must be disposed of correctly, using authorised waste carriers.
Regulatory Reform (Fire Safety) Order (RRO) 2005	Aims to reduce death, damage and injury caused by fire by placing legal responsibilities on employers to carry out a fire risk assessment; requires all organisations to have procedures for evacuation in the event of a fire	+ Premises must reach required fire safety standards. + Employees must have fire safety training – at induction and regular updates.
Manual Handling Operations Regulations 1992, as amended by the Health and Safety (Miscellaneous Amendments) Regulations 2002	Require employers to assess and minimise the risk to employees' health involved in the manual handling, moving and positioning of an object, person or animal and workplace ergonomics	Manual handling must be avoided as far as is reasonably practical, for example encourage service users to move themselves and use equipment for repositioning and lifting.

> **Revision activity**
>
> Create a set of revision cards on each piece of legislation or set of regulations, with two examples of them being implemented in practice.

> **Typical mistake**
>
> COSHH regulations do not just apply to chemicals and gases. Biological agents, such as bacteria and viruses, are also considered substances hazardous to health. Anything that is or could be contaminated with a body fluid, such as sharps (for example needles and scalpels), wound dressings or even bedsheets, is covered by COSHH regulations.

Check your understanding and progress at www.hoddereducation.co.uk/myrevisionnotes

Legislation	Purpose	Examples
Health and Safety (Display Screen Equipment) Regulations 1992	Define employers' responsibilities in carrying out risk assessments of workstations used by employees, including the use of display screen equipment, to minimise identified risks	+ Employers should ensure regular breaks are taken away from screens. + Employers should provide an eye test if requested by an employee.

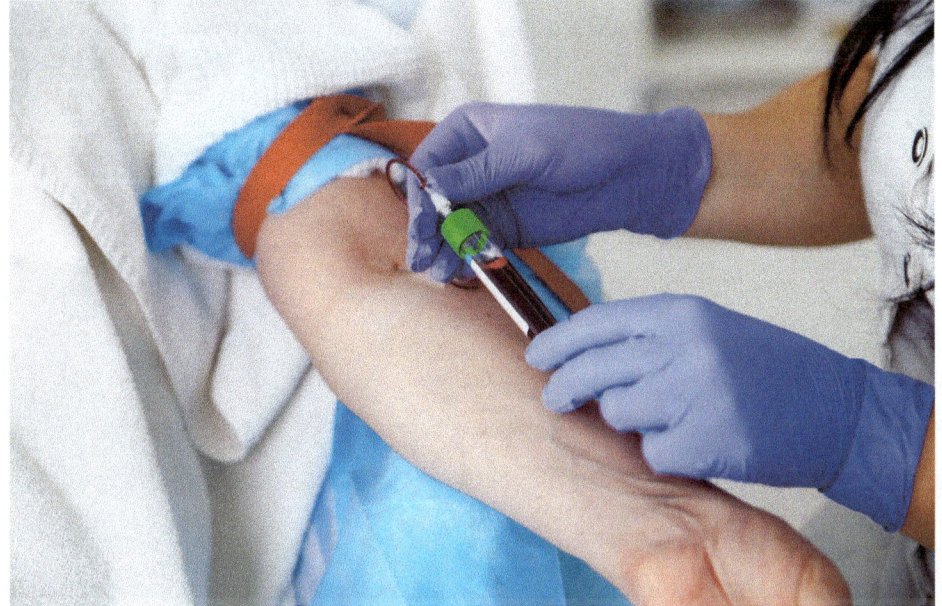

Figure 3.1 Under COSHH regulations, biological agents such as viruses and bacteria, that may be found in blood, are considered hazardous substances

> **Now test yourself**
> 1. Name **two** sets of regulations that control how waste is handled.
> 2. What is the purpose of COSHH regulations?
> 3. What does RIDDOR stand for and when might it be used?
>
> TESTED

A3.2 How to assess and minimise potential hazards and risks, including specific levels of risk, by using the Health and Safety Executive's 5 Steps to Risk Assessment

REVISED

The Health and Safety Executive (HSE) is the national regulator for workplace health and safety.

The 5 Steps to Risk Assessment (Table 3.2) set out how employers can fulfil their obligations under the Health and Safety at Work etc. Act 1974, and the resulting Management of Health and Safety at Work Regulations 1999, to be responsible for the health and safety of employees and visitors by assessing and controlling risk.

Table 3.2 The 5 Steps to Risk Assessment

Step 1	Identify **hazards**	Look at what could cause harm: + objects such as equipment + processes such as manual handling + activities such as outdoor sports + people/behaviours.
Step 2	Assess **risks**	Decide who might be harmed and how: + How likely is it that the harm will occur? + How serious would it be if the harm occurred?
Step 3	Control the risks	Evaluate the risks and decide on precautions: + Can the hazard be completely removed? + If not, how can the risk be controlled so the harm is unlikely?

> **Hazard** An event, object, substance, condition or activity that has the potential to cause harm.
>
> **Risk** The likelihood of harm occurring and the possible seriousness of that harm.

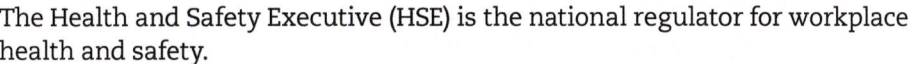

| Step 4 | Record findings | Record findings and implement them, including completing risk assessment documentation. Record:
+ the hazards
+ who might be harmed and how
+ what is being done to control the risks. |
| Step 5 | Review the controls | Review your assessment (as required) and update if necessary.
Review:
+ whether controls are still effective
+ changes in staff
+ changes in process
+ changes in substances or equipment used
+ changes in environment
+ whether any problems are spotted, or accidents or near misses occur. |

> **Typical mistake**
>
> When completing a risk assessment, it can be tempting to merge the first three steps. However, it is vital that all potential hazards are identified first, the risks associated with each one considered in turn and then the control measures for each hazard decided. One activity may have multiple hazards, each one with a different level of risk and a different method of controlling that risk.

> **Revision activity**
>
> Think of a simple activity you have observed in your work placement, for example a service user being helped to stand up from a chair by a healthcare assistant.
>
> Can you use the 5 Steps to Risk Assessment to risk assess this activity? This will help you remember the steps in your exam.

> **Now test yourself** TESTED
>
> 1 What is a hazard?
> 2 How do you assess risk?
> 3 What needs to be considered in Step 3 of the 5 Steps to Risk Assessment?
> 4 What findings should be recorded as part of the risk assessment process?
> 5 List **three** occasions when risk assessment should be reviewed.

A3.3 How health and safety at work is promoted

REVISED

Health and safety is a collective responsibility and it requires everyone to work together to promote safe ways of working. Every health setting will have a health and safety policy that sets out how to promote health and safety in the workplace.

Table 3.3 shows how health and safety at work is promoted.

Table 3.3 Ways health and safety at work is promoted

Method	Example
Encouraging individuals to take reasonable care of their own and others' safety	Wearing PPE provided
Modelling good practice	Washing hands and wearing appropriate PPE
Following organisational policies and standard operating procedures (SOPs), including site-specific emergency procedures	Knowing how to evacuate the building in case of a fire
Ensuring there is clearly visible information and guidance	Displaying the HSE health and safety law poster (as is mandatory)

> **Making links**
>
> Standard operating procedures (SOPs) are covered in more detail in A7.

Check your understanding and progress at www.hoddereducation.co.uk/myrevisionnotes

Method	Example
Following processes for recording and reporting issues and concerns	Completing the accident book when appropriate
Maintaining equipment and removing faulty equipment	Reporting to healthcare science staff working in medical engineering when equipment requires maintenance or repair
Following correct manual handling techniques	Following a specific manual handling policy
Ensuring working environments are clean, tidy and hazard free	Disposing of waste immediately and appropriately
Appropriately storing equipment and materials	Keeping cleaning chemicals in a locked cupboard
Completing **statutory training**	Completing moving and handling training to comply with the Manual Handling Operations Regulations 1992

> **Statutory training**
> Training that is required for legal compliance. For example, fire safety training is a requirement of the Regulatory Reform (Fire Safety) Order (RRO) 2005.

> **Revision activity**
> 1 Create a concept map on promoting health and safety.
> 2 For each row of Table 3.3, see if you can link to a real-life example, as well as a law or regulation.

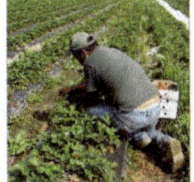

Figure 3.2 It is mandatory to display the HSE health and safety law poster

A3 Health, safety and environmental regulations in the health and science sector

My Revision Notes: Health T Level

Now test yourself TESTED

1. List **three** ways that health and safety can be promoted by employers.
2. Why is it important that employers provide clearly visible information and guidance on health and safety?
3. List **three** ways that health and safety can be promoted by employees.
4. Why is it important for employees to complete statutory training?

A3.4 How to deal with situations that can occur in a health or science environment that could cause harm to self or others (for example spillage of hazardous material)

REVISED

The process for dealing with health and safety incidents will be covered by the health and safety policy and, in the case of spillage of hazardous material, underpinned by COSHH regulations.

The process will include:

+ following organisational health and safety procedures, for example what signs to display, who should clear up and how
+ keeping yourself and others safe, including evacuation as appropriate
+ securing the area to prevent anyone from being exposed to potential harm
+ reporting and/or escalating as appropriate, for example completing an incident form or alerting someone more senior (who may need to make a report under RIDDOR regulations)
+ debriefing and reflecting on the root causes, to prevent the situation from recurring, which will also include reviewing the current risk assessment and associated controls.

Other incidents that can be handled following the principles above would include fire, or damage to the built environment caused by explosion or impact.

> **Exam tip**
>
> When an exam question asks about a process, such as dealing with health and safety incidents, it is particularly important to ensure your answer follows a logical order. This is also important when there are marks for the quality of your written communication.

Now test yourself TESTED

1. Smoke is coming out of the bin in the reception area of a hospital. What is the process that should be followed?
2. A spillage of water occurred in a busy medical ward and a nurse slipped and fractured their wrist. After first aid has been given, what paperwork needs to be completed?
3. Six weeks ago, hazardous chemicals were spilled in a GP surgery. How can the practice manager learn from this incident?

Exam practice

1. Aleesha is the manager of an outpatient clinic where blood samples are routinely taken. She needs to ensure her staff are not exposed to any risk when taking blood from patients.
   a. Identify **one** piece of legislation that Aleesha should be aware of when creating the health and safety policy for her clinic. [1]
   b. Outline the purpose of that legislation. [1]
2. Farah is the manager of a hospital ward. The ward has recently been refurbished and new equipment has been installed. Discuss the importance of assessing risk in this situation and the steps Farah should follow to carry out a risk assessment. [6]
3. Rupa is the nurse in charge of a residential nursing home for elderly people. She has a lot of new staff joining the organisation.
   Give **two** ways that Rupa can promote health and safety to new employees. [2]
4. Gurinder has knocked over a bottle of chemical cleaning agent in the hospital reception.
   Give **two** ways he should deal with this situation to reduce harm to himself and others. [2]

Check your understanding and progress at www.hoddereducation.co.uk/myrevisionnotes

A4 Health and safety regulations applicable in the healthcare sector

A4.1 The purpose of workplace health and safety regulations in the health sector

REVISED

There are some regulations specific to health and safety in the health sector. Their purpose is to:
+ maintain the safety and wellbeing of both the individual and healthcare workers
+ reduce risk to the individual and healthcare workers
+ provide a duty of care to the individual and healthcare workers.

Duty of care A moral or legal obligation to ensure the safety or wellbeing of others. In this context, employers such as the NHS have a duty of care to their employees.

Social care The provision of services that offer practical support to individuals who require it because of illness or disability.

Making links
A3 explores ways that health and safety is maintained and promoted. Thinking about this will help you understand the purpose of regulations explored in A4. You can also link this to learning from A9, which focuses on the health and wellbeing of individuals.

Now test yourself
TESTED

1 What are the purposes of having workplace health and safety regulations in the health sector?

A4.2 The purpose of specific health and safety regulations, guidance and regulatory bodies in relation to the health sector

REVISED

Health and Safety (First-Aid) Regulations 1981
These regulations set legal guidelines for employers to provide adequate and appropriate equipment, facilities and personnel (trained first aiders) to ensure employees receive immediate attention if they are injured or taken ill at work.

Making links
The responsibilities of trained first aiders are covered in A4.3.

Care Act 2014
The Care Act 2014 sets out how adult social care in England should be provided. The purpose of this legislation is to promote and improve people's independence and wellbeing.

Making links
The key principles of the Care Act 2014 are covered in more detail in A8.2.

Under the Act, local authorities must provide or arrange services that help to:
+ prevent people developing needs for care
+ prevent deterioration of people's situations that could result in a need for ongoing care and support.

Ionising Radiation Regulations 2017
The purpose of these regulations is to impose duties on employers to protect employees and members of the public from:
+ radiation arising from work (for example from operating or being in the vicinity of X-rays, CT scans or radiotherapy)
+ radioactive substances (for example radioactive substances used as a treatment to kill cancerous tissue (brachytherapy) and radioactive tracers used in diagnostic imaging)
+ any other forms of ionising radiation (for example when working on the preparation or disposal of radioactive treatments).

Ionising radiation Radioactive particles, X-rays or gamma rays with sufficient energy to cause damage when passing through something, such as cells in the body, due to ionisation.

My Revision Notes: Health T Level

Medicines and Healthcare products Regulatory Agency (MHRA)

The purpose of the MHRA is to ensure medicines and medical devices (including stethoscopes, syringes and X-ray machines) work, are safe for use and meet quality and efficacy standards. This responsibility also extends to blood components for transfusion.

> **Revision activity**
>
> Create a set of revision flashcards to help you remember the purpose of health and safety legislation. Add key health and safety legislation to your cards as you progress through this section.

> **Now test yourself** TESTED
>
> 1 What is the purpose of the Health and Safety (First-Aid) Regulations 1981?
> 2 Give **two** ways that the Care Act 2014 provides health and safety guidance.
> 3 What is the purpose of the Ionising Radiation Regulations 2017?

A4.3 The overarching responsibilities of trained first aiders

REVISED

First aid is immediate attention given to a person that becomes injured or is taken ill, until full medical treatment is available (if it is necessary).

A first aider should have completed training appropriate to the level identified in the organisation's first-aid needs assessment.

Trained first aiders will have completed either the First Aid at Work or the Emergency First Aid at Work course.

Responsibilities

The responsibilities of a trained first aider are shown in Figure 4.1.

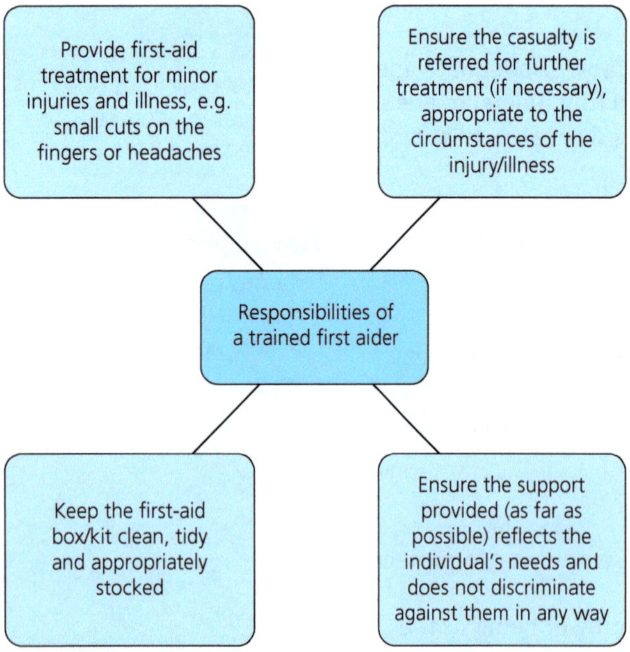

> **First aid** Help given immediately after an injury or illness occurs often at the location where it occurred.
>
> **Needs assessment** A systematic process for deciding how to meet a need, for example how much first-aid provision is required in a workplace.

> **Typical mistake**
>
> To give first aid in the workplace, you must be a trained first aider. The extent of aid given is dependent on the scope of training received. No first-aid training gives the first aider the authorisation to administer medications.

Responsibilities of a trained first aider:
- Provide first-aid treatment for minor injuries and illness, e.g. small cuts on the fingers or headaches
- Ensure the casualty is referred for further treatment (if necessary), appropriate to the circumstances of the injury/illness
- Keep the first-aid box/kit clean, tidy and appropriately stocked
- Ensure the support provided (as far as possible) reflects the individual's needs and does not discriminate against them in any way

Figure 4.1 The responsibilities of a trained first aider

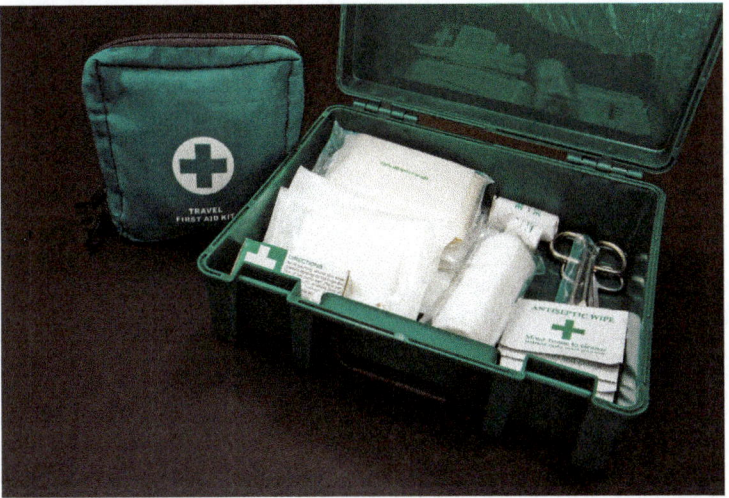

Figure 4.2 A first aider must ensure the first-aid kit for which they have responsibility is kept clean, tidy and appropriately stocked; this may include travel kits if work involves leaving a usual premises, for example on a trip or during an activity

> **Revision activity**
>
> Think of two healthcare settings, either where you have worked or where you have received care yourself. What first aid is likely to be required in these settings? What would the first-aid kit need to contain? Remember, first aid may be required by anyone in the setting – service users, family members or staff.

> **Now test yourself** 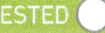 TESTED
>
> 1 What is first aid?
> 2 What is a first aider?
> 3 List **two** responsibilities of a first aider.

A4.4 The purpose of guidelines produced by the Resuscitation Council (UK)

 REVISED

Resuscitation Council

The Resuscitation Council is the national expert in resuscitation and is committed to improving survival rates for respiratory and cardiac arrest.

The role of the Resuscitation Council is to:
+ promote and publish high-quality scientific resuscitation guidelines
+ develop educational materials for resuscitation
+ support research into resuscitation.

Resuscitation guidelines

The Resuscitation Council guidelines are based on the best available scientific data.

The purpose of the guidelines is to provide detailed information about basic life support (BLS) and advanced life support (ALS) for adults, children and newborns.

The guidelines also include an algorithm, which is a simple flowchart showing the steps required to resuscitate an adult, a child or a newborn. This makes it easier to remember the necessary steps in an emergency.

> **Resuscitation** To revive someone from unconsciousness. It may be used interchangeably with the term *cardiopulmonary resuscitation* (CPR).
>
> **Respiratory arrest** Respiratory arrest is when a person stops breathing but their heart is still beating. Without rapid intervention, respiratory arrest will quickly lead to cardiac arrest.

Information for the use of an external defibrillator

The guidelines also have information on the use of cardiopulmonary resuscitation (CPR) and external defibrillators.

Defibrillators are used in clinical settings, but they are also available in many public spaces (such as schools and community centres) and private spaces (such as supermarkets and offices).

> **Cardiac arrest** When the heart suddenly stops. Blood stops being pumped around the body and the brain becomes starved of oxygen. This causes the person to become unconscious and stop breathing. Death occurs within minutes of the heart stopping.
>
> **Basic life support (BLS)** Uses CPR and/or external defibrillation for resuscitation. Anyone can be trained to use BLS.
>
> **Advanced life support (ALS)** Advanced clinical skills for resuscitation. Only professionals that hold, or are in training for, a professional healthcare qualification may be trained in ALS.
>
> **Cardiopulmonary resuscitation (CPR)** Hands-only CPR is giving chest compressions to a person in cardiac arrest to keep them alive until emergency help arrives. CPR with rescue breaths includes respiratory support.
>
> **External defibrillator** A medical device used outside of the body to give a person in cardiac arrest a jolt of energy to the heart to re-establish a normal rhythm. Also known as a defib, an AED (automated external defibrillator) or a PAD (public access defibrillator).

> **Exam tip**
>
> A defibrillator might also be known as a defib, an AED (automated external defibrillator) or a PAD (public access defibrillator).

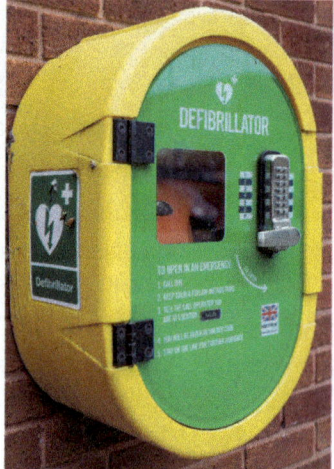

Figure 4.3 An AED in a lockbox on the wall in a public space; the code to access the defibrillator is acquired by calling 999

> **Typical mistake**
>
> Students often confuse heart attack and cardiac arrest. They are not the same. A heart attack occurs when one of the arteries that supplies the heart muscle with blood becomes blocked. This causes chest pain and damage to the muscle. A heart attack may cause cardiac arrest, but cardiac arrest is not the inevitable outcome of a heart attack.

> **Now test yourself**   TESTED
>
> 1. Which **three** elements form the role of the Resuscitation Council?
> 2. What is the purpose of the resuscitation guidelines?
> 3. How are resuscitation guidelines used?

A4.5 The purpose of manual handling regulations and training, and why it is important to follow policy and guidance when moving and positioning people, equipment or other objects safely

REVISED

Manual handling includes moving objects, moving and operating equipment, carrying out tasks such as bed making or disposing of waste, as well as assisting individuals to reposition or move.

The primary purpose of manual handling regulations and training is to prevent injury or harm. Policies and guidance set out how manual handling can be carried out safely. If not performed correctly, manual handling can lead to serious injury to service users and service providers.

> **Making links**
>
> This links directly to A3.1, which sets out the purpose of key health and safety legislation and regulations.

Following policy and guidance is important as it ensures:
+ protection from harm for individuals and healthcare professionals
+ compliance with mandatory requirements – carrying out legal responsibilities
+ conditions of insurance are met – in case of accident or injury, insurance cover will be invalid if policies and guidelines have not been followed.

Typical mistake

Remember that manual handling applies to both objects and people. It is a routine part of all healthcare sector work. Proper manual handling keeps service users *and* service providers safe.

Now test yourself

TESTED

1 What is the primary purpose of manual handling regulations and training?
2 Give **two** reasons why following manual handling guidelines and policies is important.

Exam practice

1 Jonti is a healthcare assistant in A&E. Portable X-ray machines are in regular use in the A&E department.
   a Identify the regulations that will keep Jonti safe when the X-ray machine is in use. [1]
   b Outline the purpose of the regulations. [1]
2 Abimbola has recently completed the Emergency First Aid at Work course.
   Identify **one** responsibility Abimbola has as the trained first aider in their workplace. [1]
3 Outline the purpose of resuscitation guidelines. [3]
4 A healthcare practitioner is working on a post-operative care ward, where the patients have limited mobility.
   State **one** reason why it is important to follow manual handling regulations. [1]

A5 Managing information and data within the health and science sector

A5.1 Common methods used to collect data

REVISED

Large amounts of data are collected within the healthcare sector. Data collection has numerous purposes, such as:
+ providing detailed information on the condition of an individual patient
+ gaining feedback on care or treatment received
+ conducting research into new ways of working.

A range of methods can be used to collect data, as shown in Table 5.1.

Table 5.1 Common methods used for collecting data in the healthcare sector

Method	Description	Example
Focus groups	A way of obtaining first-hand information from a group of people purposely selected to provide their opinion or experience An opportunity to gather detailed, descriptive data, as they usually provide **qualitative data**	A GP practice may use a patient focus group to generate feedback on their experience. An example of **primary research**
Open-question surveys	Questions without a predefined set of possible answers Invite detailed responses that may give opinion or experience Usually provide qualitative data	A healthcare worker may use open-question surveys to find out why patients choose whether or not to comply with treatment or advice. An example of primary research
Closed-question surveys	Surveys that have a predefined set of answers for each question from which the participant chooses Usually provide **quantitative data**	A GP may ask new patients to complete a survey on their lifestyle, including questions on physical activity levels or units of alcohol consumed. An example of primary research
Interviews	Face-to-face discussions between two or more individuals Can use predetermined questions (structured interview) or be a free-flowing conversation (unstructured interview) Usually provide qualitative data	A midwife may interview pregnant women about their experiences of screening tests in pregnancy. An example of primary research
Observation	Involves watching a process, activity or interaction being carried out and recording what is seen May provide quantitative or qualitative data	Observation could be used to audit compliance with handwashing guidelines. An example of primary research

> **Primary research** Gathering data that has not been collected before.
>
> **Qualitative data** Data that describes qualities or characteristics, or comments on opinion or experience.
>
> **Quantitative data** Numerical data that expresses how many or how often.

Check your understanding and progress at www.hoddereducation.co.uk/myrevisionnotes

Method	Description	Example
Public databases	Organised collections of data accessed electronically Most often provide quantitative data	A healthcare researcher interested in **morbidity data** and mortality data linked to alcohol-related behaviours could use a public database. An example of **secondary research**
Journals and articles	Journals publish primary research and articles written by professionals. May provide quantitative or qualitative data	A student healthcare worker may search through journals to read other people's research on a topic of interest, such as vaccine trials. An example of secondary research
Carrying out practical investigations	May range from taking samples from a patient for testing, imaging patient bodies or carrying out experiments or clinical trials Usually provides quantitative data	Clinical trials are carried out to test the safety and efficacy of new treatments or drugs. An example of primary research
Official statistics	Numerical data collected by local authorities, regional or national governments, as well as other interested agencies such as charities Provide quantitative data	A healthcare worker that wants to know how many people have accepted a COVID-19 vaccination could use official government statistics. An example of secondary research

Morbidity data Rates of a disease, medical condition or set of symptoms in a population.

Secondary research Collating or analysing data that has already been collected.

Revision activity

Look again at Table 5.1. Extend the table to give more examples for when to use each data-collection method.

Now test yourself — TESTED

1. List **two** methods of data collection that provide quantitative data.
2. List **two** methods of data collection that provide qualitative data.
3. Explain how data can be collected through observation.
4. Explain how data can be collected from:
    a. open-question surveys
    b. closed-question surveys.

A5.2 The considerations to make when selecting a range of ways to collect and record information and data

REVISED

There are numerous points to consider when selecting the method to collect and record information and data:
+ The type of data required:
    + Is detailed and descriptive qualitative information or numerical quantitative data required? This will depend on the intended purpose or use of the data.
+ The most appropriate method of data collection:
    + Manual data collection by an individual or team versus automated collection
    + Choice of method depends on whether you want qualitative or quantitative data; some methods of data collection only produce one type of data and not the other
    + Can depend on what resources you have (time, staff, budget) to complete the data collection.

- The most appropriate way to present the information or data:
  - Transcripts of interviews can be used for qualitative data.
  - Graphs and charts (for example scatter graphs, line graphs, bar graphs/histograms, pie charts) and tables are easiest for quantitative data.
- The type and depth of analysis required:
  - Quantitative data can be extracted from spreadsheets and databases and analysed via computer software.
  - Qualitative data needs to be interpreted by a human and categorised before any analysis can take place.
- The intended audience:
  - Information and data presented to the public need to be easy to understand.
  - Data presented to healthcare professionals can be more complex.
- The storage method:
  - Will this be digital or paper-based?

> **Exam tip**
>
> Make sure you are confident about the differences between quantitative and qualitative data in terms of: methods used, data generated, analysis of data, presentation and usefulness of results.

> **Revision activity**
>
> Create a list or table of information and data that may be collected in the healthcare sector using your knowledge from A5.1. Use the bullet points from A5.2 to help you decide what data-collection method is most appropriate and the best method to present the data.
>
> For example:
>
> | Data example | Appropriate method | Appropriate presentation |
> |---|---|---|
> | Age of patients admitted to A&E with alcohol-related illness or injury (quantitative data) | Statistics harvested from hospital administrative and patient data that has already been collected | Spreadsheet or graph |

> **Now test yourself**
>
> 1. Why do you need to decide whether you want quantitative or qualitative data before selecting your data-collection method?
> 2. Why do you need to know who the intended audience for your information or data is before selecting a method of collection and recording?
>
> TESTED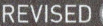

A5.3 The importance of accuracy, attention to detail and legibility of any written information or data

REVISED

When recording information and data, it is vital that it is:
- accurate – correct in all details
- thorough – pays attention to relevant detail
- legible – clear enough to be read.

Table 5.2 shows the importance of accuracy, attention to detail and legibility of any written information or data.

Table 5.2 Importance of accuracy, attention to detail and legibility of any written information or data

Reason	Example
Ensures compliance with legal requirements	For example, UK General Data Protection Regulation (UK GDPR)
Limits **liability**	If we record that we have gained informed consent, we are limiting the risk of organisations or people being open to a claim or prosecution.
Provides an accurate account of events	This protects from harm, for example by recording drug dosages accurately so overdoses do not occur.
Informs integrated working and data sharing	Different members of a multidisciplinary team may need to refer to the same record.
Ensures accurate analysis of findings	When research data is recorded accurately, we can depend on the results of any analysis.

> **Liability** The state of being legally responsible for something.

Check your understanding and progress at www.hoddereducation.co.uk/myrevisionnotes

Reason	Example
Provides support with audit trails	Accurate records can prove compliance with guidelines and protocols.
Ensures reproducibility of results	If data is not collected with precision and recorded accurately, and the method is not recorded clearly, **reproducibility** of the method or the results is impossible.

Reproducibility The extent to which consistent results are obtained when a study or experiment is repeated.

> **Now test yourself** — TESTED
>
> 1 When completing a patient record, what **three** things should you ensure about the information recorded?
> 2 Why is it important to record data accurately? Give **three** reasons.
> 3 Why is it important to record information legibly? Give **two** reasons.

A5.4 The strengths and limitations of a range of data sources when applied in a range of health and science environments

REVISED

Once you have selected your method of data collection, it is important to consider the strengths and limitations of your data source. This is shown in Table 5.3.

Table 5.3 Strengths and limitations of data sources used in health and science environments

Data source	Strength	Limitation
Results of investigations	Consistent results should be produced if the investigation is carried out under **controlled conditions**.	There is the possibility of **over-extrapolation**.
Patient history	This provides detailed information over time.	It may not be accurate or complete.
Patient test results	Tests (for example blood tests) should produce accurate and consistent data because the test method is standardised. The **reliability** of the resulting data is increased.	Results may be open to personal interpretation or inaccuracy if methods of sample collection and testing are not followed correctly.
Published literature	If the literature is **peer reviewed**, this improves validity.	It could be based on small-scale/biased research or come from fraudulent (obtained by deception) sources. The smaller the population size in any study, the less valid and reproducible the data is and the less applicable the data is to other contexts.
Real-time observation	This provides immediate data.	It can be subjective or have low **validity**, for example people might behave differently if they know they are being watched.

Controlled conditions Ensuring extraneous variables (those not being studied) are controlled so they do not affect results.

Over-extrapolation To extrapolate (draw conclusions) excessively or well beyond known values.

Reliability How consistently a method measures something.

Peer review When the data/literature is evaluated by other experts in the same field.

Validity How accurately a study or method measures what it intends to measure.

> **Exam tip**
>
> Do not just learn the strengths and limitations of each data source in isolation. Context is everything. Certain data sources are more suitable for certain contexts, for example blood cholesterol levels cannot be observed in real time but they can be tested.

My Revision Notes: Health T Level

> **Typical mistake**
>
> The concepts of reliability and validity are tricky to understand. As such, students may use them incorrectly or interchangeably. Ensure you learn both definitions and then use the phrase 'reliability requires reproducibility' to help you get the right definition for each term.

> **Now test yourself** TESTED
>
> 1 Give **one** strength and **one** limitation of a practical investigation such as a laboratory-based vaccine trial.
> 2 Explain how a blood test result could be inaccurate.
> 3 Explain why peer review is a strength of published literature.

A5.5 How new technology is applied in the recording and reporting of information and data

REVISED

New technology can be used to record and report data.

AI

- AI (artificial intelligence) is useful for recording, analysing and reporting on very large data sets.
- AI can sift through thousands of electronic health records (EHRs) to pinpoint and report on specific items.
- Bioinformatics tools can be used to examine large amounts of biological data, such as that generated by genome sequencing.

Mobile technology and applications

- Smartphones, smartwatches and wearable devices can collate, record and report health informatics, such as steps walked, hours slept, pulse, blood pressure and blood glucose levels.
- This can be used for self-management by patients with diagnosed conditions or simply to improve their lifestyle.
- The information can also be shared with healthcare professionals.
- These devices are also capable of providing location data via GPS. During the COVID-19 pandemic, the NHS COVID-19 app alerted people when they had close contact with another person with the virus, as part of the wider NHS Test and Trace programme.

Cloud-based systems

- The use of databases of information hosted on the internet that can be accessed via a connected device.
- EHRs are stored on a private system, which requires users to submit a data access request service (DARS) to NHS Digital.
- The use of cloud-based systems such as EHRs enables easy data sharing and analysis between healthcare professionals.

Digital information management systems

- Computer software that enables settings such as hospitals to manage all the digital information generated within the setting.
- This sophisticated approach enables EHRs, appointment scheduling, bed management, clinical records and more to be brought together into one system.
- An advantage of such systems is the ability to generate a complete digital audit trail for each patient journey.

Check your understanding and progress at www.hoddereducation.co.uk/myrevisionnotes

Data-visualisation tools

+ Data visualisation analyses large amounts of data and communicates the results in a visual context, making them quick and easy to comprehend.
+ This is particularly useful for showing anomalies or outliers, as well as patterns and trends.
+ Various sources of data can be consolidated (combined) into one visualisation.
+ Data visualisation uses graphs, charts or maps, and if an interactive dashboard is used, data can be updated in real time.

> **Making links**
>
> Data stored on cloud-based systems and digital information management systems is subject to data protection and confidentiality principles. This is covered in A5.6.

> **Exam tip**
>
> You may be asked about the advantages or disadvantages of new technology used for recording and reporting data.

> **Now test yourself** — TESTED
>
> 1 Why is AI useful for data recording and reporting?
> 2 What can mobile technology and applications be used for?
> 3 How are cloud-based systems accessed?
> 4 What is a digital information management system? Why are these systems advantageous?
> 5 What is data visualisation and what are its benefits?

A5.6 How personal information is protected by data protection legislation, regulations and local ways of working/organisational policies

REVISED

Data Protection Act 2018 and UK GDPR

The General Data Protection Regulation (GDPR) 2016 is a European Union (EU) regulation. GDPR provides a set of principles with which any individual or organisation processing sensitive data must comply.

In the UK, this regulation is implemented by the Data Protection Act 2018. This Act established strict rules called data protection principles that control the use of personal information by organisations, businesses or governments.

Under the Data Protection Act 2018, individuals have the right to:
+ be informed about how their data is being used
+ access their personal data
+ have incorrect data updated
+ have data erased
+ stop or restrict the processing of their data
+ port their data (allowing people to get and reuse their data for different services)
+ object to how their data is processed in certain circumstances.

> **Exam tip**
>
> You are expected to be familiar with all aspects of the GDPR and Data Protection Act 2018 that are referred to in this section. Make sure you know all the ways in which personal information is collected, used, stored and protected in the healthcare sector, as referred to in this and the next section.

> **Personal information** Any information where the person can be identified, directly or indirectly, including a person's name, address or date of birth. Also called personal data.

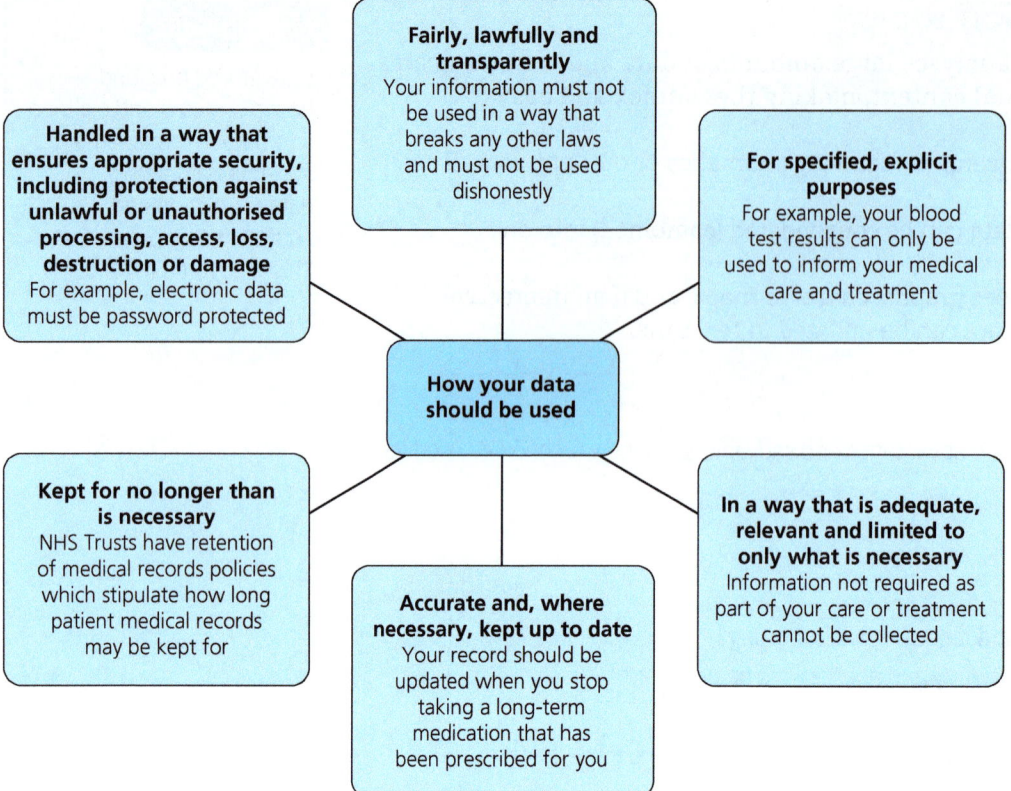

Figure 5.1 How personal information must be used

Local ways of working/organisational policies

Healthcare organisations have additional agreed ways of working written into their organisational policies, which ensure compliance with GDPR principles and reflect the context of healthcare settings. These are shown in Table 5.4.

Table 5.4 Local ways of working/organisational policies to ensure compliance with legislation and regulations

Agreed way of working written into policy	Explanation
Ensuring data is stored securely	Electronic data is only to be saved on organisational devices and with password protection. Paper-based data, such as care plans, must be stored in locked cabinets and/or rooms.
Restricting the use of mobile devices to ensure confidentiality	Personal mobile devices should not be used in healthcare settings. This ensures patient images, voices and data cannot be recorded or passed on by accidental or deliberate means.
Preventing potential conflicts of interest	Every organisation must have a data protection officer (DPO) to ensure compliance with data protection legislation. The DPO must not also hold a position or perform tasks that may lead them to influence the use of personal data.

Now test yourself TESTED

1. What law governs the protection of personal information?
2. What are the data protection principles?
3. What rights do you have regarding any personal data kept by organisations?
4. Why is the use of mobile phones and devices restricted in healthcare settings?

Check your understanding and progress at www.hoddereducation.co.uk/myrevisionnotes

A5.7 How to ensure confidentiality when using screens to input or retrieve information or data

REVISED

Healthcare workers are required by law to maintain confidentiality and the security of information. Table 5.5 shows how to maintain confidentiality when using computers or tablets.

Table 5.5 The actions to ensure confidentiality when using screens and why they are important

Method	Explanation
Log out of a system when leaving the screen	Every time a screen is left unattended, even for just moments, you should log out or lock the screen to prevent unauthorised access.
Protect login and password information	Login information and passwords must not be disclosed, written down, shared or easy to guess. This prevents unauthorised use or access. Only the individual to whom the username is allocated should use that username.
Be aware of your surroundings	Computers and tablets may be used in patient-facing settings or busy areas. It is important to be aware of who is around you when accessing confidential data and ensure no one is looking over your shoulder. Do not look at confidential information when others are present.
Use secure internet connections	This helps to prevent information being hacked or compromised by breaches. Specific email programmes, such as NHSmail, may be used. This has an optional encryption service as an additional security tool.
Use privacy screen filters where appropriate	Privacy screen filters that clip over computer screens only permit normal vision from a position directly in front of the screen. This prevents the screen being read from sideways glances or over the shoulder.

Revision activity

Create a concept map on A5.6 and A5.7. Demonstrate how these two areas of content link to one another. For example, when taking a patient history, what does the patient need to know about the information you are collecting? What are your responsibilities when collecting this information? And how can you ensure confidentiality when inputting this information into a computer?

Now test yourself

TESTED

1. How can you protect your username and password login details?
2. Why should you only use secure internet connections?
3. How can you stop people accidentally or deliberately seeing confidential information on a screen while you are using it?
4. What should you do when you leave a screen unattended?

A5.8 The positive use of, and restrictions on the use of, social media in health and science sectors

REVISED

Positive uses

Social media can be used positively by the healthcare sector in several ways:
+ Awareness campaigns, disseminating (spreading) information, correcting misinformation and crisis communication:

- During the COVID-19 pandemic, Public Health England (now replaced by the UK Health Security Agency, UKHSA) used all major social media channels to provide information on COVID-19 protection measures (spreading information and correcting misinformation), symptoms (awareness campaigns), rules and restrictions (crisis communication) and vaccination programmes.
+ Monitoring public health and data gathering:
  - It might be possible to observe an increase in people reporting on social media that they are experiencing a particular set of symptoms.
  - It can also be used in a more targeted way, by requesting certain populations to complete online surveys, or express interest in joining research studies, which ultimately lead to data gathering.
+ Establishing support networks:
  - Formal professional bodies, such as the Royal College of Nursing (RCN), have a social media presence which can be used to support members and colleagues.
  - Informal networking opportunities also exist, for example midwives may self-organise into networking groups, where CPD or journal articles are discussed online.
+ Recruitment and marketing:
  - Social media can be used to advertise job vacancies and services.

Restrictions on use

It is important that the healthcare sector places some restrictions on social media use. When acting in a professional capacity or representing their organisation, healthcare workers should:
+ refer to the organisation's code of conduct regarding social media use
+ not post personal or sensitive information about themselves or others
+ maintain professional boundaries when interacting with others
+ avoid sharing inaccurate or non-evidence-based information.

> **Revision activity**
>
> 1 Create a table of the positive uses of social media. For each positive use, give a real-world example. For example: awareness campaigns – social media was used to raise awareness during the COVID-19 pandemic.
> 2 Now create a spider diagram on restrictions on social media use. Include the possible negative impacts of unprofessional use of social media – on patients, family members/carers, staff, organisations and the public.

> **Now test yourself** TESTED
>
> 1 Give an example of how social media can be used to disseminate information in the healthcare sector.
> 2 Give an example of how social media can be used to support research.
> 3 Give an example of how social media can be used to support CPD.
> 4 List **two** ways that social media use should be restricted in the healthcare sector.

A5.9 The advantages and risks of using IT systems to record, retrieve and store information and data

REVISED

The recording of most information and data in the healthcare sector is now performed using IT systems. There are advantages and risks to this, as shown in Table 5.6.

Table 5.6 The advantages and risks of recording information and data using IT systems

Advantages	+ Easily accessible – all computers connected to a network can access data stored on the network + Makes sharing and transferring data easy + Contributes to speedy data analysis – computer software can be used to interrogate and report on data + Offers security via secure servers, password protection and encryption + Enables data to be standardised – data is entered into specific categories in a database, which means specific data can be retrieved easily + Enables continuous and real-time monitoring of data – as soon as data is entered, it can be interrogated, analysed and reported + Is cost and space efficient compared to large archives of paper records + Contributes to integrated working, as data is accessible and can be shared and transferred + Supports safeguarding practice, as professionals can access patient history and records to see a full picture
Risks	+ Security breaches, either accidental or malicious; for example, if systems are hacked or passwords are compromised, confidential information may be leaked and data could be used in unauthorised or unlawful ways + Potential for corruption of data; errors that occur during reading, writing, storage, transmission or processing of data may mean the data becomes incomplete or unusable + Lack of access due to system failure, for example due to power failure, hardware failure or malicious events (hacking)

Exam tip

Most of your exam questions are presented with a context or scenario and require you to apply your knowledge to that context or scenario. Make sure you can apply these advantages and risks of using IT systems to specific healthcare sector contexts. For example, the benefit of easy data sharing means that multiple healthcare professionals on multiple sites can see a patient's test results. On the other hand, corruption of data could mean that a patient's test results are lost.

Now test yourself

1 Give **three** advantages of using IT systems to record data.
2 Give **two** potential risks of using IT systems to store data.

TESTED

A5.10 How security measures protect data stored by organisations

REVISED

Organisations implement security measures to protect data that is stored. Table 5.7 shows some of these.

Table 5.7 Security measures to protect stored data

Security measure	Reason
Controlling access to information	Having usernames and passwords, as well as security or authority levels, ensures individuals have access to the minimum amount of data and information required for their job.
Only allowing authorised staff into specific work areas	The use of security passes and door codes, combined with security or authority levels, means that only specific individuals with clearance can access certain work areas.
Regular and up-to-date staff training	This ensures staff know exactly how to comply with data security measures. This can be tailored to the level of access to data and information that the employee has.
Back-up systems	Back-up systems make a copy of all data. This is important in case original data becomes corrupted or is stolen.
Cyber security strategies	Threats to cyber security change all the time, so the most up-to-date strategies must be used to prevent unintended and malicious data breaches. There are several NHS and governmental cyber security agencies that organisations can consult for support in this area.
Storing back-up externally	Using off-site, external or cloud-based back-up services adds an additional layer of data security should there be an event such as fire or flood that could damage servers.

Now test yourself

TESTED

1 How can organisations control access to information?
2 How can organisations work with staff to protect stored data?
3 What is a back-up system and why is it important?

Revision activity

Make a concept map to cover all the ways in which these types of security measures improve working practices and have positive impacts on individual service users.

My Revision Notes: Health T Level

A5.11 What to do if information is not stored securely

REVISED

Step 1: When possible, secure the information by following any relevant protocols

For example, if a paper record is left on a desk, move it to a locked cupboard or room; if a screen is left unattended by a colleague, log them out or lock the screen.

Step 2: Record and report the incident to the designated person, following organisational policy and procedure

This is particularly important if you discover a breach; for example if you accidentally sent confidential information to the wrong person or did not use secure or encrypted email, you must report this.

> **Now test yourself**
>
> 1 If you find unsecured data, what should your:
>   a first action be?
>   b follow-up action be?
> 2 Where will you find guidance on how to act in this type of situation if you are unsure?
>
> TESTED

Exam practice

1 Describe **two** methods of data collection. [4]
2 A GP practice wants to know how satisfied its patients are with the care and treatment they receive.
   a Identify **two** appropriate methods for collecting this data. [2]
   b Explain why each method is appropriate. [4]
3 A nurse is working in the high-dependency unit, caring for patients with complex medical needs. An emergency occurs and the nurse completes a record of what happened.
   a State **one** reason why it is important that the record is legible. [1]
   b Explain a possible impact of not doing this. [2]
4 Jensa has been asked to observe nurses as they administer medicine on a hospital ward. This is part of an audit to check that staff are always complying with policy.
   Explain **one** limitation of direct observation in this context. [2]
5 A ward manager has been asked to share key performance indicators for the ward with staff and patients. These indicators include: average length of stay, bed occupancy rates, staff-to-patient ratio and patient satisfaction.
   Explain how data visualisation could be used for this and why this approach would be advantageous. [3]
6 A GP practice usually records patient data on organisational computers. There is a power cut and the practice manager advises all staff to use pen and paper to record any new data.
   Discuss the implications for data protection when records are paper-based. [6]
7 Ren is working at the nurses' station on a busy hospital ward. There are three computers and a tablet for staff to use.
   a State **one** way to reduce unauthorised access to computers and electronic devices in healthcare settings. [1]
   b Explain a possible impact of not doing this. [2]
8 Explain **one** responsibility healthcare workers have when using social media in a professional capacity. [2]
9 Describe **two** benefits of using IT systems to retrieve data. [4]
10 Brad is working as a healthcare assistant in a community mental health team. Part of his job is to enter patient data into the computer.
   Outline how the data can be protected from accidental deletion or loss. [2]
11 A member of staff has left a computer screen unattended in a busy clinic. It is possible that the information displayed on screen may have been seen by multiple patients.
   Explain what action must be taken. [4]

Check your understanding and progress at www.hoddereducation.co.uk/myrevisionnotes

A6 Managing personal information

A6.1 Your role in relation to record keeping and audits

REVISED

Record keeping

Keeping records of patient care and treatment is essential and required by law. Written records, whether paper-based or electronic, must:
+ be accurate
+ be timely – completed as soon as possible and always before the end of a shift
+ provide detail on the care provided for each individual
+ be factual and recorded according to legislative requirements (for example UK GDPR and the Data Protection Act 2018)
+ be free from abbreviations (where possible) and jargon.

You must ensure:
+ familiarity with and competence in using all systems used to record information – seek training as necessary
+ confidentiality and data protection by using secure storage systems and passwords and never leaving information unattended
+ never to disclose information in public spaces.

> **Making links**
>
> A5.6 covers requirements of UK GDPR and the Data Protection Act 2018. Refer back to that section to check legal requirements for record keeping.

Audits

Audits involve tracking activities and behaviours to see whether they comply with workplace policies and procedures. Most audit activities have some element of reviewing recorded data and information. Complaint investigations may also involve audits of records.

You must ensure:
+ handwritten records are legible and completed in black ballpoint pen (so they cannot be erased, and can be read if photocopied)
+ care is taken to enter the data accurately when records are completed electronically
+ all entries in a record have a date, time and signature to confirm when they were completed, to provide a detailed timeline, and to confirm who completed them.

> **Exam tip**
>
> When asked to 'identify', simply provide a brief one- or two-word answer; you do not need to write in sentences. For example, 'Identify two requirements of handwritten records'. Any two of the following answers would be appropriate and gain marks:
> + written in black pen
> + legible
> + signed with date and time.

> **Now test yourself** TESTED
>
> 1 What are the key principles you must adhere to when making patient records?
> 2 To enable an audit to take place, how should handwritten records be completed?
> 3 When entering data into a system, what important consideration should you take?

A6.2 Why personal information is collected, stored and protected

The purpose of collecting personal information

Personal information is collected in the healthcare sector to:
+ create a personal history
+ inform the diagnosis of a condition or an illness
+ inform the treatment to be given
+ inform follow-on care to be provided.

The purpose of storing personal information

Personal information is stored so that it can be:
+ shared (as appropriate) with the wider multidisciplinary team involved in diagnosis, treatment and care
+ used in the future, for example for future diagnosis or treatment of the individual or as part of research (anonymised and/or with consent).

Individuals have the right to access their data and records and to ask how they are being used, for example through the Freedom of Information Act 2000. They also have certain rights to withdraw consent for their data to be used for purposes such as audit and research (see information governance below).

> **Making links**
>
> See A5.6 for more on how personal information is protected by data protection legislation and Figure 5.1 for how personal information should be used.

How personal information is protected

Data protection regulations

GDPR is a set of rules enacted in the UK through the Data Protection Act 2018 to protect personal information.

Information governance

Information governance describes the complex legal framework that governs the use of personal confidential information in healthcare.

It establishes that personal information may be shared among organisations and professionals giving direct patient care, but it also protects patients' confidentiality when information about them is used for other purposes.

These other purposes, or secondary uses, include:
+ reviewing and improving the quality of care provided (for example through audit)
+ researching the treatments that work best
+ commissioning clinical services
+ planning public health services.

When personal information is used for these purposes, it must either be anonymised or, if it will identify an individual patient, their consent must be obtained.

> **Exam tip**
>
> Some questions require you to give examples. You should make your examples directly relevant to any scenario or context given in the question and be as specific as possible. Ask yourself, 'Does my example answer the question by showing how or why something is done?'

> **Now test yourself**
>
> 1. Why does the healthcare sector collect personal information?
> 2. Why does the healthcare sector store personal information?
> 3. What is the purpose of information governance?

Check your understanding and progress at www.hoddereducation.co.uk/myrevisionnotes

A6.3 The types of information needed when obtaining a client history

REVISED

The types of information needed when obtaining a client history are listed in Table 6.1.

Table 6.1 The types of information needed when obtaining a client history

Information needed	Reason
Name	Patient identification can be confirmed and their records maintained and tracked.
Date of birth	Patient identification can be confirmed and their records maintained and tracked. Age can increase the risks of certain conditions and diseases and can be important in determining treatments and drug dose calculations. In children and young people, age is important regarding capacity and consent.
Individual NHS or hospital number	Patient identification can be confirmed and their records maintained and tracked.
Health status	It is important to establish details regarding the patient's current health, as this may influence care and treatment decisions.
Medication/treatment history	This concerns what medications or treatments the patient has received, either to relieve a new or pre-existing condition.
Family history	Individuals may have a genetic predisposition to certain conditions (for example diabetes) or may even have a genetically inherited condition (for example Huntington's disease).
Social history	This refers to whom the individual lives with, their job and lifestyle factors such as diet, exercise and substance use.
Social care involvement	For example, whether the individual has a named social worker, or whether they receive any care and support services from social care agencies.

> **Typical mistake**
>
> Students often confuse genetic predisposition to disease and genetic inheritance of disease. Being predisposed to a disease or condition does not guarantee that you will develop it.

> **Exam tip**
>
> Most exam questions require application of your knowledge to a given scenario. This means you should practise putting your knowledge into context, for example knowing what elements of taking a client history would be important in different scenarios.

> **Now test yourself** TESTED
>
> 1 What is the shared purpose of recording patient name, date of birth and NHS or hospital number?
> 2 Why is it important to take a medication/treatment history?
> 3 What is a social history and what information might you record as part of that?

> **Making links**
>
> Remember that children and young people may have the capacity to make their own decisions and provide their own consent. See A1.3.

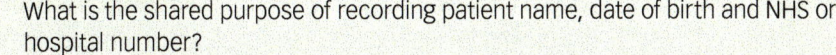

My Revision Notes: Health T Level

A6.4 The purpose of common abbreviations used in the healthcare sector

REVISED

The purpose of common abbreviations

Common abbreviations can be used to:
+ facilitate shorter written accounts of care and treatment
+ ensure standardisation across staff and organisations.

Common abbreviations

Table 6.2 A list of common abbreviations used in the healthcare sector

Abbreviation	Meaning
PRN	*Pro re nata* – meaning 'as needed' or 'as required' – is used in reference to certain medications.
BP	Blood pressure
MAR	Medication administration record: the MAR records all medications given (dose, date and time, and signature of the person administering them).
DNR	Do not resuscitate or a do-not-resuscitate order: in the case of cardiac arrest, CPR will not be attempted.
MST	Malnutrition screening tool: a 5-step tool used to identify adults that are malnourished or at risk of becoming so.
NEWS 2	National early warning score: a chart used to record adult patient physiological observations. It calculates a score based on these observations and provides an algorithm for subsequent action.
PEWS	Paediatric early warning score: a chart used to record paediatric patient physiological observations. It calculates a score based on these observations and provides an algorithm for subsequent action.

> **Making links**
>
> A6.1 covers the principles of good record keeping, which include the avoidance of abbreviations and jargon whenever possible.

> **Exam tip**
>
> Always write out a term in full, with the abbreviation in brackets, the first time you use it in your exam. After that you can use the abbreviation without explaining it.

> **Now test yourself** TESTED
>
> 1 Where might you see the abbreviation PRN used?
> 2 What is a MAR used for?
> 3 What is the difference between a NEWS 2 and a PEWS?

A6.5 The advantages of reporting systems for managing information with regards to incidents, events and conditions

REVISED

Computer software reporting systems enable healthcare staff to report incidents, events and conditions.

There are advantages of using such systems:
+ They prevent misinterpretation of information.
+ They allow timely reporting of information by someone who witnessed or discovered the event or incident.
+ They provide easy access to information for ongoing tracking or monitoring.

> **Now test yourself** TESTED
>
> 1 Why are reporting systems quick and easy to use?
> 2 What are **two** advantages of providing a reporting system?

Check your understanding and progress at www.hoddereducation.co.uk/myrevisionnotes

A6.6 When it may be appropriate to share information and the considerations that need to be made when sharing data

REVISED

When it is appropriate to share information

In some circumstances, it may be appropriate to share information. These circumstances are outlined in Figure 6.1.

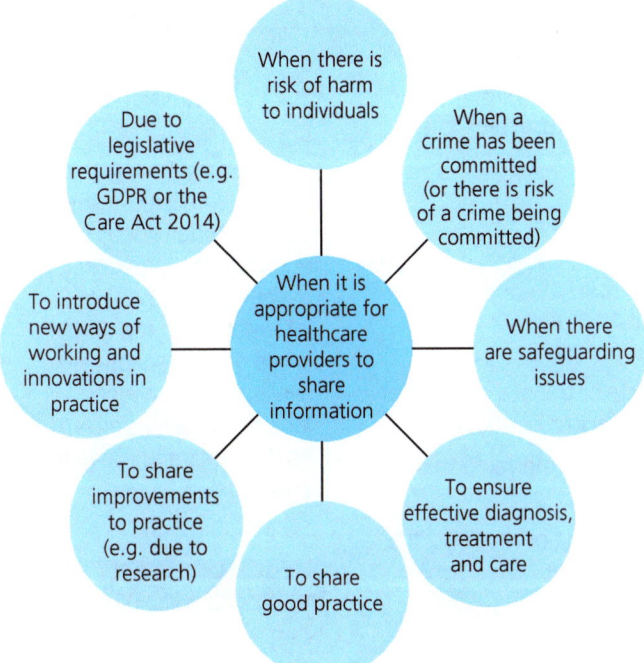

Figure 6.1 Circumstances when it is appropriate for healthcare providers to share information

Considerations when sharing data

Before data is shared, the following should be considered:

+ protecting the individual's identification, for example using the Caldicott principles
+ using the individual's NHS number instead of their name so they are not as easily identifiable
+ informing the individual and gaining consent to share their data, unless it is required by law to share or the benefit in sharing it outweighs keeping it confidential (for example safeguarding risks)
+ ensuring the individual's information and confidentiality requirements are followed as set out in relevant regulations
+ informing an appropriate adult or advocate if sharing the individual's information where the age or mental capacity of the individual is an issue
+ who the intended audience is, for example the individual or other health professionals
+ why the information is being shared, for example is it to support the individual's care or to present the outcomes of a project?

> **Caldicott principles**
> Eight principles to ensure people's information is kept confidential and used appropriately.

> **Making links**
> How personal information is kept confidential and the relevant regulations surrounding this are covered in A5.6.

> **Exam tip**
>
> Six-mark 'discuss' questions are usually accompanied by the statement: 'Your response should include reasoned judgements'.
>
> This requires you to provide reasons why something should be done in a particular way, or reasons why a particular outcome might be expected. This could include consideration of the importance or impact of something. For example, if you state that an individual's information should be shared because there are safeguarding concerns, you should explain what the safeguarding concerns are, why it is important to share some specific piece of information and what the expected outcome of that will be.

> **Revision activity**
>
> Use the internet to find out what the eight Caldicott principles are. Draw up a table that lists each principle and gives an example of how it could be followed in a healthcare setting you know well.

My Revision Notes: Health T Level

> **Now test yourself** TESTED
>
> 1 What are the Caldicott principles used for?
> 2 When sharing best practice or research findings, how should patient confidentiality be protected when sharing their data?

A6.7 The different formats for the sharing of information

REVISED

When sharing information, the most appropriate format should be chosen. This will be based on what information is to be shared, the purpose of the information and who the intended audience is. Table 6.3 summarises the different formats.

Table 6.3 The different formats for the sharing of information

Format	Example
Oral reports	Giving immediate verbal information or answering questions to support an individual's care
Written reports	Completing change-of-shift reports or transfer reports, or other reports where a permanent record is required
Forms and documents	Completing a report-of-injury form or a referral form from a GP to social care children's services
Presentations	Sharing good practice in a team meeting or reporting the findings of a research project
Graphs and tables	Summarising an individual's information or the findings of a research project
Leaflets or posters	Providing information about treatment options
Web pages and social media	Providing information about health promotion initiatives

> **Revision activity**
>
> For each format of information sharing, think of an example in healthcare practice when it would be appropriate. For example, a leaflet would provide information on the different types of contraceptives available to someone looking to start using contraception to prevent pregnancy.

> **Typical mistake**
>
> Oral reports provide immediate verbal information. However, as they are not formally recorded anywhere, do not use oral reports to share important information that is not also recorded somewhere in writing or digitally. For example, a test result may be reported orally from the laboratory to the healthcare professional but should be accompanied by a written report.

> **Now test yourself** TESTED
>
> 1 When is an oral report most appropriate?
> 2 When is a written report more appropriate than an oral one?
> 3 There has been an accident in the workplace and a paramedic has attended after the first aider made a 999 call. Which format of information sharing would be best when the first aider informs the paramedic what has happened, and why?
> 4 When would leaflets and posters or web pages be used to share information?

A6.8 The reasons for record keeping and how this contributes to the overall care of the individual

REVISED

Reasons for record keeping

Record keeping provides:
+ an overview of an individual's medical history
+ an overview of an individual's care needs
+ access to an individual's information for all multidisciplinary teams
+ a record of all services accessed.

Record keeping supports:
+ continuity of care – smooth and co-ordinated care across and between services and professionals

Check your understanding and progress at www.hoddereducation.co.uk/myrevisionnotes

- protection of the individual – accurate records ensure care will be safe and effective (for example avoidance of drug errors)
- protection of healthcare and social care professionals – accurate records show that professionals acted with competence and integrity to give safe and effective care.

How record keeping contributes to the overall care of the individual

Record keeping:
- ensures uniform care is given by professionals across services, as care needs are clearly established
- provides an accurate record of:
  - what has been discussed
  - what took place at each interaction
  - agreed next steps.

> **Exam tip**
>
> Ensure you are confident in explaining the reasons why record keeping is such an important part of working in the healthcare sector. If you are asked to explain its importance in a particular context, it may be helpful to consider what the impact would be (on service user, service provider and organisation) if record keeping was not completed to the required standard.

> **Now test yourself**
>
> 1. Give **three** reasons for record keeping.
> 2. Give **two** ways that record keeping contributes to overall care of the individual.
>
> TESTED

A6.9 The responsibilities of employees and employers in relation to record keeping and when to escalate issues

REVISED

Responsibilities

Legal requirements and inspections
- The Care Quality Commission (CQC) is responsible for the inspection of healthcare settings.
- Records are one of the data sources that the CQC uses to inform these inspections.
- Records contribute to decisions made by the CQC about the standard of care being delivered.

Duty of care
Record keeping is one of the ways of demonstrating that duty of care is being fulfilled.

> **Making links**
>
> In A4.1 you learned the meaning of 'duty of care'. If you are not sure what it means, you should go back and remind yourself.

Duty of candour
- Duty of candour is a responsibility to be open and honest.
- This includes making individuals aware when mistakes are made in their care or treatment, apologising for these mistakes and, when possible, putting things right.
- If records are not accurate, duty of candour requires that you are open and honest with service users about this.
- If a mistake in care is discovered, accurate records need to be kept of any subsequent actions and conversations about this.

> **Making links**
>
> Duty of candour is also important when supporting and communicating with individuals who are bereaved. See A8.14.

Investigating and tracking incidents and accidents
- Accurate and legally compliant record keeping is an essential part of investigating and tracking incidents and accidents.
- Records should accurately demonstrate care given and actions carried out – they enable the causes and contributory factors in incidents and accidents to be found.

Accountability

- This refers to responsibility for actions.
- Organisations and the individuals who work in them are accountable for their actions to employers or governing bodies, professional bodies and the public.
- Record keeping provides an audit trail and is one way of demonstrating accountability.

When to escalate issues

Employees and employers have a duty to escalate (take further action) when there are:
- safeguarding concerns (for example suspected abuse)
- radicalisation concerns.

If anyone working in the healthcare sector is not assured that sufficient action is being taken in such cases, they can use whistleblowing. Every organisation in the healthcare sector must have a whistleblowing policy and associated procedures.

> **Radicalisation** The process by which an individual or a group becomes increasingly extreme in their views in opposition to political, social or religious norms in a society.
>
> **Whistleblowing** When an employee passes on a concern of wrongdoing in the workplace that is causing or may cause harm. Or, if an employee has already tried to raise a serious concern about something they have seen but they do not feel it is being dealt with.

Typical mistake

Taking action and following escalation procedures is important when record keeping is not carried out correctly and may result in disciplinary action for an individual, but it is not just about the disciplinary action. Reporting and investigating incidents are key ways that organisations are able to learn from their mistakes and make improvements in how they deliver care.

> **Making links**
>
> Safeguarding is covered in more detail throughout A11. Whistleblowing procedure is covered in A11.7.

Now test yourself   TESTED

1. Why is record keeping linked to CQC inspections?
2. How does record keeping relate to duty of care?
3. How does record keeping relate to duty of candour?
4. What does accountability mean?
5. Define the term *escalation*. When should an employee escalate an issue?

Exam practice

1. You are working as a healthcare assistant in a GP practice and you have taken a patient's blood pressure.
   Describe your record-keeping role when entering this information onto an IT system. [2]
2. Explain why personal information on patients is collected and stored in the healthcare sector. [3]
3. Describe **three** important details taken as part of a client or patient history. [3]
4. The abbreviation DNR is recorded on the notes of an elderly patient.
   a Identify what DNR stands for. [1]
   b Explain what would happen if this patient had a cardiac arrest. [1]
5. Discuss why a healthcare setting should consider using a reporting system for managing information with regards to incidents, events and conditions.
   Your answer should consider the advantages of these systems. [3]
6. The community nurse is with a patient at home with worrying symptoms. They have requested a home visit from the GP and will need to inform the doctor about their concerns.
   a Identify **one** format for sharing this information. [1]
   b Explain why this format would be appropriate. [2]
7. A healthcare assistant is recording information on an individual.
   a Identify **one** reason for record keeping. [1]
   b Explain why that reason is important. [2]
8. A healthcare assistant has observed a young adult in the care of a hospital viewing extremist material online using their smartphone.
   a Identify the concern. [1]
   b State what action the healthcare assistant should take. [1]

Check your understanding and progress at www.hoddereducation.co.uk/myrevisionnotes

A7 Good scientific and clinical practice

A7.1 The principles of good practice in scientific and clinical settings

The principles of good practice in scientific and clinical settings are:
- using standard operating procedures (SOPs)
- effectively managing calibration and maintenance of equipment and work areas
- effectively managing stock
- appropriately storing products, materials and equipment.

The rest of this section will go through these principles in more detail.

A7.2 What an SOP is

A standard operating procedure (SOP) is a set of sequential steps or instructions designed to standardise the approach to a process or an action. An example would be the process for calibrating a set of weighing scales.

A7.3 Why it is important for everyone to follow SOPs

SOPs are based on evidence and industry standards, and are therefore proven to be safe, effective and reliable.

SOPs are important because they:
- maintain health and safety – they are established on proven safe practice
- enable a consistent approach – everyone does each task in the same way
- meet any legal or organisational requirements – for example for health and safety or testing standards
- uphold professional standards – they use evidence-based practice
- demonstrate compliance for audit purposes.

> **Revision activity**
>
> Create a concept map with as many SOPs as you can think of that are relevant in a healthcare setting. SOPs may include how to clean the environment, how to maintain personal hygiene, how to move or handle objects, how to carry out clinical tasks and so on.

A7.4 How to access SOPs for a given activity

You must know how to access a SOP for any given activity. This is done by:
- completing detailed staff inductions and ongoing training on the use of SOPs
- carrying out detailed index searches for specific SOPs, for example via your organisation's intranet or the relevant manual.

When an appropriate SOP is located, it is important to ensure:
- it is the most up-to-date version by checking the published and proposed review dates
- all relevant documentation has been completed, dated and signed.

> **Now test yourself** TESTED
>
> 1. What are the **four** principles of good scientific and clinical practice?
> 2. What is an SOP?
> 3. Give **two** important reasons to follow SOPs.
> 4. Give **one** way to access the appropriate SOPs for a given activity.

A7.5 The potential impacts of not regularly cleaning and preparing work areas for use

REVISED

Clinical and laboratory areas must be cleaned regularly. Substances that are hazardous to health are handled in these areas, and even non-infectious or non-hazardous substances can cause contamination issues.

The potential impacts of not cleaning regularly include:
+ Risks to health and safety:
    + spread of infection from contaminated surfaces or aerosols (coughing, sneezing) – for example from patient samples to members of staff
    + production of toxic/dangerous by-products – for example during laboratory tests if equipment is not cleaned properly
+ Invalid results:
    + contamination or cross-contamination, for example from environmental samples, reagents (substances used to examine chemical reactions) or DNA, can invalidate test results
+ Inefficient working practices:
    + this leads to increased costs and timescales
+ Damage to equipment:
    + this leads to increased costs and timescales.

Contamination The unwanted pollution of something by another substance.

Cross-contamination When microorganisms such as bacteria are accidentally transferred from one substance or object to another.

Exam tip

It is important to be aware of scientific practice in clinical science settings, as clinical scientists are part of the multidisciplinary team that healthcare professionals work with every day. Issues such as contamination of patient samples may take place at any point in their processing, from a clinician taking the sample to a scientist testing it.

> **Now test yourself** TESTED
>
> 1. Give **two** ways that failing to clean regularly risks health and safety in a clinical setting.
> 2. How can failing to clean regularly lead to invalid results in a laboratory setting?

A7.6 The potential impacts of not maintaining, cleaning and servicing equipment

REVISED

Just as work areas must be kept clean, equipment must also be kept clean. It should also be maintained and serviced as necessary.

Failing to maintain, clean or service equipment could lead to:
+ Risks to health and safety:
    + increased risk of injury due to malfunctioning equipment
    + spread of infection due to unclean equipment
+ Invalid results:
    + contamination or cross-contamination of equipment (for example environmental samples, reagents)
+ Reduced function of equipment:
    + decreased lifespan of equipment – if it is not maintained and serviced, it is more likely to malfunction or stop working altogether
    + increased costs and timescales (for example equipment needing repair or being out of service).

Check your understanding and progress at www.hoddereducation.co.uk/myrevisionnotes

> **Typical mistake**
>
> While a healthcare assistant may not be directly responsible for the maintenance and servicing of equipment, health and safety legislation states that taking action to reduce hazards is a universal responsibility. If a healthcare assistant notices that equipment is faulty and may risk safety, they must take action to ensure the person responsible is alerted. This links to A7.7.

> **Now test yourself**   TESTED
>
> 1. Give **one** way that failing to service and maintain equipment regularly risks health and safety in a clinical setting.
> 2. How can failing to clean equipment regularly lead to increased costs and timescales?

A7.7 Why it is important to calibrate and test equipment to ensure it is fit for use

REVISED

Regular testing of equipment checks its quality, performance or reliability prior to use. Testing and calibration of equipment is required to ensure:

+ measurements are accurate – if measuring equipment is not regularly tested and calibrated, the data will be invalid
+ the life of equipment is maintained or prolonged – testing means that faults can be prevented or identified and fixed
+ legal requirements are met – calibration against industry-set standards ensures validity and quality.

> **Calibration** Checking that equipment is operating correctly against a required standard and making any adjustments to return it to the standard.

For example, a calibration weight can be used to ensure scales are still weighing accurately and precisely.

A system for recording when equipment has been serviced, tested or calibrated is used. Most often this will be a sticker on the equipment which is dated and signed.

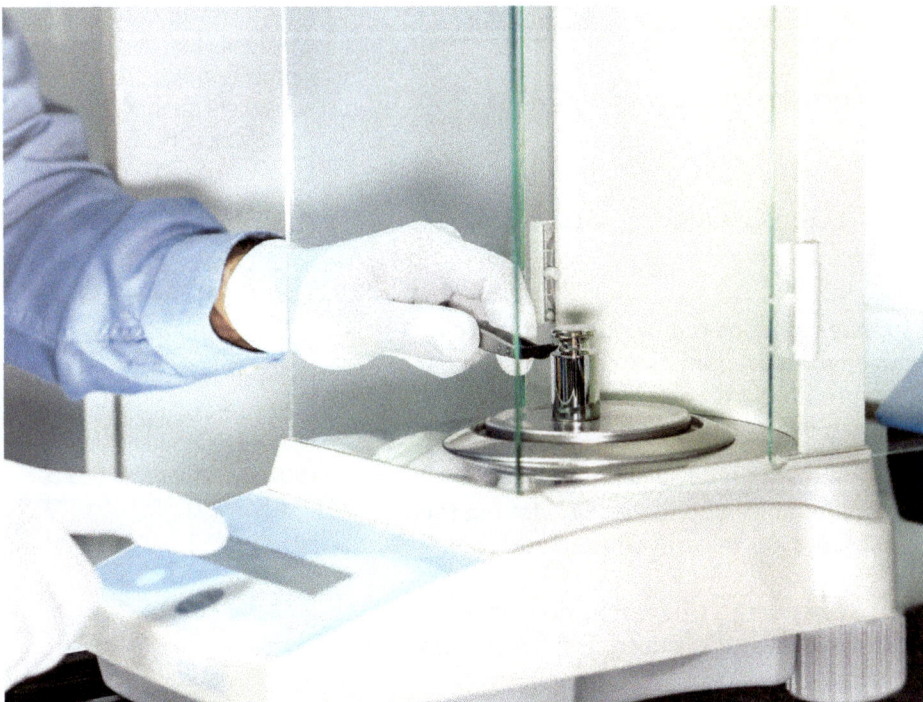

Figure 7.1 Scales are calibrated using calibration weights. This ensures they continue to measure precisely.

> **Revision activity**
>
> Make a list of equipment that you might find in clinical settings, such as a medical ward in a hospital, that would require regular testing and calibration. For each piece of equipment listed, make a note of any potential impacts of not testing and calibrating the equipment.
>
> One full example has been completed for you in the table. Copy the table, complete the second entry and then add to the table with your own settings, equipment and impacts.
>
> | Setting | Equipment | Impact of not testing and calibrating regularly |
> |---|---|---|
> | Medical ward | Blood pressure monitor | Blood pressure may be measured inaccurately, leading to a failure to spot a deteriorating patient or abnormal measurement requiring treatment. |
> | | Weighing scales | |

> **Now test yourself**
>
> 1 What is the difference between testing and calibration?
> 2 Give **one** example of a piece of equipment used in clinical settings that should be tested and calibrated regularly.
> 3 List **two** potential impacts of not testing and calibrating equipment.
>
> TESTED

A7.8 How to escalate concerns if equipment is not correctly calibrated/unsuitable for intended use

REVISED

Any concerns regarding equipment that is found to be incorrectly calibrated or otherwise unsuitable for use must be escalated.

This can be done by:
+ taking the equipment out of action – removing it from the setting
+ labelling the equipment as being out of use, if appropriate – particularly useful if it is not possible to remove it from the setting
+ reporting concerns to the relevant person, in line with organisational policies and procedures
+ recording concerns according to organisational procedures.

> **Exam tip**
>
> Remember, there will be an SOP that states clearly how to escalate concerns if equipment is not correctly calibrated or is otherwise unsuitable for use. Similarly, if reports of unsuitable equipment are not acted upon, whistleblowing procedures can be used. See A11.11.

A7.9 Why it is important to order and manage stock

REVISED

Stock of clinical and laboratory supplies must be managed using a stock control system. These systems can be used to monitor stock levels of materials and consumables and ensure timely reordering, while avoiding having too much stock that is not often used.

Ordering and managing stock will ensure:
+ a sufficient supply of required consumables and materials – for example knowing how many gloves, masks and aprons are required and then ordering to meet demand
+ the use of materials before their expiry date – this can be done by having regular stock checks and ensuring oldest stock is used first (for example by putting the newer stock to the back of the shelf)
+ reduced costs by not ordering excess stock, which may go to waste if it expires prior to use
+ efficiency and productivity, as stock is available when needed rather than waiting for reorders and restocking
+ the safety of stock, for example by checking that bottles and containers are not damaged or degraded.

> **Consumables** Items used by healthcare providers to treat people that are usually single-use products, for example bandages.

Check your understanding and progress at www.hoddereducation.co.uk/myrevisionnotes

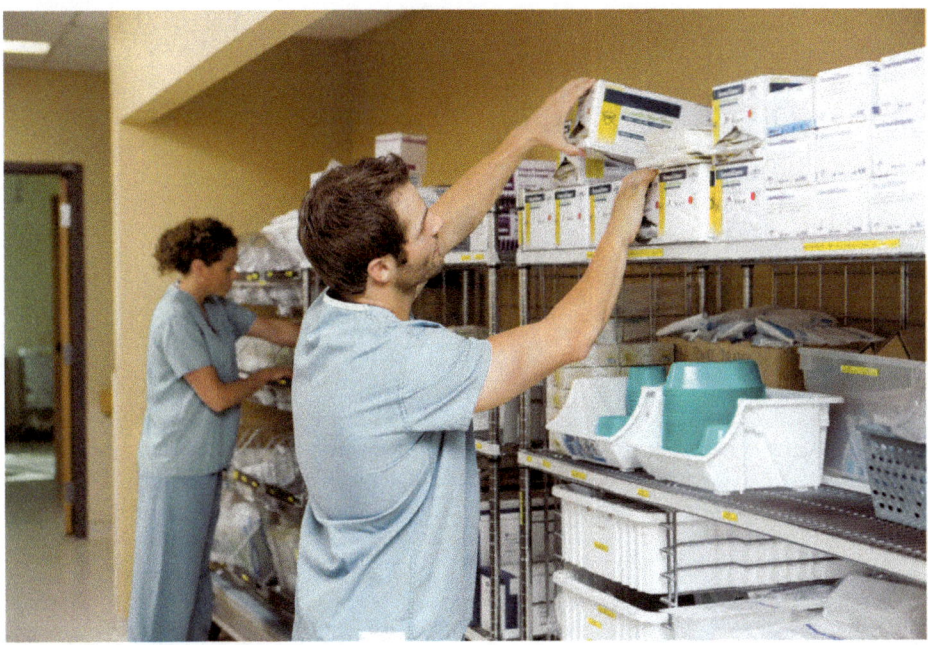

Figure 7.2 It is essential that stock is ordered and well managed.

> **Now test yourself** TESTED
> 1 What is a stock control system?
> 2 List the benefits of having a stock control system for ordering and managing stock.

A7.10 The potential consequences of incorrectly storing products, materials and equipment

REVISED

Products, materials and equipment used in clinical and laboratory settings must be stored correctly and according to the manufacturer's instructions. The consequences of incorrect storage are detailed in Table 7.1.

The original containers that stock is supplied in will list any storage requirements (manufacturer's instructions) and expiry dates. For this reason, all stock should be stored in original containers.

Table 7.1 The consequences of incorrect storage of products, materials and equipment

Consequence	Explanation
Cross-contamination	A damaged bottle may allow other materials to enter, such as glass or plastic fragments (physical contamination), bacteria (biological contamination) or other substances (chemical contamination). This would mean the contents are now contaminated and cannot be used.
Breakdown of limited stability products	Some chemicals and medications may become unstable if stored incorrectly – they may become corrosive, explosive or reduced in efficacy.
Products exceeding expiry dates	Expiry dates set the limit of safe and efficacious use of products. For example, gloves may become stiff and prone to breakage when used past their expiry date and will therefore not provide the required protection.
Loss of samples or degradation of reagents not stored at the correct temperature (−20°C, −4°C, 4°C or room temperature)	Certain products must be stored in an appropriate, temperature-controlled environment. Regular checks should be carried out to ensure the temperature is being maintained, otherwise the products can no longer be used.
Risks to health and safety	These could include spread of infection, release of dangerous chemicals or heavy items not stored at correct height.
Stock being difficult to locate	This wastes time and may lead to unnecessary restocking.
Financial loss	If stock becomes unstable, degrades or expires, it will have to be disposed of and replaced, incurring costs.

My Revision Notes: Health T Level

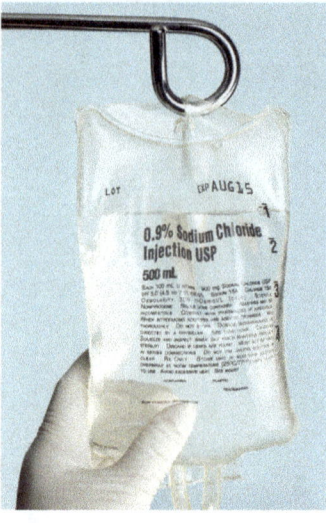

Figure 7.3 This bag of saline lists storage instructions and expiry date. Incorrect storage of products such as this may cause direct harm to patients.

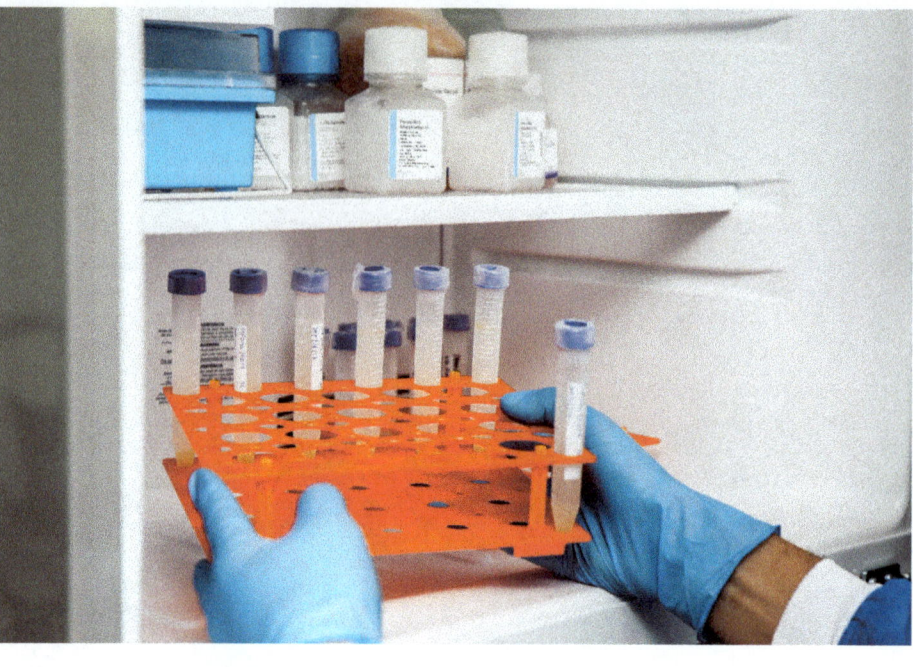

Figure 7.4 Some products and materials must be stored at the correct temperature.

Typical mistake

The safety risks associated with storing items are not limited to harmful chemicals or the shelf life of products. Large, awkward or heavy items need to be stored so they do not pose a risk of falling onto, or tripping, people. They should also be at a height where they can be manoeuvred without causing musculoskeletal injuries.

Now test yourself

TESTED

1 What is meant by 'manufacturer's instructions'?
2 How might a bag of saline solution become contaminated if stored incorrectly?
3 Why could poor storage practices lead to stock expiring?
4 Why might an organisation experience financial losses due to incorrect storage of stock?

Exam practice

1 Simeon is doing work experience in a hospital pathology laboratory. He is told he should familiarise himself with the standard operating procedures (SOPs) for testing patient samples.

   Explain **three** reasons why it is important for everyone to follow SOPs in a laboratory setting. [6]

2 Hanna has been asked to clean down the work surfaces in the clean utility room of a hospital ward.
   a Give **one** reason why it is important to regularly clean clinical work areas. [1]
   b Explain the potential impact of not doing this. [2]

3 A heart-rate monitor has been sent for servicing.
   a State **one** reason why it is important to service equipment regularly. [1]
   b Explain the potential impacts if this is not done. [2]

4 It is Pavel's first day of his new job. He has been asked to weigh a patient. Pavel checks to see if there are any calibration stickers on the scales prior to using them.

   Explain why Pavel is checking if the scales have been calibrated. [2]

5 Staff on a hospital ward have noticed that one of the glucometers is not working correctly and there is no record of when it was last calibrated.

   Outline what action should be taken. [3]

6 A stock check has been carried out at a GP surgery and there are many products that have expired.

   Identify **one** way that this could be avoided in future. [1]

7 A new hospital department has opened and is being stocked with products and materials.
   a Identify **two** ways that the stock can be managed correctly. [2]
   b For **one** way identified in **a)**, explain the impact of not managing that stock correctly. [2]

Check your understanding and progress at www.hoddereducation.co.uk/myrevisionnotes

A8 Providing person-centred care

A8.1 The purpose of the Mental Capacity Act 2005 plus Amendment (2019) in relation to healthcare

REVISED

The Mental Capacity Act 2005 plus Amendment (2019) applies to:
+ anyone over the age of 16 whose mental capacity to make their own decisions around care and treatment may be limited
+ everyone delivering or responsible for the care and treatment of over 16s who have potentially limited mental capacity.

The purpose of the Act
The Act protects rights and safeguards and supports people to make their own decisions where at all possible, providing a decision-making framework.

If an individual lacks the mental capacity to make choices about their own treatment or care, the Act lays out who can make decisions in the person's best interests and how these decisions should be made.

> **Exam tip**
> When planning your revision, allow sufficient time to learn this section thoroughly. Person-centred care is a fundamental concept and underpins all patient-facing activities in the healthcare sector. Person-centred care is the focus of section D on your exam paper.

> **Mental capacity** The ability to make decisions, by being able to understand information and remember it for long enough to make the decision and then communicate it to others.

> **Now test yourself** TESTED
> 1 Who does the Mental Capacity Act 2005 apply to?
> 2 What is the principal purpose of the Act?

A8.2 The key principles of the Care Act 2014

REVISED

The Care Act 2014 is the most significant piece of legislation governing the provision of adult social care in England. It requires local authorities to provide:
+ resources and services to help prevent, reduce or delay the development of care and support needs
+ information and advice that individuals need to make good choices about care and support
+ a range of high-quality and appropriate services to choose from when need arises.

The key principles of the Care Act 2014 are shown in Table 8.1.

Table 8.1 The key principles of the Care Act 2014

Principle	Explanation
Empowerment	Individuals should be supported to make their own decisions based on best possible information.
Protection	Protection should be provided for service users who are in greatest need of support and protection.
Prevention	Action should be taken to prevent harm before it occurs.
Proportionality	Any protective or preventative actions should be proportionate to the risk: being overprotective can disadvantage service users to be able to make their own decisions.
Partnership	Working with a range of professionals, groups and communities is required to prevent, detect and report neglect or abuse.
Accountability	Healthcare and social care professionals need to be accountable for any activities in relation to safeguarding.

My Revision Notes: Health T Level

> **Exam tip**
>
> When asked to *explain*, you are required to give a justification for an action. For example, if asked to explain why proportionality is important in safeguarding, your explanation should give a clear motivation for using this concept. If you simply describe or define proportionality, you will not gain marks.

> **Making links**
>
> The legal framework of the Care Act 2014 is also covered in A11.2.

> **Now test yourself** TESTED
>
> 1 What are the six key safeguarding principles of the Care Act 2014?
> 2 Explain the Care Act principle 'proportionality'.
> 3 How does proportionality relate to the remaining five key principles?

A8.3 The role of a range of regulatory bodies within the health sector

REVISED

Regulatory bodies and their role

Regulatory bodies are appointed by the government. The specific role of each of the healthcare regulators is underpinned by legislation.

The primary purpose of the regulation of healthcare activities is to limit risks and protect the public. The regulators in the health sector are split into those that regulate professionals and those that regulate activities.

Regulation of professionals

General Dental Council (GDC)
The GDC is the UK-wide statutory regulator of dental professionals, such as dentists, dental hygienists and dental nurses.

Health and Care Professions Council (HCPC)
The HCPC is the UK-wide statutory regulator of 15 health and care professions, known as allied health professionals, including:
+ occupational therapists
+ prosthetists
+ orthotists
+ speech and language therapists
+ dieticians
+ physiotherapists.

Nursing and Midwifery Council (NMC)
The NMC is the UK-wide statutory regulator for nurses and midwives. In England, the NMC also regulates nursing associates.

> **Exam tip**
>
> You are expected to be familiar with the names of regulatory bodies and what they do. Make sure you understand clearly the role of bodies that regulate professionals (such as the NMC) and the role of bodies that regulate activities (for example the CQC).

> **Regulator/statutory regulator** An organisation appointed by the government to control an area of activity, such as healthcare, by means of rules.
>
> **Statutory regulation** Regulation required by law.
>
> **Occupational therapist** An allied healthcare professional that supports people of all ages to overcome challenges in their daily life, through assessment, goal planning and targeted adjustments to environment and activities.
>
> **Prosthetist** An allied healthcare professional that provides engineered solutions to people with limb loss, for example by designing, making and fitting prosthetic legs.
>
> **Orthotist** An allied healthcare professional that provides engineered solutions to people experiencing issues with their neuro, muscular and skeletal systems. For example, by designing, making and fitting braces, splints, callipers and so on.
>
> **Nursing associate** A nursing role that bridges the gap between healthcare assistants and registered nurses.

Check your understanding and progress at www.hoddereducation.co.uk/myrevisionnotes

The roles of the GDC, HCPC and NMC are shown in Figure 8.1.

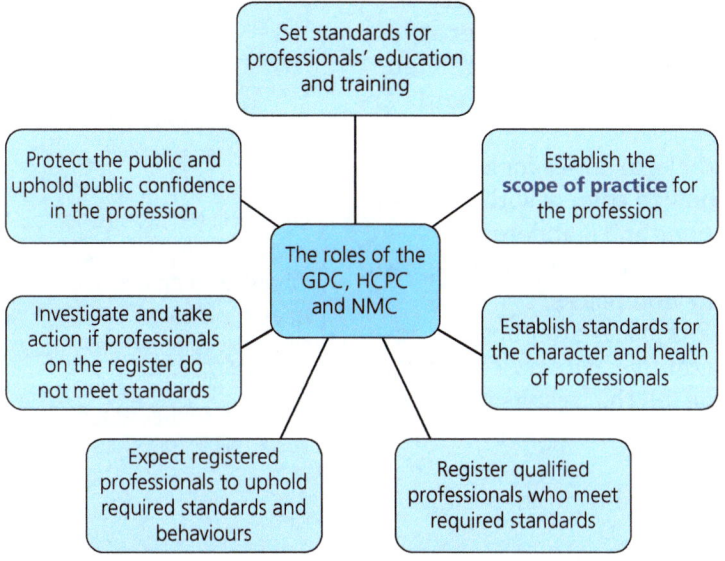

Figure 8.1 The roles of the GDC, HCPC and NMC

Regulation of activities

Care Quality Commission (CQC)

The CQC is an independent regulator with an independent voice. It publishes views on quality issues in health and social care services in England, with a focus on service improvement.

It exists to ensure that services provided are safe, effective, compassionate and high quality.

Any individual, partnership or organisation in England that provides any of the 14 regulated activities specified in the Health and Social Care Act 2008 must register with the CQC.

Regulated activities include:
+ treatment of disease, disorder or injury
+ accommodation for persons who require nursing or personal care
+ maternity and midwifery services
+ nursing care.

Hospitals, GPs, residential nursing homes and other health and care services must be registered with the CQC.

A key role of the CQC is to monitor, inspect and rate services. All inspections and ratings are published, so the public can see how safe and effective the provided care is.

If failings in service provision are found, an extension of the CQC role is to take action to protect people who use services, including:
+ recommendations for change
+ fines
+ legal action
+ closing services.

> **Revision activity**
>
> Create a concept map on regulation of professionals. Include:
> + names of regulatory bodies and who they regulate
> + how they carry out their regulatory role.

> **Exam tip**
>
> Although outside the scope of your T Level Health specification, it is important to know that to be on a professional register as a dental professional (GDC), allied health professional (HCPC) or nursing and midwifery professional (NMC), you must also:
> + have a professional indemnity arrangement (all)
> + make an annual CPD statement (GDC)
> + make a declaration every two years that you continue to meet professional standards (HCPC)
> + revalidate every three years.

> **Scope of practice** The limit of a professional's knowledge, skills and experience. Comprises the activities they carry out within their professional role.

> **Making links**
>
> A1.2 covers the importance of adhering to quality standards to facilitate continuous improvement and objective, independent reviews of care and care practice.

Health and Safety Executive (HSE)

The HSE is the national independent regulator for health and safety in the workplace, including public and private healthcare services. It improves health and safety in the workplace – preventing work-related death, injury and ill health – by ensuring health and safety standards are adhered to.

+ It publishes extensive guidance on how to fulfil legal duties for keeping employees and the public safe. For example, how to comply with first aid, fire safety and manual handling laws, regulations and standards.
+ It works to raise awareness of health and safety issues and priorities, with the objective of improving health and safety in workplaces.
+ It inspects and investigates health and care workplaces after health and safety incidents of a non-clinical nature. For example, if a service user that had been assessed as being at risk of falls has a fall that results in serious injury or death (reportable under RIDDOR), the HSE will inspect the service and investigate the incident.
+ It takes enforcement action against organisations failing in their duties.

Office for Standards in Education, Children's Services and Skills (Ofsted)

The Care Standards Act 2000 gave Ofsted responsibility for inspecting and regulating services that care for children and young people by providing regulated activities. An example of this is a residential children's home.

Where children's homes and similar services provide regulated activities (for example personal care) under the Health and Social Care Act 2008, the provider must be registered with and subject to inspection and monitoring by the CQC.

Ofsted's objective is to improve lives by raising standards.

Information Commissioner's Office (ICO)

The ICO is the independent regulator for data protection and its role is to promote and support information rights in the public interest.

The ICO does this by:
+ carrying out audits of and advisory visits to health organisations in relation to personal data
+ encouraging transparency on data usage and data privacy for individuals
+ providing information, resources and guidance on how to comply with data protection and information rights law.

> **Typical mistake**
>
> While Ofsted inspects and regulates schools and education facilities, this is not directly relevant to your T Level Health qualification. What is relevant, however, is that Ofsted also inspects and regulates settings where children and young people are cared for through regulated activities, such as giving personal care. For example, agencies responsible for adoption.

> **Now test yourself** TESTED
>
> 1. What does the term *statutory regulation* mean?
> 2. What does regulation mean in the context of the health sector?
> 3. Name **three** regulatory bodies for health professionals.
> 4. List **two** ways that regulatory bodies regulate professionals.
> 5. Give **two** examples of regulated activities governed by the Health and Social Care Act 2008.
> 6. Give **two** examples of health sector services that are regulated by the CQC.
> 7. How does the CQC regulate health sector services?
> 8. What is the role of the HSE?
> 9. In what circumstances can the HSE inspect a service within the health sector?
> 10. Apart from schools and colleges, what else does Ofsted regulate?
> 11. What is the role of the ICO?

> **Revision activity**
>
> Create a concept map on regulation of health sector activities. Include:
> + names of regulatory bodies and what activities they regulate
> + how they carry out their regulatory role.

A8.4 How physical and mental function across the lifespan impacts on care needs and informs person-centred care

REVISED

Typical care needs
Typical care needs common across the lifespan include:
- nutrition and hydration
- personal care
- general health and wellbeing
- positive relationships
- self-esteem
- personal growth
- independence.

Stages of human development across the lifespan

Birth and infancy, 0–2 years
- Human infants are completely dependent on others for survival.
- They require intervention from others to remain healthy and to grow and develop.
- Infants flourish in an environment where they receive emotional security, from caregivers who demonstrate responsive and predictable behaviour.

Early childhood, 3–8 years
Children require additional support for social and emotional health, for example support to:
- develop independence and begin to meet their own physical needs
- learn, play and develop social skills
- explore and establish their own identities and develop their self-esteem.

Adolescence, 9–18 years
Adolescence is a transitionary period involving:
- puberty
- emerging sexuality and intimate relationships
- increasing independence.

Early adulthood, 19–45 years
Early adulthood involves:
- completion of physical growth and sexual maturation
- sexual and reproductive health.

Lifestyle and behavioural choices can impact health status, for example:
- physical activity levels
- dietary choices
- use or misuse of substances such as tobacco, alcohol and drugs.

Middle adulthood, 46–65 years
Here the ageing process commences with:
- deterioration of sense organs
- perimenopause and menopause in females
- increased susceptibility to conditions such as cardiovascular disease and type 2 diabetes.

Later adulthood, 65 years onwards
For later adulthood, ageing degenerates the cells across all body systems, increasing susceptibility to a wide range of diseases and conditions that may limit normal physiological functioning. Person-centred care in later adulthood can contribute to personal fulfilment and improved quality of life.

As the immune system weakens, older adults are also more likely to develop and be more seriously affected by illness.

Older adults may become dependent on others for support with hydration, nutrition, personal care and mobility.

> **Exam tip**
> The scenarios in exam questions provide important contextual information that you should use in your answers. If you are told that an individual is of a particular age, you are expected to consider what this means for any care or treatment, support, procedure or service you discuss in your answer.

> **Menopause** When menstruation ceases. This usually occurs in middle adulthood.
>
> **Perimenopause** The period immediately prior to the occurrence of menopause. May start at the end of early adulthood.

> **Typical mistake**
>
> It is possible to live well and in good health in later adulthood. Factors that are protective of health earlier in the lifespan, such as regular physical activity, good social connections and healthy lifestyle habits (such as reducing alcohol consumption and avoiding smoking), contribute to good health and wellbeing and reduce the negative impacts of ageing.

> **Revision activity**
>
> Create a concept map for each life stage.
>
> Add specific notes on the physical and mental function relevant to the life stage. Make links to any related care and support needs.

> **Now test yourself** TESTED
>
> 1 List **three** requirements of physical health that infants are dependent on others for.
> 2 List **three** social and emotional support requirements of children.
> 3 List **three** of the transitions common in adolescence and identify linked support needs.
> 4 Identify **three** possible physical and mental support needs in adulthood.
> 5 List **three** features of later adulthood that result in an increased need for care and support.

A8.5 The key values of the healthcare sector when providing care and support

REVISED

NHS core values

The NHS Constitution sets out rights for patients, the public and the staff to ensure the NHS operates safely and effectively. It is underpinned by the NHS core values, shown in Table 8.2. Adhering to these values will ensure the best care for individuals.

Table 8.2 NHS core values

Value	Example
Compassion	Treating everyone with kindness and humanity, to meet their needs and reduce any anxiety, pain, fear or distress
Improving lives	Working to improve the health and wellbeing of everyone
Respect and dignity	Valuing every person – patients, family members, staff – and respecting their needs, wishes and preferences
Commitment to quality of care	Working continually and proactively to provide safe and effective care
Working together for patients	Putting individuals at the centre of care and bringing together multidisciplinary and multi-agency teams to meet their needs
Everyone counts	Maximising benefit for everyone, ensuring equality of access to services and **anti-discriminatory practice**

> **Anti-discriminatory practice** Practice which aims to undermine, reduce or prevent discrimination.

Check your understanding and progress at www.hoddereducation.co.uk/myrevisionnotes

Six principles produced by the People and Communities Board

The People and Communities Board (PCB) was established as part of the NHS Five Year Forward View programme. Part of the work of the board was to establish six principles that set out the basis of good, person-centred, community-focused health and social care, as shown in Figure 8.2.

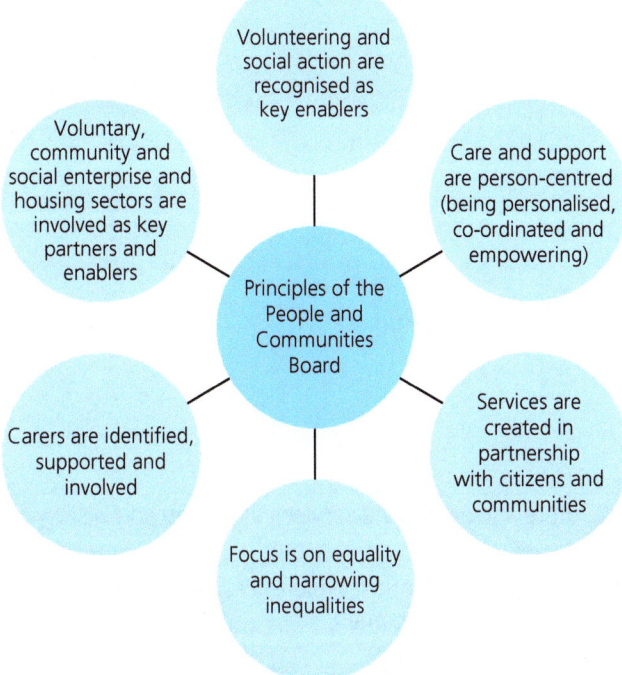

Figure 8.2 The six principles produced by the PCB

> **Revision activity**
> 1 Create a way to remember the NHS values. Perhaps you could think of a rhyme or a mnemonic.
> 2 Think of examples of how the six principles could be used to develop community-focused health care. Choose a service user or health need to focus on and draw a concept map. You can then create a set of flashcards.

> **Now test yourself**
> 1 What is the purpose of the NHS values?
> 2 Define the **two** values: 'compassion' and 'respect and dignity'.
> 3 Give an example of 'everyone counts' being put into practice in a health setting.
> 4 What is the purpose of the six principles established by the PCB?
>
> TESTED

> **Exam tip**
> If you are asked about NHS core values, you will almost certainly be expected to explain how they can be used or why they are important. Make sure you can give real-life examples of each value being used in a practical way.

A8.6 The purpose of the Personalisation Agenda 2012 and the importance of using holistic approaches in order to place individuals, their carers and significant others at the centre of their care and support

REVISED

Purpose of the Personalisation Agenda 2012

The purpose of the Agenda is to put the individual first in the process of planning, developing and providing their care.

Care for those with long-term illnesses and conditions is tailored to their individual needs and desires.

This means the service user is provided with greater choice and more information, including a choice of care provider.

Holistic approaches

Holistic care approaches consider the whole person and their life and do not simply focus on a diagnosis or set of physical symptoms.

> **Holistic** Considering the whole person; acknowledging that physical health cannot be separated from other elements of the person (such as psychological wellbeing) and their environment.

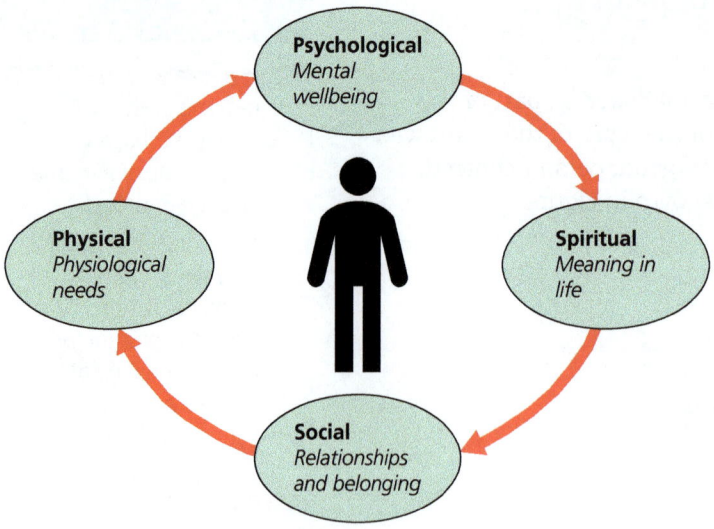

Figure 8.3 Holistic care requires consideration of the whole person when managing and preventing ill health

Table 8.3 details a range of holistic approaches.

Table 8.3 Holistic approaches

Person-centred planning (PCP)	Enables individuals to plan their own future and access the services they need and wish.
Person-centred care (PCC)	Focuses care on the needs of individuals, by asking for their preferences, needs and values to guide all decisions made regarding their care and treatment.
Hierarchy of the individual's needs (Maslow's hierarchy of needs theory)	Provides a framework for meeting needs in a holistic way. The hierarchy shows that while meeting physiological needs (for example food and shelter) is a prerequisite for health, more is needed to enable full psychological wellbeing and quality of life. This requires meeting needs for safety and security, love and belonging, and self-esteem.
Advanced care planning	Enables individuals to plan their future care, including any medical treatment, while they have the capacity to do so. For example, individuals in the early stages of terminal illness can be involved in making decisions about their end-of-life care while they are still able to do so. This ensures the choices and wishes of the individual will continue to be met even when they can no longer express them directly.
Integrated working	When all agencies, professionals and systems work together to consider the needs of a population and plan for person-centred care.
Do Not Resuscitate directive (DNR)	In collaboration with a doctor, an individual can decide that if their heart or breathing stops, their healthcare team will not attempt to restart it.

> **Typical mistake**
>
> Remember in A6.4 it was pointed out that an individual with a DNR has not had all treatment withdrawn, only that CPR will not be used if their heart or breathing stops.

The importance of holistic approaches

Holistic approaches are important for several reasons:
+ They ensure all individual needs are met and any care provided is in the individual's best interest.
+ They respect individual autonomy, as they respect an individual's rights to make decisions for themselves.
+ They encourage engagement with healthcare and social care professionals and organisations, as they contribute to trusting and respectful relationships between service provider and service user.

Check your understanding and progress at www.hoddereducation.co.uk/myrevisionnotes

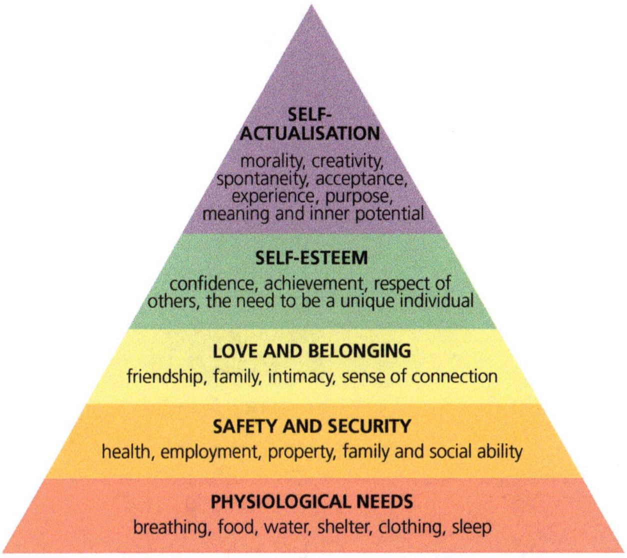

Figure 8.4 Maslow's hierarchy of needs

> **Revision activity**
> 1 Create a set of flashcards to help you learn and remember the six holistic approaches to personalised care.
> 2 Sum up the Personalisation Agenda 2012 in three sentences.

> **Now test yourself** TESTED
> 1 Describe how person-centred care can be planned and given.
> 2 Give an example of advanced care planning.
> 3 What is meant by a 'holistic approach'?

> **Making links**
> A2.10 covers how multidisciplinary and multi-agency teams work together. It might be useful to recap that section now.

A8.7 A range of verbal and nonverbal communication techniques, potential communication barriers and how to overcome them to support an individual's condition

REVISED

Communication techniques

Effective communication enables healthcare workers to be clearly understood by everyone. As communication is a shared relationship, the quality of a service provider's communication technique also affects the quality of communication they receive back.

Techniques include verbal and nonverbal communication, as shown in Table 8.4. Nonverbal communication is an important way to show that you are genuinely listening to others.

> **Makaton** A language programme that uses a combination of symbols, basic signs and speech to enable people to communicate. It is most often used with individuals with learning disabilities.

Table 8.4 Communication techniques

Communication technique	Ways of communicating	Example
Verbal	Involves speech and sound Possible to vary pitch, tone, volume and pace	+ Taking a formal tone when communicating with colleagues in a professional capacity + Using a gentle tone when breaking bad news
Nonverbal	Conveying information without speech	+ Gestures involving hands, arms or head to express meaning + Facial expressions + Body language + Eye contact + British Sign Language (BSL) + Makaton

> **Typical mistake**
>
> BSL is a complete language and is not easy to learn. It is typically learned and used by children and adults that identify as being deaf as their first language. This means it is not usually a suitable communication method for someone experiencing hearing loss in later adulthood because of ageing.

> **Exam tip**
>
> The way in which we communicate verbally and nonverbally can both improve and worsen the effectiveness of the message we are trying to communicate.

> **Revision activity**
>
> Figure 8.5 shows an interaction between a healthcare professional and an individual.
>
> List all the ways that the healthcare professional is showing effective communication.

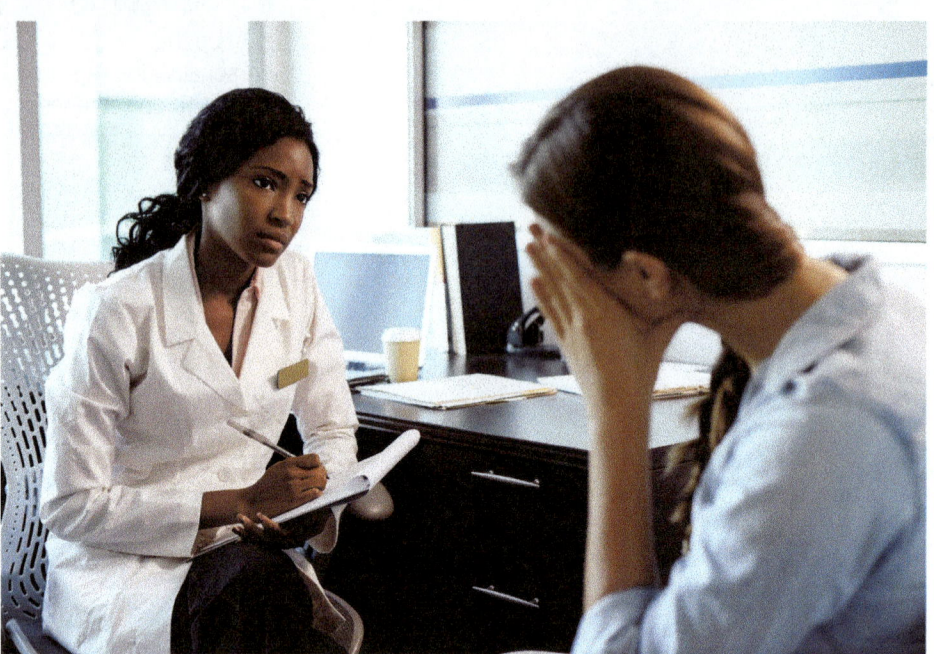

Figure 8.5 Nonverbal communication is an important way to show that you are genuinely listening to others.

Barriers to communication

Barriers to communication are factors that disrupt or prevent effective communication. They include:
+ sensory disorders (for example speech, hearing or sight)
+ mental health conditions
+ language barriers (for example jargon, spoken language or accents)
+ time pressures
+ noisy environments
+ poorly lit environments
+ positioning of the individual from the healthcare professional (for example proximity)
+ tension or conflict.

Overcoming barriers to communication

An important part of person-centred care and anti-discriminatory practice is actively working to remove as many communication barriers as possible.

This can include:
+ actively asking about and listening to the individual about their communication needs or preferences
+ providing access to a range of support options and choices – such as the use of advocates or foreign language or BSL interpreters
+ active involvement from the individual in how, when, where and in which way they are communicated with to meet their needs
+ providing access to information that is understandable to the particular individual
+ providing a choice of communication aids or supports that match the needs and preferences of the individual.

Check your understanding and progress at www.hoddereducation.co.uk/myrevisionnotes

> **Revision activity**
>
> 1 Create a concept map of verbal and nonverbal communication techniques. Use a different colour to indicate settings or situations where healthcare workers might need to use specific techniques.
> 2 Create a table of specific communication barriers, matched to ways to overcome them. Give examples of specific settings and service users where issues may arise and suggest what could be done to improve communication.

> **Exam tip**
>
> Tablets, computers and mobile phones can be used to aid communication. For example, professional foreign language interpretation services can be accessed via the phone.

> **Now test yourself** TESTED
>
> 1 List the **four** parts of verbal communication that can easily be adapted.
> 2 Summarise how gestures and facial expressions can be used to enhance meaning.
> 3 When you first meet a service user, what can you do to minimise any potential communication barriers?

A8.8 The application of relevant legislation, including Mental Capacity Act 2005 plus Amendment (2019) and Liberty Protection Safeguards (LPS) on the provision of person-centred care

REVISED

Mental Capacity Act 2005

The Mental Capacity Act (MCA) 2005 plus Amendment (2019) gives protection to vulnerable adults (aged 16 years and over) around decision-making.

Every adult, whatever their ability, has the right to make their own decisions wherever possible, from everyday decisions (for example clothing choices) to very difficult decisions around treatment and the end of life.

The Act promotes person-centred care because it gives healthcare workers a legal responsibility to support individuals to be empowered to make their own decisions as much as possible.

There are five principles of the Act:
1 Begin by assuming the individual has capacity, unless it is proven otherwise.
2 Support individuals to make their own decisions.
3 Recognise that unwise decisions do not mean the individual lacks capacity.
4 If decisions must be made for someone, they must be in the individual's best interests.
5 When someone does lack capacity, consider whether a decision can be made in a way that is least restrictive of their freedom.

> **Making links**
>
> Remember, A8.6 covers the Personalisation Agenda 2012, which promotes person-centred care through holistic approaches.

Liberty Protection Safeguards

The 2019 Amendment to the MCA proposed that Liberty Protection Safeguards (LPS) be introduced to replace the previous system of Deprivation of Liberty Safeguards (DoLS).

The purpose of the LPS (like DoLS) is to ensure anyone lacking capacity and experiencing deprivation of liberty is still placed at the centre of all decision-making. An individual may be deprived of their liberty because they would be unsafe without continuous supervision, for example an individual with advanced dementia. The arrangements must be proportionate to the likelihood and severity of harm.

> **Deprivation of liberty**
> This is when an individual is not free to go anywhere without permission or close supervision and lacks capacity to consent to this. This is against the law unless done under the rules of the Mental Capacity Act 2005.

> **Now test yourself** — TESTED
>
> 1. Who does the Mental Capacity Act (MCA) 2005 apply to?
> 2. What is the purpose of the MCA?
> 3. What is the first principle of the MCA?
> 4. What is the purpose of Liberty Protection Safeguards (LPS)?

> **Exam tip**
>
> In 2023, the introduction of LPS was put on hold indefinitely, therefore the DoLS system remains.

A8.9 The considerations when providing person-centred care to people with pre-existing conditions or living with illness

REVISED

Conditions or illnesses

When providing person-centred care to people with pre-existing conditions or illnesses, a range of considerations must be made.

Medical conditions, for example cancer
+ Individuals will experience a range of symptoms caused by the cancer and the side effects of treatment.
+ Diagnosis and treatment can be frightening and distressing.
+ Cancer has physical, psychological and financial implications.
+ Wider effects include the impact on family.

Neurological conditions, for example dementia
+ Individuals will experience progressive cognitive and, eventually, physical decline.
+ Diagnosis and symptoms may cause distress to individuals and their families.
+ Family members may become significantly burdened with caring responsibilities.
+ Carers' assessments and mental capacity assessments will be required at the appropriate time.

Physical disabilities, for example a wheelchair user
The extent to which ability is affected varies but may include
+ restricted mobility
+ decreased stamina
+ support with personal-care tasks.

Considerations

Consideration must be given to various factors when providing person-centred care to people living with long-term illnesses and pre-existing conditions, such as those detailed above.

Consideration must be given to:
+ the social model of disability and inclusion
+ ongoing treatments
+ overall wellbeing
+ following the person-centred plan
+ co-morbidity
+ assessment of need
+ discharge planning
+ mental capacity
+ individual's rights and wishes
+ access to community provision
+ access to relevant additional secondary services
+ financial circumstances
+ carer's assessment.

> **Social model of disability** The idea that people are disabled by barriers within society, rather than an individual impairment or difference. These barriers are seen not just in the physical environment but also in terms of the way that society is organised and operates.
>
> **Co-morbidity** The presence of two or more diseases or conditions in one patient.

Check your understanding and progress at www.hoddereducation.co.uk/myrevisionnotes

> **Now test yourself** TESTED
>
> 1. List **two** considerations when providing person-centred care to people living with illness.
> 2. What does co-morbidity mean?
> 3. What is the social model of disability?
> 4. How can you make sure you give person-centred care to an individual with a physical disability?

> **Revision activity**
>
> List all the considerations for providing person-centred care to people with pre-existing conditions or living with illness. Use a different colour pen to make notes to indicate considerations that apply to specific groups of people.

A8.10 How mental health conditions, dementia and learning disabilities can influence a person's needs in relation to overall care

REVISED

Individuals with mental health conditions, dementia or learning disabilities experience fluctuations in their capacity to make decisions and care for themselves.

Increased support requirements

Individuals with mental health conditions, dementia or learning disabilities might have increased support requirements, as shown in Table 8.5.

Table 8.5 Increased support requirements for people with mental health conditions, dementia or learning disabilities

Increased support requirements	Example of support
Physical support	+ Shopping and preparing meals + Obtaining and taking medication + Travelling to and attending appointments + Assistance to participate in social or leisure activities
Communication support and behaviour support	+ Easy-read information + **Advocacy services** + Communication/**hospital passport** + Adapting communication style, for example speaking clearly, in short sentences and allowing processing time
Support with self-care	+ Provision of personal care + Support with healthcare needs, for example taking medication, applying creams or lotions, changing dressings or catheters
Support with social inclusion	+ Provision of activities which encourage social interaction + **Befriending services**
Support with monitoring	+ Regular healthcare appointments, for example with learning disability nurse and/or GP

> **Advocacy services** Services that provide an advocate for an individual, to help them express their opinions and get their voice heard.
>
> **Hospital passport** A document that individuals with a learning disability create and carry with them. It explains their healthcare and support needs, learning disability, communication preferences and how to make things easier for them.
>
> **Befriending service** The organised provision of supportive and reliable friendships, usually through volunteer networks.

Behavioural factors

Behaviour that challenges (for example violence, aggression or self-harm) may arise, particularly when an individual is distressed or does not understand what is happening.

Care given needs to be compassionate and understanding and aim to reduce distress and incomprehension wherever possible, to reduce the likelihood of behaviour that challenges.

Individual care plans and documents such as hospital passports should record strategies and supportive approaches to use with individuals who may experience behaviour that challenges.

Comprehension factors

The following factors may affect someone's ability to understand that they require care:
+ Individuals may have difficulty understanding their condition or the care and treatment being offered.
+ They may have decreased rationality about their condition (be in denial) or develop anxiety about the care.
+ Some mental ill-health conditions can be dissociative (when an individual feels disconnected from reality), so they cannot relate to what is happening.
+ Limited comprehension may also result in an individual being unaware when they are in abusive situations.
+ Individuals living with mental ill health, dementia or learning disabilities may refuse care or treatment. The best interests of the individual must always be considered and the Mental Capacity Act 2005 plus Amendment (2019) used as required when supporting individuals to make decisions about their care.
+ Individuals' judgement about their condition or care options may be altered or influenced by perceived stigma attached to certain conditions and disabilities.

> **Exam tip**
>
> Most individuals with a mental health condition, dementia or a learning disability will be influenced by one or more comprehension factors. When discussing conditions and treatment with these individuals, practitioners must consider the most appropriate types and methods of communication, to reduce these barriers to understanding.

> **Making links**
>
> When supporting individuals with mental ill health, dementia or learning disabilities, the principles of the MCA must be adhered to (see A8.8).
>
> The Equality Act 2010, which is covered in A1.1, places a duty on health and social care services to make reasonable adjustments to ensure individuals with mental ill health, dementia or learning disabilities have fair and equitable access to services.

> **Now test yourself**   TESTED
>
> 1 List practical support that an individual with dementia may require.
> 2 List ways to support an individual with a learning disability to communicate their wishes and preferences.
> 3 What is meant by the term *dissociative condition*?
> 4 Write **two** sentences that explain the link between person-centred care and reasonable adjustments, with reference to learning disability, mental ill health or dementia.

A8.11 How to promote independence and self-care and the positive impact on the healthcare sector

REVISED

How to promote independence and self-care

Independence and self-care can be promoted in the following ways:
+ Individuals should be involved and given choice and control over their own self-care. This can be adapted to suit the capacity and ability of the individual.
+ Individuals should have access to support networks, appropriate information and a range of learning and development opportunities, and understand the range of options available to them.
+ Offering support with risk management and risk taking, to maximise independence and choice. For example, supporting individuals to take part in activities as desired that may involve an element of risk.
+ Individuals should be supported to identify their strengths, assess their needs and gain the confidence to self-care.
+ Assistive technology should be made available to support an individual's ability to live independently.

Check your understanding and progress at www.hoddereducation.co.uk/myrevisionnotes

Positive impact on the healthcare sector

The benefits to the healthcare sector of increased independence and self-care include:
- improved self-esteem and independence of the individual, which may reduce demand on services
- improved partnership working between service providers and service users, which improves clinical outcomes
- improved efficiency of staff time within healthcare services, as service users can do more for themselves.

> **Revision activity**
>
> Make a list of service-user groups and, for each, list the assistive technology that can contribute to independent living.
>
> For example, for vision-impaired service users: service dogs, canes, screen readers, magnifiers, audio description, high-resolution images, high-contrast display, alt text, large format text/paper, auditory feedback, specialist lighting, tactile materials, braille.

> **Now test yourself**
>
> 1. List **three** ways that an individual's independence and self-care can be promoted.
> 2. Link each way you listed above to a different benefit to the healthcare sector.
>
> TESTED

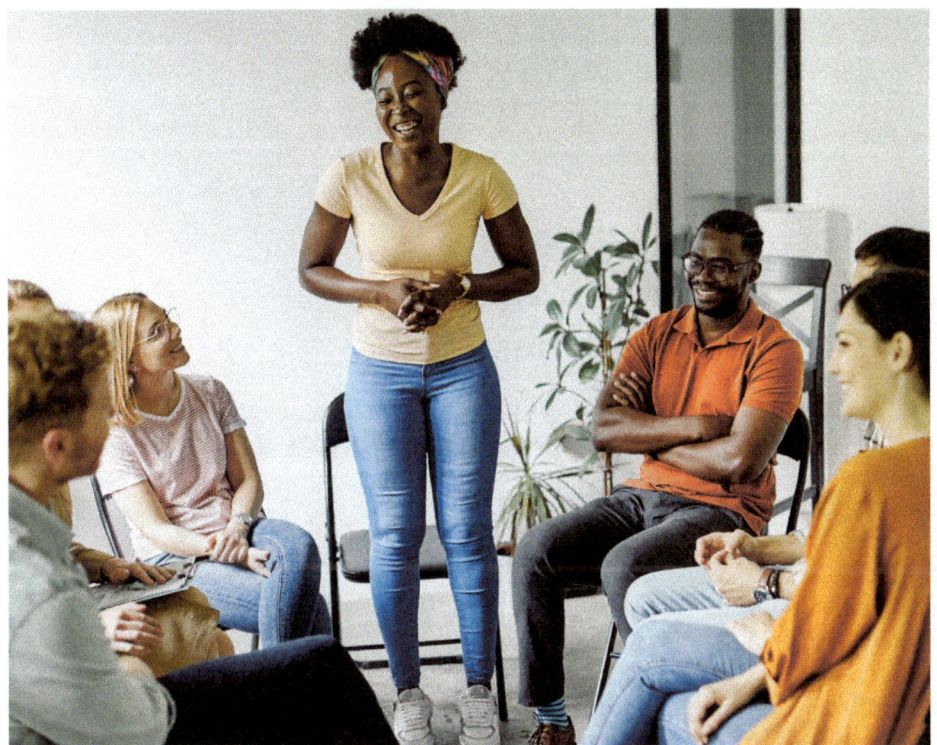

Figure 8.6 Support networks, such as patient groups, can help individuals develop independence and self-care strategies by learning from others

A8.12 The range of terms used in the healthcare sector in relation to death and bereavement, including their meaning

REVISED

Table 8.6 Terms used in the healthcare sector in relation to death and bereavement and their meaning

Terms	Meanings/usage
End-of-life care	+ Care provided to those who are in the last months or years of their life + Care provided when the efforts made to successfully treat or control a disease have ceased (stopped)
Palliative care	+ Symptom management and improving quality of life for those with progressive, life-threatening illness by relieving suffering
Hospice	+ Place or organisation that provides care for people who are dying + Hospice care can be given within the individual's own home
Expected death	+ Result of acute or gradual deterioration in an individual's health + Often due to advanced disease or terminal illness
Sudden or unexpected death	+ Death without warning, for example due to an accident, a heart attack or an act of violence
Grief	+ A response to loss and often described as intense sorrow + Used in the context of having lost a person who has died
Bereavement	+ Sense of loss when someone close passes away

> **Now test yourself** `TESTED`
>
> Complete the passage by inserting the correct terms.
>
> Care that is provided to someone to improve their quality of _____ by managing the symptoms of long-term illness is known as _____ care.
>
> Care that is given in the last _____ of life or when death is _____ is known as _____ of _____ care. This type of care is provided when it is no longer possible to _____ or control a disease.
>
> Care for those who are dying may be provided by a _____. Care may either be given in a special setting or the individual's own _____.
>
> Whether death is _____ or _____, those who knew the individual will feel a sense of loss and intense sorrow known as _____. Individuals may need support when they experience _____.

> **Typical mistake**
>
> Palliative care is suitable for anyone with compromised quality of life due to long-term illness and not just those with a terminal (life-limiting) diagnosis.

A8.13 The role of healthcare professionals in providing person-centred care for the individual during the active dying phase

`REVISED`

Healthcare professionals can provide support to both the individual and to family/carers by:
+ providing information on what they might expect during this time
+ addressing questions and concerns honestly
+ taking time to be an active listener
+ understanding the stages of grief (for example the Kübler-Ross model – see Figure 8.7) and providing emotional support or advice
+ recognising when someone may be entering the last few days and hours of life
+ involving the individual and families in decisions about their care and wishes; this may include specific wishes in relation to culture and religion
+ involving multi-agency teams where required in the care of the individual
+ advocating for the patient's rights and wishes
+ safeguarding the individual from harm, abuse and neglect.

> **Typical mistake**
>
> It should be noted that although the Kübler-Ross model suggests there are five stages of grief, these will not necessarily present in a linear sequence. Individuals may experience these aspects of grief at different times, or together, or may not experience some of these stages at all.

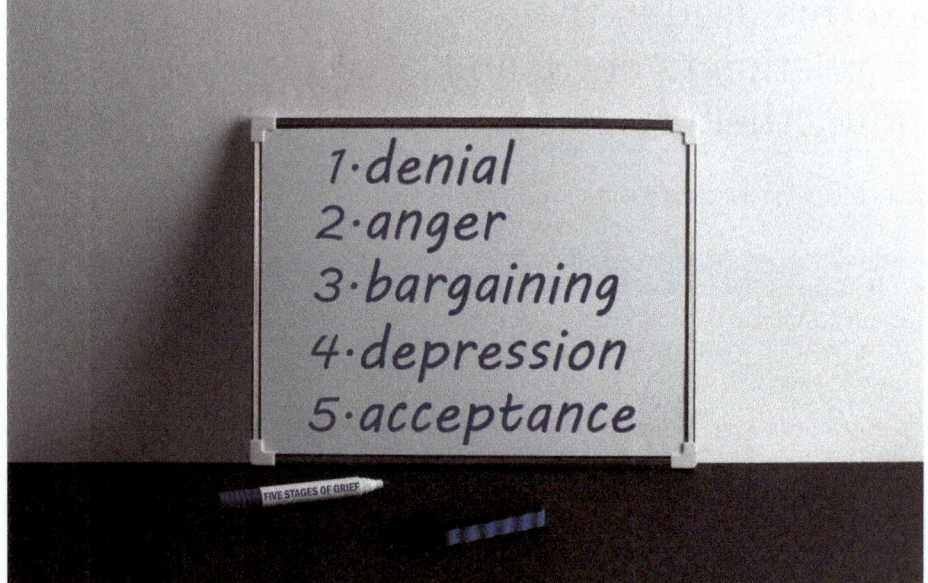

Figure 8.7 Kübler-Ross model: the five stages of grief

> **Now test yourself**
>
> 1 List **three** ways you can support an individual who is in the active dying phase.
>
> 2 List **three** ways you can support the family of an individual during the active dying phase.
>
> `TESTED`

Check your understanding and progress at www.hoddereducation.co.uk/myrevisionnotes

A8.14 How to support people with bereavement and how to communicate with families

REVISED

There are many ways to support people with bereavement, including:
+ providing a safe and comfortable environment and suitable resources, such as tissues and refreshments
+ providing emotional support, for example by listening or allowing the person to talk/cry
+ understanding families may have an emotional reaction and how to handle those situations, for example anger or aggression
+ remembering the duty of candour, for example accurately representing the situation
+ acknowledging cultural/religious rituals with a bereaved individual
+ signposting applicable services, for example bereavement care and national charities for bereaved people.

> **Revision activity**
>
> Make a list of bereavement charities and the support they can provide to individuals experiencing grief and loss.

> **Now test yourself** — TESTED
>
> 1 List **three** ways you can support people experiencing bereavement.
> 2 List **two** ways you should communicate with bereaved families.

A8.15 What the 6Cs are in relation to person-centred care

REVISED

The 6Cs are a set of values required of all patient-facing health and social care staff, shown in Table 8.7. Putting these values into practice ensures person-centred care will be given.

Table 8.7 The 6Cs in relation to person-centred care

Principle	Explanation
Care	This means putting individuals at the centre of care, acknowledging their needs and preferences, and ensuring the care given is appropriate for them.
Compassion	This means providing care that is based on empathy, respect and dignity for individuals and their personal situation.
Communication	Listening is vital to person-centred care, as it enables individuals to be involved in decisions made about their care and treatment. Person-centred care also requires openness and honesty in all communication, so individuals are well informed and have trust in their caregivers.
Courage	This enables care providers to speak up when person-centred care is not given, as well as to welcome new or different ways of working.
Commitment	Commitment to the highest standards of care ensures individuals will experience the best possible outcomes.
Competence	This means ensuring everyone providing care is appropriately trained to do so and given adequate opportunities to continue their development, so that individuals receive the best care from them.

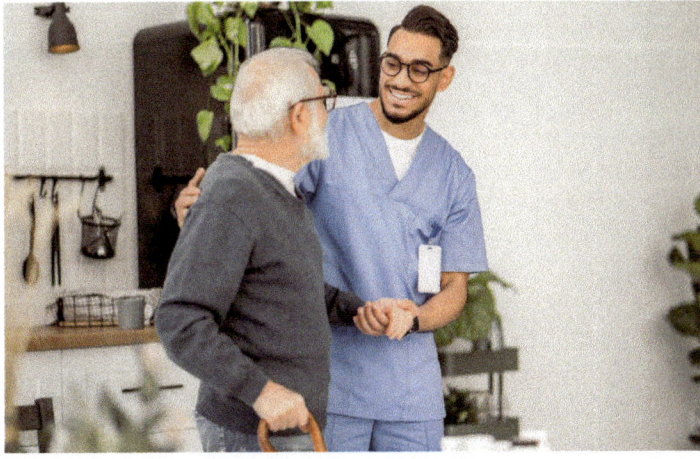

Figure 8.8 It is important to show care and compassion, particularly when supporting vulnerable individuals with intimate and personal care.

> **Revision activity**
>
> Create a flashcard for each of the 6Cs and write on it your own definition of each term.

My Revision Notes: Health T Level

> **Now test yourself** — TESTED
>
> Complete the passage by inserting the correct 6C principle.
>
> Using effective _____ enables you to understand an individual's needs and preferences, which shows that you _____. Respecting these preferences and acting in an empathetic way demonstrates _____.
>
> Knowing your legal obligations and undertaking regular training and development maintains your _____ and shows your _____ to the health and wellbeing of individuals in your care.
>
> If you are concerned about poor practice or suspect a safeguarding issue, you should act with _____ and take appropriate action.

> **Exam tip**
>
> Use context to describe or explain the 6Cs if asked in a question. Make sure you can give practical (and different) examples of healthcare professionals demonstrating each of the 6Cs. This will also help you to be sure of the differences between the meanings of each term.

A8.16 The importance of practising and promoting the 6Cs in relation to demonstrating person-centred care skills, through own actions and promoting the approach with others

REVISED

Practising and promoting the 6Cs

To practise and promote the 6Cs when giving person-centred care, it is important to act in the ways described in Table 8.8.

Table 8.8 Practising and promoting the 6Cs

How to practise and promote the 6Cs	Notes
Provide choice and gain consent	+ To demonstrate care and compassion, it is essential to ask about and respect an individual's choices. + Gaining consent supports care and compassion, however it is also vital to competence, as informed consent is required by law and professional codes of conduct. + These actions are underpinned by effective communication skills.
Ensure privacy and dignity	+ Care and compassion are needed to protect individuals' rights to privacy and to maintain their dignity. + Ensure you listen to and consider the views and circumstances of individuals. + Maintaining dignity and privacy may call for courage, for example if a practitioner is not working in a way that upholds this, it should be challenged. + These actions require effective communication skills.
Respect individuals	This refers to: + equality, diversity and inclusion + sexuality + faith, cultural needs and preferences + rights + confidentiality. Each of these points requires: + care, compassion and communication, for example to ask about and respond to individual preferences and circumstances + competence, for example to know legal and moral obligations to maintain confidentiality and legal rights to equal and fair treatment + courage, perhaps; for example if discrimination occurs, it is essential that this is challenged.

Check your understanding and progress at www.hoddereducation.co.uk/myrevisionnotes

How to practise and promote the 6Cs	Notes
Follow duty of care	Duty of care incorporates all the 6Cs: + Ensuring the safety and wellbeing of others requires care and compassion for their individual wishes and circumstances. + Competence and courage are required to take appropriate action when an individual's safety or wellbeing is compromised. + Commitment is needed to maximise the best possible outcomes for individuals. + Good communication ensures effective working practices between colleagues and with service users and their families.
Deal with conflicts between rights and duty of care	+ Courage, competence and commitment are required when conflict arises between an individual's rights and a wider duty of care. + To assist the decision-making process, care and compassion are needed. + At all times, communication needs to be open and effective.
Ensure partnership working	+ Individuals will feel more relaxed when they are treated with care and compassion, and will therefore be more willing to work with healthcare providers. + Using effective communication, which demonstrates competence, commitment and courage, ensures trustworthiness, as individuals will feel confident in their care providers.
Ensure honesty	+ Communication must be transparent. + Courage may be needed if others are dishonest.
Prevent discrimination through promoting inclusion and an inclusive environment	+ Care, compassion and commitment establish an inclusive environment. + Competence ensures staff know what their legal responsibilities are. + Courage enables individuals to work in new ways and to challenge discrimination.
Escalate concerns	+ Competence is required to know when something is not right. + Courage is needed to speak out and act. + There must be commitment to the safety and wellbeing of individuals. + Communication ensures information is passed on accurately and effectively.

Exam tip

You can link your knowledge from other areas of the specification in any questions about the 6Cs. For example, demonstrating competence links to professional accountability and regulation (A8.3). Demonstrating commitment to safety and wellbeing links to the Health and Safety at Work Act (A3) and safeguarding responsibilities (A11). Demonstrating courage and speaking out links to whistleblowing, safeguarding and professional accountability (A8.3 and A11). Be prepared to make links like this in your answers, particularly when asked to discuss or evaluate in extended responses.

Revision activity

On each of the flashcards you created for the definitions of the 6Cs, add an example of how you could put that 'C' into practice.

Now test yourself

TESTED

1 List **two** ways the 6Cs can be used when gaining consent.
2 List **two** ways the 6Cs can be used when following duty of care.
3 List **two** ways the 6Cs can be used to ensure partnership working.

A8.17 The concept of safeguarding in relation to providing person-centred care

REVISED

Safeguarding is keeping individuals protected from harm, abuse or neglect. It is central to high-quality, person-centred care. It enables individuals to live independent, fulfilled lives and experience the best health outcomes.

Safeguarding as a key part of person-centred care is enabled by:
+ actions that protect people's health and wellbeing
+ allowing people to live free from harm, abuse or neglect and protecting their human rights
+ health services and healthcare professionals enacting their duty to safeguard all service users.

Making links

For more on safeguarding, see A11.

A8.18 The importance of managing relationships and boundaries, and how to work within parameters, when providing person-centred care

REVISED

The importance of managing relationships and boundaries

The ability to build meaningful relationships with others is a key skill in the healthcare sector. However, it is important that all relationships remain professional.

The relationship between service provider and service user is established to provide healthcare and to promote the health and wellbeing of the service user; this is not a friendship.

The relationship between colleagues is established so that they can work safely and effectively together to deliver healthcare and to meet the health and wellbeing needs of service users.

Colleagues may become friends, however the working relationship must remain professional.

Care providers must manage their professional relationships with service users and colleagues and observe the boundaries of these relationships.

Managing relationships and boundaries is important because it:
+ protects those providing and receiving care
+ avoids misinterpretation of roles
+ helps prevent potential abuse.

How to work within those parameters

To guide work within these parameters, regulatory bodies such as the CQC and the NMC provide standards and codes of conduct which must be adhered to. These standards and codes govern how to form and maintain professional relationships and boundaries.

When working with colleagues, it is essential to use professional conversation. The content of the conversation should be focused and limited to work. The language used should remain formal and professional.

> **Making links**
>
> The full role of professional regulators such as the CQC and NMC is covered in A8.3.

> **Revision activity**
>
> Create a mini-quiz for your study partner on professional relationships and boundaries. Create a mark scheme so you can assess their answers.

> **Now test yourself** TESTED
>
> 1 Write **one** sentence to describe how safeguarding promotes person-centred care.
> 2 Write your own definition of 'professional relationship'.
> 3 Give **two** reasons why boundaries are important when forming a professional relationship with a service user.
> 4 Give **two** reasons why a professional relationship is important between colleagues.
> 5 List the key features of professional conversation.

Check your understanding and progress at www.hoddereducation.co.uk/myrevisionnotes

Exam practice

1. Grant is 25 years old and has an acquired brain injury. This affects his ability to make decisions. Outline how the Mental Capacity Act 2005 safeguards individuals like Grant when they require healthcare treatment. [3]

2. Explain why the principle of partnership is important in adult safeguarding. [2]

3. Marianne is a midwife with 15 years' experience. She trained, qualified and practised as a midwife in France. She is going through the process of registering as a midwife with the Nursing and Midwifery Council, so she can work for the NHS.

   Explain the importance of professional regulation for a midwife like Marianne, giving examples of the purpose of **three** elements of the process. [6]

4. Jacinta is starting her first job as a healthcare assistant in a residential nursing home for elderly people.

   Identify **four** areas where the elderly residents may require care and support due to ageing. [4]

5. Gretchen is being interviewed for a job as a healthcare assistant. She has been asked to discuss how she would demonstrate the NHS values.
   a. Explain the purpose of the NHS values. [2]
   b. Outline **two** of the values. [2]

6. Outline the purpose of the Personalisation Agenda 2012. [2]

7. Henry has a moderate learning disability which affects his speech and means he takes longer to understand information. He has an appointment at the hospital.

   Discuss how communication barriers can be reduced or overcome for individuals like Henry. [6]

8. Gail is 28 years old and she has been admitted to hospital with a respiratory illness. She also has a serious mental health condition. Gail has declined multiple medical treatments, although her doctor has said this is a risky and unwise decision.

   Discuss how the Mental Capacity Act 2005 plus Amendment (2019) can be used to support Gail. [6]

9. Darcus is 84 years old and he has a recent diagnosis of dementia. He also has some left-sided weakness after a stroke last year. He takes medication to control his hypertension.

   Outline why it is important to consider co-morbidities when giving person-centred care. [3]

10. Sadie is 23 years old and has a learning disability. She is attending the hospital for a routine appointment with the cardiology team because she has a congenital heart defect. Sadie is feeling anxious about her appointment.

    Discuss the factors that will influence Sadie's overall care needs that should be considered by the hospital staff. [6]

11. Explain why you should consider ongoing treatment for pre-existing conditions when giving person-centred care. [2]

12. Explain how someone's overall wellbeing can be affected by a condition like dementia. [2]

13. Georgie has a visual impairment and a learning disability. She is an inpatient on the medical ward of the hospital. Georgie has a few assistive devices with her that enable her to eat her own meals, pour her own drinks and move around the ward and go to the bathroom independently.

    Outline the benefits to the healthcare service of individuals like Georgie being independent and carrying out their own self-care. [3]

14. Chi is working as a healthcare assistant on the oncology ward at the hospital. She has heard staff discussing the referral of patients for palliative care and for end-of-life care. Chi thought these were the same but now she is not sure.

    Outline the difference between palliative care and end-of-life care. [2]

15. Jakob is supporting the family of an individual who died suddenly. The family are in denial about what has happened.
    a. State why the family may be in denial. [1]
    b. Describe how Jakob could support and communicate with the family. [4]

16. Student nurse Radhika is starting her first shift on a women's health ward in a busy hospital. She is keen to show that she knows what the 6Cs are.

    Radhika's mentor has asked her to answer the patient call bells.

    Describe how Radhika can demonstrate each of the 6Cs when carrying out this task. [6]

17. Rashid is a healthcare assistant working on a surgical ward in the hospital. At handover, he hears several staff joking about a patient that wears a wig.

    Outline how Rashid could respond using each of the 6Cs. [6]

18. Anatoly is training as a nursing associate. He is working in a service that provides healthcare to young adults that are similar in age to him.

    Explain how Anatoly can develop and maintain a professional relationship with the young adults in his care. [4]

A8 Providing person-centred care

A9 Health and wellbeing

A9.1 Changes in the approach to healthcare and how to support a person's health, comfort and wellbeing

REVISED

Changes in the approach to healthcare

Policy changes to focus on the promotion of health and wellbeing and the prevention of ill health

The NHS Long Term Plan was published in 2019, setting out how world-class care would be achieved for everyone over the following 10 years.

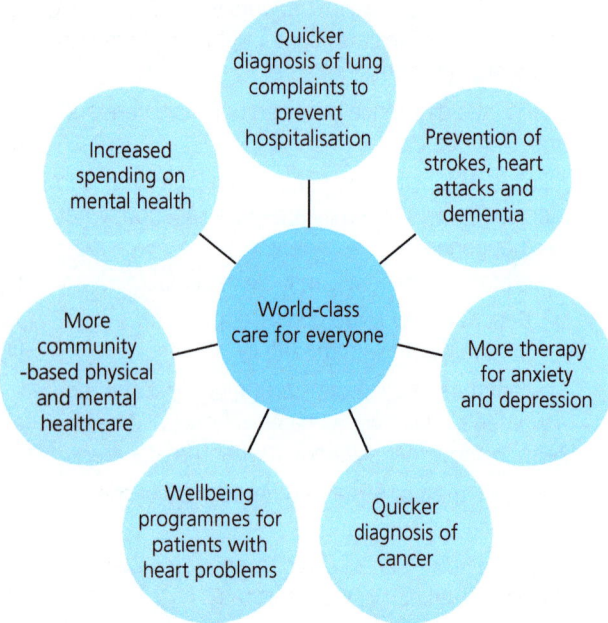

Figure 9.1 NHS Long Term Plan: world-class care for everyone

This plan acknowledges that health inequalities exist in the social and economic environments in which we are born, grow, live and work.

Health inequalities include:
+ poor living environments
+ poverty
+ reduced life chances
+ poor educational opportunities.

The plan includes the concepts of 'starting well' and 'ageing well', which represent a life-course approach to promoting health and wellbeing and preventing ill health.

Change in approach from treating illness to promoting wellbeing

Encouraging individuals to choose healthy lifestyles and to take responsibility for managing their own health and wellbeing is critical to promoting health and wellbeing. This can be supported for example by:
+ stop-smoking services – smoking is a direct cause of respiratory diseases such as chronic obstructive pulmonary disease (COPD) and lung cancer

Check your understanding and progress at www.hoddereducation.co.uk/myrevisionnotes

+ social prescribing schemes – enabling individuals to access community services such as exercise groups can reduce risks of cardiovascular diseases and diabetes
+ digital tools, such as smartphone apps, to enable more individuals to access NHS services and self-manage their condition.

Improved multi-agency working to support individuals' health and social care needs

A variety of agencies must work together to provide a seamless response that meets the multiple or complex needs of individuals.

Many individuals with health needs, such as those with long-term diseases, will also require support to maintain their independence at home.

In specific circumstances, other agencies must also collaborate to support health, comfort and wellbeing, such as the police, courts and schools.

> **Making links**
>
> Multi-agency working is vital to successful care of individuals and is a feature of both A2.5 and A2.10.

How to support a person's health, comfort and wellbeing

Supporting an individual to have good health and wellbeing and to live in comfort is achieved through:
+ **collaborative approaches** across the healthcare and social care sectors, including with communities and individuals
+ encouraging active involvement of individuals to **self-manage** their health and wellbeing, taking into account lifestyle choices
+ encouraging individuals to make decisions about the care, support and treatment they receive
+ adopting a person-centred approach to support an individual's physical, intellectual, emotional and social wellbeing.

> **Collaborative approach**
> Healthcare professionals and agencies, community groups and interest groups such as charities, governmental agencies and individuals all co-operating to improve health.
>
> **Self-management**
> Services that encourage, support and empower people to manage their own physical and mental health conditions themselves. Known in the NHS Long Term Plan as 'supported self-management'.

> **Making links**
>
> Person-centred care is a holistic approach to healthcare, covered in more detail in A8.6.

> **Revision activity**
>
> Create a concept map of ways that people can self-manage their health. Make your examples as specific as you can by linking them to a health concern or condition. Extend your revision by annotating your diagram in a different colour to explain how the method will manage or even improve health.

> **Now test yourself** TESTED
>
> 1 Write your own definition of the term *health inequalities*.
> 2 Explain why stop-smoking services are an important element of preventing ill health.
> 3 List **two** ways that wellbeing can be promoted.

A9.2 How to recognise the signs and symptoms of a person who is experiencing pain and discomfort and/or whose health and wellbeing is deteriorating

Physical signs and symptoms

Physical tics
Physical tics are repetitive muscle movements and can be involuntary. They can be linked to pain, stress or fatigue.

Altered baseline observations
Observations should be taken as directed by qualified medical or nursing staff. Any deviation from the individual's baseline observations and/or normal ranges should be reported by following local procedure.

Changes to observations can indicate discomfort, pain and/or deterioration in health, as shown in Table 9.1.

Table 9.1 Observations and what abnormal readings may indicate

Observation	Normal range (adults)	Indications of abnormal readings (examples)
Respiratory rate	12–20 breaths per minute at rest	Raised respiratory rate may be due to pain or infection.
Oxygen saturation	95–100%	Reduced oxygen saturation indicates poor lung function.
Blood pressure	90/60 to 120/80 mmHg	Raised blood pressure may be due to pain or infection.
Heart rate	60–100 beats per minute	Raised pulse rate may be due to pain or infection.
Consciousness	Alert	Confused individuals may be experiencing pain or infection; unconsciousness indicates a serious deterioration in health and immediate action should be taken.
Temperature	36–37°C	Both reduced temperature and raised temperature can indicate infection.

Oxygen saturation A measure of the percentage amount of oxygen that is bound to the haemoglobin in the blood.

> **Making links**
>
> B1.29 covers normal expected ranges for physiological measurements and the factors which may affect these measurements.

Skin condition
When assessing skin colour, the observer should consider the usual skin colour for the individual and remember that conditions may present differently on different skin colours. Table 9.2 shows some skin conditions and what they may indicate.

It is important to note that these observations of skin colour may be limited when applied to individuals from Black, Asian and minority ethnic groups. The very latest national and local guidelines on skin condition observations must be followed.

Table 9.2 Skin colour, temperature and moisture observations and possible health implications

Skin condition	Observation	Indication
Skin colour	Blueish/purple	Indicates lack of oxygen
	Paler than usual	May indicate dehydration, shock or blood loss
	More flushed than usual	May indicate hypertension, fever or a temporary hot flush
Skin temperature	Cool	May indicate hypothermia
	Hot	May indicate infection or fever
Skin moisture	Wet	Can indicate infection, hypoglycaemia, shock or heart attack
	Very dry	Dehydration

> **Hypoglycaemia** When the blood glucose concentration falls below the normal or optimal level.

Repeatedly touching or guarding part of the body
When a part of our body is in pain, guarding is a way to protect from further pain.

Moving slowly
Moving slowly and with care is a way to minimise pain or can show that a person has low energy or consciousness.

Wringing or clenching
Wringing the hands or clenching the hands or jaw/teeth can be a method individuals use to distract from or control pain.

Verbal signs
Verbal signs include:
+ self-reporting pain – the person feeling the pain tells the healthcare professional they are in pain
+ crying out in pain
+ groaning or grunting – if a person has reduced consciousness or communication challenges, they may groan or grunt when in pain.

Nonverbal signs
A person's facial expressions may show pain, for example:
+ grimacing
+ frowning
+ looking sad.

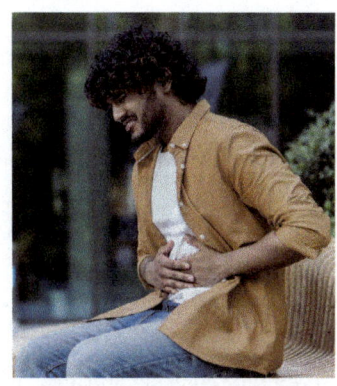

Figure 9.2 Individuals in pain may show multiple signs, for example guarding the part of the body where the pain is felt and facial grimacing.

Behavioural signs and symptoms
Pain can significantly change a person's behaviour, ranging from:
+ altered energy levels – pain can leave an individual lethargic and low on energy
+ altered disposition or character – pain can make people confrontational, aggressive or withdrawn
+ changes in usual eating/sleeping patterns – it can be difficult to eat when experiencing pain and it can cause problems with getting to sleep and staying asleep.

> **Disposition** A person's usual way of feeling or behaving, for example a person's tendency to be happy and optimistic.

> **Typical mistake**
> Each individual experiences pain differently and may exhibit multiple signs of pain, or very few. Healthcare workers must use skills of observation and questioning, as well as physical examination, to determine the type and level of pain a person is experiencing.

My Revision Notes: Health T Level

> **Now test yourself** — TESTED
>
> 1. What is the normal range for pulse?
> 2. What can a raised resting pulse rate indicate?
> 3. What can changes to the usual colour of a person's skin indicate?
> 4. Why do people move slowly when they are in pain?
> 5. What verbal signs can indicate a person is feeling pain?

> **Revision activity**
>
> Create a concept map for signs and symptoms of pain and deterioration in health. Fill it with as much information as you can without looking at your notes.

A9.3 How to work in a person-centred way, to ensure adequate nutrition, hydration and care are provided to prevent deterioration in the individual's wellbeing

REVISED

Ensuring effective nutrition and hydration

It is important to ensure individuals are supported to meet their nutrition and hydration needs, while also ensuring the care and support given are person-centred. This is shown in Table 9.3.

Table 9.3 How person-centred care ensures adequate nutrition, hydration and care

Person-centred care	How this ensures adequate nutrition, hydration and care
Provide food and drink that meets individual needs (considering preferences, beliefs and medical conditions)	Individuals are more likely to consume required levels of food and drink if it is palatable and enjoyable for them.
Ensure food and drink provided does not have **contraindications**	This ensures individuals will not become unwell due to interactions between food/drink and their treatment.
Support individuals who might experience difficulties in eating or drinking	This ensures individuals are physically able to take in required food and fluids and empowers the individual.
Provide equipment where appropriate to help individuals to eat and drink independently	This makes it easier for individuals with additional needs to eat and drink, for example by providing two-handled cups for those with weak hands.
Ensure sufficient time to eat and drink	This ensures individuals do not feel rushed with their meals and have sufficient time to eat to meet their needs.
Closely monitor nutrition and fluid intake	This means it is clear when an individual is under- or over-nourished, well hydrated or dehydrated.
Communicate with individuals to identify any barriers	Explore individuals' needs (for example for appropriate equipment) and preferences (for example for certain foods they find palatable).
Promote the value and importance of effective nutrition and hydration to overall wellbeing	Individuals who are aware of the benefits of good nutrition and hydration for their recovery and wellbeing are more likely to adhere to any nutrition and hydration plans.
Work with carers or family members	This ensures individuals' needs and preferences can be met and any difficulties with eating and drinking can be understood and accounted for.
Work with other healthcare professionals	For example, it may be necessary to report to a dietitian or therapist that the individual is not enjoying a specific diet plan, or report to a nurse or doctor if the individual is becoming dehydrated.

> **Contraindication** When a medication or treatment should not be used because it may cause harm, for example if it interacts with food or drink taken, or another medication or treatment being taken.

> **Revision activity**
>
> Create a concept map on this topic:
> + Map out all the ways you should support hydration and nutrition.
> + For each way, give an example of a particular service user you may encounter.
>
> For example:
> Working in partnership with family to ensure an individual eats and drinks appropriately; for instance, when working with young children, involve the parents or guardians.

> **Now test yourself** TESTED
>
> 1 List **two** ways that you could demonstrate a person-centred approach when providing food and drink to individuals.
> 2 When providing food and drink, why do you need to consider any potential contraindications?
> 3 How can you ensure that individuals in your care can access adequate nutrition and hydration?
> 4 Who should you work in partnership with when supporting individuals with nutrition and hydration?

A9.4 The purpose of the prevention agenda and the concept of preventative approaches for moving towards good health and wellbeing

REVISED

The prevention agenda

The 'prevention agenda' refers to the concept that preventing ill health from occurring is preferable to waiting for ill health to occur and then treating it.

The prevention agenda is incorporated into the NHS Long Term Plan and the Department of Health and Social Care policy paper 'Prevention is better than cure: our vision to help you live well for longer'.

Preventative approaches

There are different ways for moving towards good health and wellbeing. These approaches are shown in Table 9.4.

Table 9.4 Preventative approaches for moving towards good health and wellbeing

Approach	Example
Helping people to stay healthy and independent for as long as possible	Using primary healthcare services, such as GPs and dentists, and through social care services, such as adult social care.
Stopping problems arising in the first place and focusing on keeping people healthy, not just treating them when they become ill	Vaccination and screening programmes can prevent diseases.
Providing people with knowledge and skills to make lifestyle choices that support them to stay healthy	Health education and health promotion on smoking and substance use can provide knowledge and life skills to help people make healthier lifestyle choices.

> **Making links**
>
> B1.27 focuses on how health promotion helps to prevent the spread of and control disease and disorder.

> **Vaccination** A treatment given via injection, orally (by mouth) or sprayed into the nose. The vaccine triggers the body's immune system to create antibodies against the target disease. Part of preventative healthcare.
>
> **Screening** The process of identifying individuals from the population who may have an increased chance of a disease or condition, so that treatment can begin early.

> **Typical mistake**
>
> Screening tests are not usually performed on individuals who present as unwell, and they do not diagnose an individual with a disease or condition. They are used to indicate whether an apparently healthy person has an increased risk of a specified disease or condition.

> **Now test yourself** TESTED
>
> 1 Summarise what is meant by the 'prevention agenda'.
> 2 Teaching people about the risks of their behaviour is an example of what?
> 3 Why is providing a vaccination programme an example of the prevention agenda?

A9.5 The ways in which health promotion is used to support the prevention agenda to support good health and wellbeing

REVISED

Social and environmental interventions to empower individuals to improve their health

National campaigns from government agencies and departments

National health promotion campaigns may be run directly by government agencies and departments, or the scientific evidence and statistics that inform these campaigns may be provided by those agencies and departments.

Table 9.5 Examples of national health promotion campaigns

Agency/department	Purpose	Example campaign
UK Health Security Agency (UKHSA)	Responsible for protecting the public from infectious diseases, and chemical, biological, radiological and nuclear incidents	Health promotion and protection messages on the COVID-19 virus: 'Hands – Face – Space'
Office for Health Improvement and Disparities (OHID)	Responsible for health protection and promotion such as: mental health, weight, diet, the health of children and families, smoking and the health of vulnerable groups	Jointly launched the *Every Mind Matters* campaign with the DHSC in 2021 to support better mental health and reduce stress and anxiety.
Department of Health and Social Care (DHSC)	Responsible for policy on health and adult social care matters in England	Launched the *Better Health* campaign in January 2022 to offer free support and guidance on losing weight, getting active, quitting smoking and drinking less

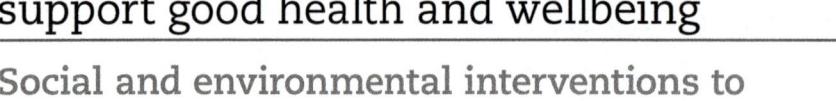

Figure 9.3 *Hands – Face – Space* was a health promotion campaign aimed at encouraging individuals to wash their hands, wear a mask and socially distance from one another, with the purpose of preventing the transmission of COVID-19

Opportunistic delivery of health promotion by all healthcare professionals

All healthcare professionals have a responsibility to deliver health promotion messages when the opportunity arises.

For example, if an individual visits the GP and smoking habits are discussed, the GP should take the opportunity to explain the risks of smoking to health.

> **Making links**
>
> Opportunistic health promotion is operationalised by the Making Every Contact Count initiative (see A9.6).

Campaigns by specific groups and charities

There are many groups and charities in the UK that carry out health promotion campaigns, for example:

+ February is always the British Heart Foundation's Heart Month. In 2024, the focus was on encouraging more people to learn CPR. (www.bhf.org.uk/how-you-can-help/support-our-campaigns/heart-month).
+ 1 December is always World AIDS Day. In 2022 the theme was *Equalize*, in recognition that health inequalities are obstructing the end of the AIDS pandemic. (www.unaids.org/en/World_AIDS_Day).

Sharing examples of health promotion activities

Health promotion activities cover a wide range of public health topics, including smoking cessation, promoting physical activity, promoting breast feeding and reducing alcohol intake.

The government and its agencies, and interest groups such as charities, provide resources for carrying out health promotion campaigns.

> **Revision activity**
>
> How many examples of national health promotion campaigns can you list? How is each one supporting the health prevention agenda?

> **Now test yourself** — TESTED
>
> 1 List the **three** government agencies and departments that carry out health promotion campaigns.
> 2 Give **two** examples of health promotion campaigns run by charities.
> 3 In your own words, define what is meant by 'opportunistic delivery of health promotion'.

A9.6 The overarching principle of the opportunistic delivery of health promotion through the Making Every Contact Count (MECC) initiative and the risk factors this initiative targets

REVISED

Making Every Contact Count (MECC) was published in 2016. It uses day-to-day interactions that individuals have with any healthcare or social care professional to help change behaviours.

MECC uses brief and very brief interventions whenever the opportunity arises, for example during routine appointments. These interventions are used to highlight risk factors, such as smoking, poor diet, alcohol consumption, physical activity levels, and mental health and wellbeing.

Health professionals can also signpost individuals to additional support and resources available.

An example of MECC with a brief intervention:

Janice is 65 years old. She attends an appointment at the health centre to have her blood pressure checked. The healthcare assistant notices that Janice seems to be quite low in mood. He chats to Janice, asking her how she is feeling and whether she sees friends and family every day. He finds that Janice is lonely, so he signposts her to the local friendship group run by Age UK by giving her a flyer.

> **Signposting**
> Recommending or providing the contact details for additional resources, services and support networks.

> **Typical mistake**
>
> MECC is not a structured intervention or health campaign. It is about healthcare workers taking any opportunity during their usual work to deliver key health messages to individuals on smoking, diet, physical activity and mental health and wellbeing.

> **Now test yourself** — TESTED
>
> 1 Write **two** sentences to describe how Making Every Contact Count (MECC) works.
> 2 Give an example of a brief intervention using MECC. Describe what might happen at a routine antenatal appointment involving someone newly pregnant and the midwife.

A9.7 How lifestyle choices impact good health and wellbeing

REVISED

Nutrition and diet choices affecting body mass index (BMI)

Obesity

Eating a balanced and healthy diet containing recommended proportions of macronutrients and micronutrients is essential for good health. The government provides the Eatwell Guide to advise the public how to eat healthily (Figure 9.4).

Body mass index (BMI) is a measure of whether an individual has a healthy weight for their height. However, a clinical judgement will need to be made regarding its accuracy; for example, a patient who has a higher than average muscle mass will weigh heavier. Table 9.6 shows BMI classifications (for most adults).

Sometimes, established health measures must be adapted. The NHS recommends that for adults with Asian, Middle Eastern, Black African or African–Caribbean family backgrounds, a lower threshold is used for overweight and obesity, as shown in Table 9.7.

> **Macronutrients** The nutrients the body requires in large quantities for energy: fat, protein and carbohydrate.
>
> **Micronutrients** The nutrients the body requires in trace (very small) amounts for normal growth and development: vitamins A, B, C, D, E, K and minerals such as calcium, copper, iodine, iron, magnesium and zinc.

Table 9.6 BMI classifications (for most adults)

Classification	BMI
Underweight	<18.5 kg/m²
Healthy weight	18.5–24.9 kg/m²
Overweight	25–29.9 kg/m²
Obese	30–39.9 kg/m²
Severely obese	>40 kg/m²

Source: www.nhs.uk/conditions/obesity/

Table 9.7 Adjusted BMI classifications for overweight and obesity for Asian, Middle Eastern, Black African or African–Caribbean adults

Classification	BMI
Overweight	23–27.4 kg/m²
Obese	>27.5 kg/m²

Source: www.nhs.uk/conditions/obesity/

> **Typical mistake**
>
> Established measures may have limitations, but this does not make them useless. For example, BMI does not measure the proportion of fat or muscle an individual has. It is possible to have a higher BMI than is considered 'healthy' but to have very little fat and a lot of muscle, as some professional sportspeople do. BMI continues to be used because it is time and resource efficient to calculate and can indicate that a person's weight might need to be looked at in more detail by a healthcare professional.

Consuming more calories than the body can burn through physiological functioning, activity and exercise leads to weight gain. Excessive weight gain causes obesity, which increases the risk of developing a range of diseases including:
+ type 2 diabetes
+ hypertension
+ heart disease.

Malnutrition risk of vitamin deficiency

Failing to consume macro- and micronutrients in proportions required for growth, development and functioning of the body can lead to malnutrition. In turn, this can lead to deficiency diseases, such as:
+ iron-deficiency anaemia
+ vitamin B9 (folate) deficiency anaemia
+ vitamin B12 (cobalamin) deficiency anaemia
+ vitamin D deficiency.

> **Deficiency diseases** Conditions that arise due to a long-term lack of a vitamin or mineral in the body.
>
> **Anaemia** When the body does not have enough healthy red blood cells.

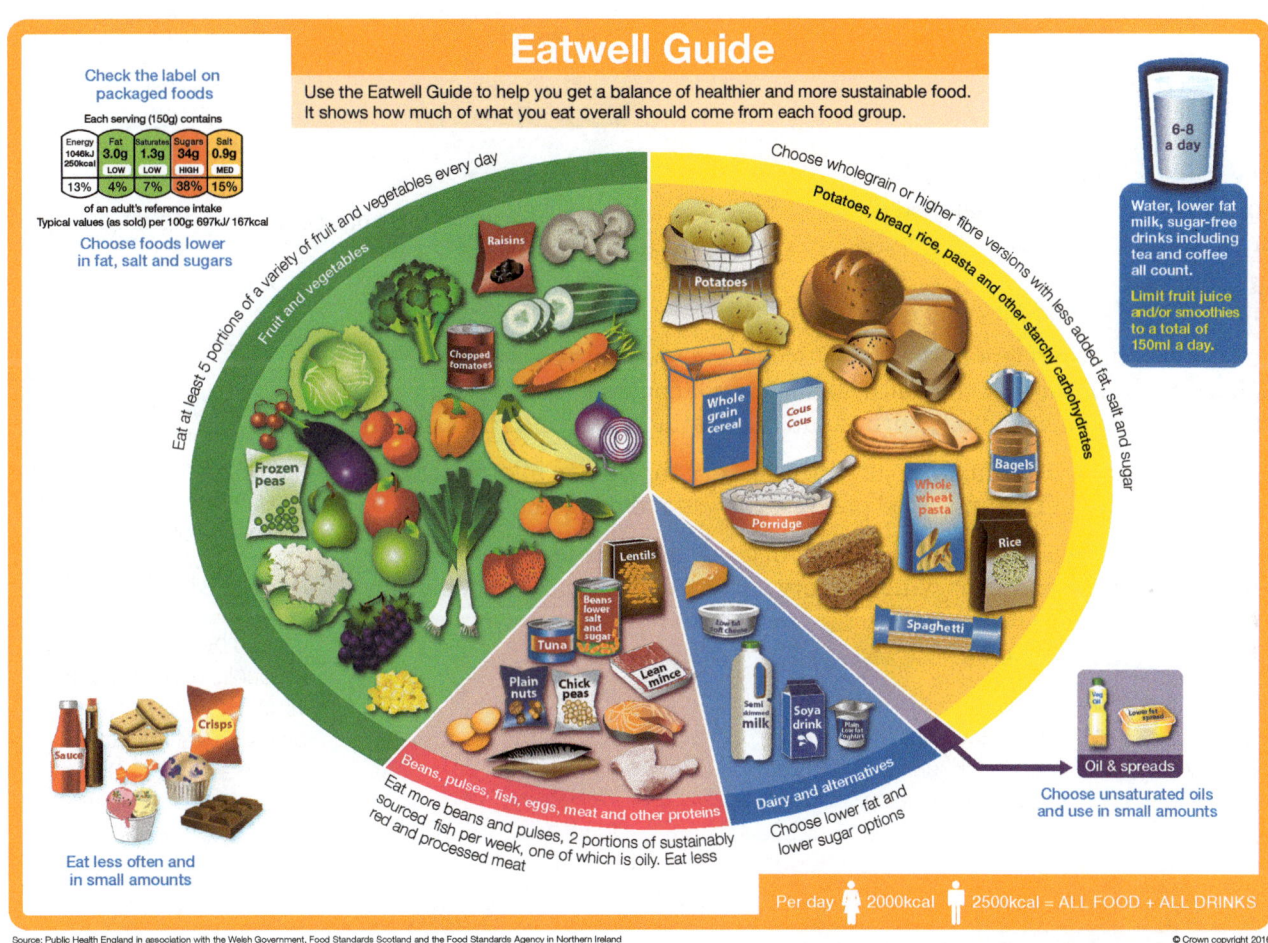

Figure 9.4 The Eatwell Guide defines government advice on healthy eating and is a visual representation of how different food groups contribute to a healthy and well-balanced diet

Smoking

Smoking is the leading preventable cause of illness and premature death in England. According to the NHS, it is responsible for approximately 76 000 deaths a year in England.

Tobacco smoke contains nicotine, carbon monoxide, tar and toxic chemicals such as benzene, arsenic and formaldehyde, increasing risks of lung and other types of cancer and heart disease.

Supporting individuals to quit smoking is a prevention priority in the NHS Long Term Plan.

> **Typical mistake**
>
> Malnutrition refers to any type of nutrition which is not optimum for healthy growth, development and functioning. It does not just mean not having enough to eat. For example, it is possible to consume enough calories but from an unbalanced range of foods, which would happen if you ate fried food for every meal.

Low physical activity

Low physical activity and sedentary lifestyles are a risk factor for a range of long-term conditions. These include cardiovascular issues such as hypertension and heart disease, as well as psychological issues such as anxiety and depression.

Physical activity is essential for the maintenance of bone density, muscle mass, balance and co-ordination. Therefore, physically active individuals maintain mobility and have a reduced risk of falls.

Consumption of alcohol

The long-term effects of alcohol consumption on the human body are listed in Figure 9.5.

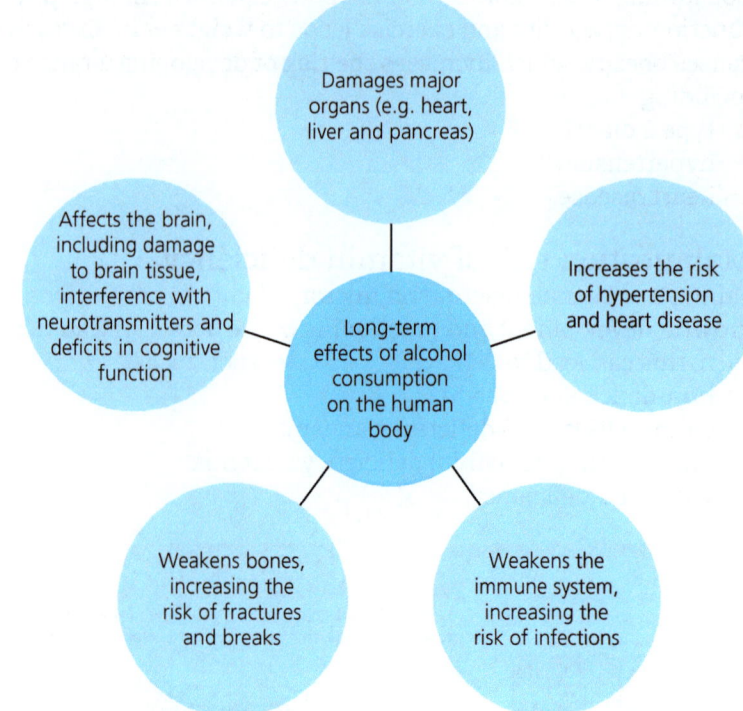

Figure 9.5 The long-term effects of alcohol consumption on the human body

Substance misuse and addiction

Substance misuse refers to the use of drugs and medication in a way that is harmful or hazardous to health. Misuse is not confined to illegal or street drugs but also includes drugs and medication prescribed by a doctor.

Harmful effects may occur after just one use. For example, an allergic reaction may occur or heart rate and blood pressure may rise to dangerous levels.

Longer-term effects include risk of heart disease, cancer and hepatitis B, C and D, along with problems with memory and concentration, and depression or anxiety.

Sedentary Spending a lot of time seated; a job that requires sitting at a desk all day can be described as a sedentary job.

Hepatitis Inflammation of the liver. It may be caused by drinking alcohol (alcoholic hepatitis) or a virus. There are several types of viral hepatitis, known as A, B, C, D and E.

Revision activity

Create a concept map for each of the five lifestyle choices above. Include:
+ any government recommendations or ambitions
+ the impact on health and wellbeing.

Now test yourself

1. Draw a table to show the BMI categories.
2. List **three** risks of obesity.
3. What is a deficiency disease?
4. Give **three** examples of deficiency diseases.
5. How does tobacco damage health?
6. Why is physical activity important? List the risks of inactive lifestyles.
7. What does the term *sedentary* describe?
8. List **three** risks of alcohol consumption on long-term health.
9. How might substance misuse impact health? Give **one** short-term and **two** long-term impacts.

Check your understanding and progress at www.hoddereducation.co.uk/myrevisionnotes

A9.8 A range of methods of taking a holistic approach to healthcare

REVISED

Holistic approaches to healthcare consider the whole person. The methods of taking a holistic approach to healthcare are listed in Table 9.8.

Table 9.8 Methods of taking a holistic approach to healthcare

Method	Example
Treating the person not just the condition	Spend time treating the social or emotional effects a condition may have on an individual, not just the physical effects.
Bespoke treatment plans that meet personal choices and needs	These should be made using the personal aims and objectives established by the individual, using person-centred care.
Understanding the individual's lifestyle	This could include the individual's commitments, such as family and work.
Understanding the individual's mental health needs	There are many mental health services that can support an individual.
Integrated working	By using a co-ordinated approach, this ensures services providing different areas of health and social care can work together with input from the individual.
The work of health and wellbeing boards (HWBs)	HWBs are responsible for promoting greater integration and partnership between the NHS, public health and local government/social care.

> **Making links**
>
> The importance of using holistic approaches for person-centred care was first introduced in A8.6.

> **Revision activity**
>
> Create your own case study on an adult with a health condition. Ensure there is at least one feature in the case study that can be linked to each of the methods of taking a holistic approach to healthcare as listed in Table 9.8. Colour code or annotate your finished case study to show exactly how a holistic approach could be taken.

> **Now test yourself** TESTED
>
> 1. List **three** methods of taking a holistic approach to healthcare.
> 2. List **three** parts of an individual's lifestyle you might need to understand to provide holistic healthcare.
> 3. Why are health and wellbeing boards important for holistic healthcare?

A9.9 The purpose of signposting individuals to interventions or other services and how this can support their health and wellbeing

REVISED

Signposting individuals

The act of signposting involves recommending or providing the contact details for additional resources, services and support networks to individuals. An example would be signposting an individual that wants to quit smoking to stop-smoking support groups.

The purpose of this is to provide the best possible care, treatment and support for an individual by determining the most appropriate services for them (this includes considering the most cost-effective approach).

> **Making links**
>
> Signposting is also covered in A9.6 as part of the MECC initiative.

How signposting can support an individual's health and wellbeing

Signposting supports an individual's health and wellbeing by providing awareness of a wider range of services available than they might be aware of and by offering alternative options, for example community-centred services.

It gives the individual choice and empowers them to make decisions about which services and approaches best meet their unique needs. For example, these services could support activities of daily living or help to provide a safe and secure home environment for an individual.

Signposting to self-help groups provides opportunities for individuals to discuss specific issues or experiences with their peers, which can be empowering and offers opportunities for learning and developing support networks.

> **Typical mistake**
>
> Signposting and referral are not the same thing. Signposting is an informal suggestion that an individual may wish to explore further sources of support or information. Referral is a formal process where a healthcare worker requests that another healthcare worker assesses an individual to see whether further treatment or support is required.

> **Now test yourself** TESTED
>
> 1 Don has been signposted to further information on elderly care options, such as domiciliary care, assisted living and residential care. How could this support his health and wellbeing?
> 2 Gemma has been signposted to a peer-support group. How could this help her health and wellbeing?

A9.10 The impact of the ageing process on health and wellbeing

REVISED

Ageing is the process of becoming older and it is associated with changes at a biological, psychological, social and emotional level.

The impact of ageing on physical health

Cellular level
Biological ageing is the accumulation of molecular and cellular damage over time. Cells become less able to divide, the cell membrane changes and there is an increase in lipids (fatty substances) within the cell.

As a result, cells either become less effective at functioning, for example they find it harder to take in oxygen and nutrients and expel waste products, or they lose their function altogether.

Body systems
The tissues formed by cells become stiffer or they lose mass (known as atrophy). These changes affect all the body systems and their organs, which results in a slow decrease in function.

Senses
Ageing leads to a deterioration in the sense organs. For example, hearing becomes impaired because of changes in the inner ear and auditory nerve. Vision can also be affected, for example by cataracts, which is when the lens of the eye becomes cloudy.

Check your understanding and progress at www.hoddereducation.co.uk/myrevisionnotes

Age-associated diseases

Ageing is associated with an increased risk of illness and disease, for example:
+ susceptibility to infection such as flu or norovirus, due to an impaired immune system
+ increased risk of heart disease, due to stiffened blood vessels and a weaker heart
+ increased risk of osteoarthritis, due to loss of cartilage between the joints
+ increased risk of neurodegenerative diseases such as Alzheimer's disease, due to accumulation of proteins in the brain and loss of brain cells.

The impact of ageing on cognitive health

Cognitive health is the ability to think clearly, learn and remember. It is an important component of performing everyday activities.

Cells and tissues of the nervous system also accumulate damage over time. This results in:
+ changes to memory and attention, for example becoming more forgetful or finding that the mind wanders
+ difficulties with reasoning and problem solving, for example finding it harder to manage a household budget
+ difficulties with information processing, which can affect reaction times, for example finding it more difficult to make quick decisions when driving.

> **Typical mistake**
>
> Age-related forgetfulness is quite different from dementia, which is pathological (caused by disease). Dementia is a progressive condition in which there is a loss of cognitive functioning to the extent that everyday life is affected. It affects memory but also how individuals speak, think, feel and behave.

The impact of ageing on emotional wellbeing

The transition into later adulthood is often marked by significant life events, for example retirement, bereavement and ill health.

Individuals often feel that they are facing their own mortality as the end of life becomes nearer, which may lead to low mood or even depression.

These transitions and life events can also lead to loneliness and social isolation, for example as family members and friends die, or as mobility and health issues make it difficult to leave the house.

> **Revision activity**
>
> Take a large sheet of paper and split it into three columns. List everything you can recall about:
> + physical effects of ageing
> + cognitive effects of ageing
> + social and emotional effects of ageing.

> **Now test yourself** TESTED
>
> 1. What is the ageing process?
> 2. What happens to cells, tissues and organs during ageing?
> 3. What illnesses and conditions are more likely due to ageing?
> 4. Summarise how ageing can affect cognitive skills.
> 5. Why does ageing impact on emotional wellbeing?

A9.11 How aspects of care requirements change throughout various life stages

REVISED

> **Making links**
>
> A8.4 describes typical care needs across the lifespan. It is helpful to review these briefly before continuing with this section.

Table 9.9 describes the potential care requirements at the various life stages.

Table 9.9 Life stages of human development and potential care requirements

Life stage	Potential care requirements
Birth and infancy (0 to 2 years)	Care requirements revolve around healthy growth and development and prevention of ill health (for example screening for hearing difficulties and general physical health, and immunisations to prevent childhood diseases). Physical growth and development (the acquisition of skills and abilities) is also monitored. Professionals and services involved include: + midwives (the first 28 days after birth) + health visitors (from birth to starting school) + general practice doctors (GPs) for all primary care needs from birth + paediatric care to meet secondary healthcare needs.
Early childhood (3 to 8 years)	Children continue to follow immunisation schedules to maintain immunity against common infectious diseases. Child growth is still measured and children are screened for obesity as part of the National Child Measurement Programme. Development also continues to be monitored, for example checking whether milestones for language acquisition and gross and fine motor skills are met. Professionals and services involved in early childhood care include: + health visitors (from birth to starting school) + school nurses (from reception to year 13) + GPs for all primary care needs from birth + paediatric care to meet secondary healthcare needs.
Adolescence (9 to 18 years)	In adolescence, children continue to follow immunisation schedules and are screened again for obesity as part of the National Child Measurement Programme. Additional care needs arise as adolescents transition through puberty and begin to explore their identity and engage in sexual relationships, for example sexual health services become important. A wide range of professionals and services can be involved in adolescent care, including: + school nurses (from reception to year 13) + GPs + sexual health services + paediatric care to meet secondary healthcare needs.
Early adulthood (19 to 45 years)	In adulthood, screening continues, for example cervical screening for people with a cervix aged 25 to 64 and diabetic eye screening for people with diabetes. As adults become sexually mature, additional care needs arise such as maternity and paternity services. During pregnancy, there is a dedicated screening and immunisation programme to ensure pregnancy is healthy and any potential problems with the foetus are either detected early or prevented from occurring in the first place.
Middle adulthood (46 to 65 years)	In middle adulthood, the ageing process begins and the risk of ill health and disease starts to increase. As a result, the screening programme provided by the NHS intensifies. For example: + NHS Health Check: this is offered to everyone over the age of 40 (without a pre-existing health condition) every five years. It is a check of overall health and looks at an individual's risk of conditions such as heart disease, kidney disease, diabetes and stroke. + Breast screening: this is offered to people aged 50 to 70 and can detect early signs of breast cancer. + Bowel cancer screening: everyone aged 60 to 74 is offered an at-home screening test kit every two years. + Abdominal aortic aneurysm (AAA) screening: this is offered to all men in the year they turn 65 and is used to detect aneurysm (bulging) in the main blood vessel that supplies blood to the lower half of the body.
Later adulthood (65 years onwards)	In later adulthood, the screening programme continues as highlighted in middle adulthood. The ageing process decreases muscle mass and bone density and, as a result, strength, mobility and balance become affected, which can lead to falls. Combined with reduced functioning of organs and body systems, older adults may become frail.

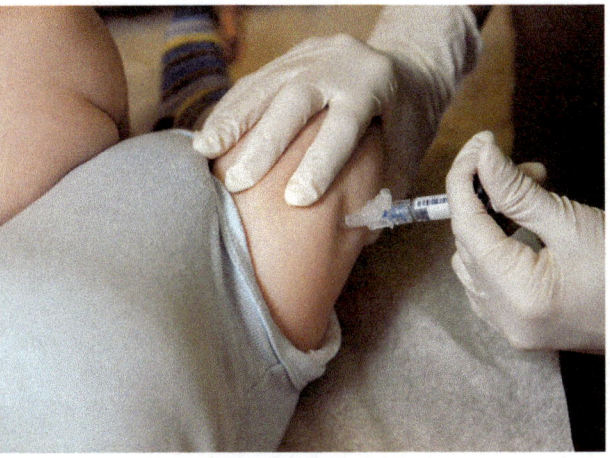

Figure 9.6 A comprehensive immunisation programme is offered to infants and children via the NHS

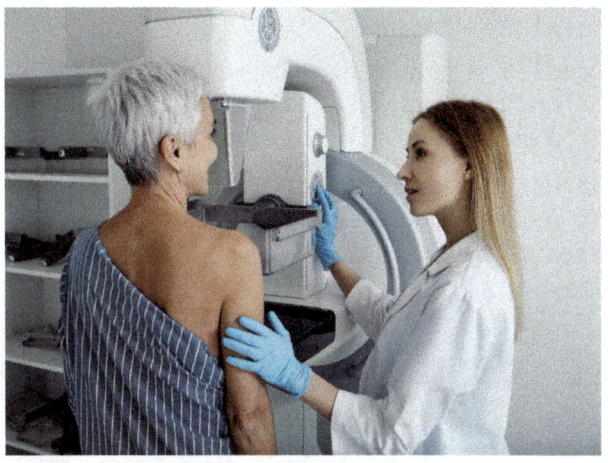

Figure 9.7 Routine breast screening is offered to people aged 50 to 70. An X-ray test called a mammogram is used to detect changes in breast tissue

> **Now test yourself** — TESTED
> 1. What is the focus of care during infancy?
> 2. Which professionals and services contribute to care of infants, children and adolescents?
> 3. Why are there more screening tests offered during middle and later adulthood?

> **Revision activity**
>
> Create a set of flashcards to cover how care requirements change over the life course.
>
> You can add more detail to them after A9.12.

A9.12 Methods of supporting individuals to look after themselves at various stages of life

REVISED

Methods of supporting individuals may vary according to life stage. They should acknowledge the preferences, values and circumstances of the individual and promote a holistic approach to health that considers physical, intellectual, emotional, social and spiritual needs. General methods can include:
+ self-care, for example taking time off work
+ taking control over lifestyle/behaviour decisions, for example quitting smoking
+ self-management of conditions, for example following a diet plan for diabetes.

Young people and healthy adults

Methods of supporting this group of people can include the promotion of:
+ healthy choices, for example avoiding smoking and alcohol consumption and making healthy sex and relationship decisions
+ self-care, for example good nutrition, exercise and good personal hygiene
+ self-awareness, for example over feelings and emotions and asserting and respecting boundaries
+ self-esteem, so that young people and adults feel they have worth and value, which underpins good mental health and wellbeing.

Adults who have health or wellbeing concerns and individuals in old age (65+)

Methods of supporting this group of people can include:
+ promoting activities of daily living, such as good sleep and nutrition
+ promoting screening programmes
+ promoting health awareness and the importance of taking prompt action regarding concerns, for example cancer red flags
+ promoting regular health check-ups
+ dispelling stereotypes, for example that all older people are frail and unwell or that people with physical or sensory impairments cannot have good quality of life.

My Revision Notes: Health T Level

End of life

Methods of supporting people at the end of life can include:
- making advanced care decisions and planning
- making end-of-life care plans.

In both cases, this support empowers an individual to consider, while they are fit and well and have capacity, how they wish to be cared for and treated in the future.

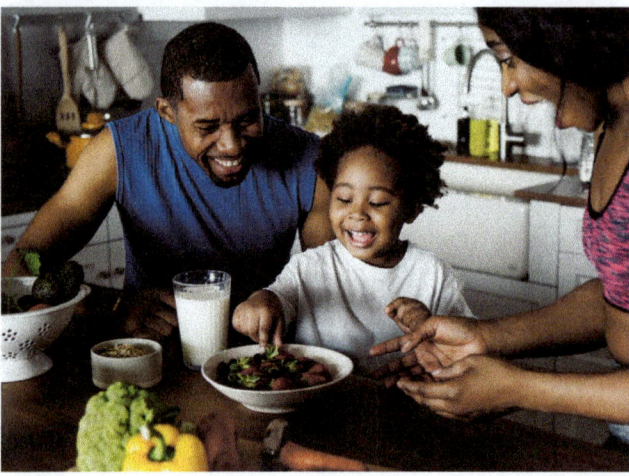

Figure 9.8 Looking after yourself by making healthy choices is an important way to ensure health and wellbeing throughout the life span

> **Exam tip**
>
> Ensure you are clear about the difference between advanced care decisions and end-of-life care planning. They are not interchangeable and mixing them up could lead to you misunderstanding the question. Refer back to A8.6 on advanced care decisions and planning and A8.12 on end-of-life care.

> **Now test yourself**
>
> 1 Give **two** examples of how to support children and young people to look after themselves.
> 2 Give **two** examples of how to support adults to look after themselves.
>
> TESTED

Exam practice

1 Janelle has booked a midwife appointment because she is 8 weeks pregnant with her first child. The midwife asks Janelle about her lifestyle, including questions on smoking, alcohol consumption and exercise.

   Explain why the midwife will encourage Janelle to be actively involved in achieving a healthy lifestyle during pregnancy. [2]

2 A patient who has recently returned from surgery is moaning and clenching their hands. Describe what might be causing these signs. [2]

3 Derek is 87 years old and has recently had a stroke. He is an inpatient on a hospital ward where he is recovering. Derek has left-sided weakness of the face and upper body. Explain **two** ways that Derek may need person-centred support with hydration and nutrition. [4]

4 Keenan is a smoker and enjoys drinking a lot of alcohol at the weekend. He has a newborn baby.

   Outline how the prevention agenda could keep Keenan and his baby healthy. [3]

5
   a Identify **one** health promotion campaign run by a government agency or department. [1]
   b State how the campaign supports the prevention agenda. [1]

6 Outline **one** way that Making Every Contact Count (MECC) can promote health and prevent ill health. [3]

7 Pablo is at his GP surgery for his NHS Health Check. He has a BMI of 32 kg/m². He enjoys drinking alcohol most nights of the week. The practice nurse calculates he consumes around 21 units of alcohol per week.

   State the possible effects of his alcohol consumption on Pablo's long-term health and wellbeing. [3]

8 Todd has a diagnosis of cancer. He is scheduled for surgery and six months of chemotherapy and he is feeling very anxious. Todd has two children and he is a single father.

   Discuss a range of holistic approaches to healthcare that could benefit Todd.

   Include in your response a recommendation for an additional service that Todd could be signposted to. [6]

9 Jagdeep is 88 years old and not as strong or mobile as he was when he was younger.
   a Outline what is meant by the ageing process. [3]
   b Describe **two** impacts of ageing on physical health. [4]

10 Describe the screening tests a woman might expect to be offered in her adulthood life stages. [4]

11 Identify one method of supporting school-aged children to look after their own health and wellbeing. [1]

Check your understanding and progress at www.hoddereducation.co.uk/myrevisionnotes

A10 Infection prevention and control in health-specific settings

A10.1 The techniques for infection control and why they are important in stopping the spread of infection

REVISED

An infection is caused by an infectious microorganism such as a bacterium or virus (also known as a pathogen).

Infection can be seen as a chain of links (Figure 10.1). If all of the links in the chain are present, infection will result. If any of the links in the chain are broken, infection can be prevented.

Infection prevention and control techniques aim to break the links in the chain of infection.

> **Infection** When pathogens enter a person's body and multiply, causing illness, organ and tissue damage, or disease.

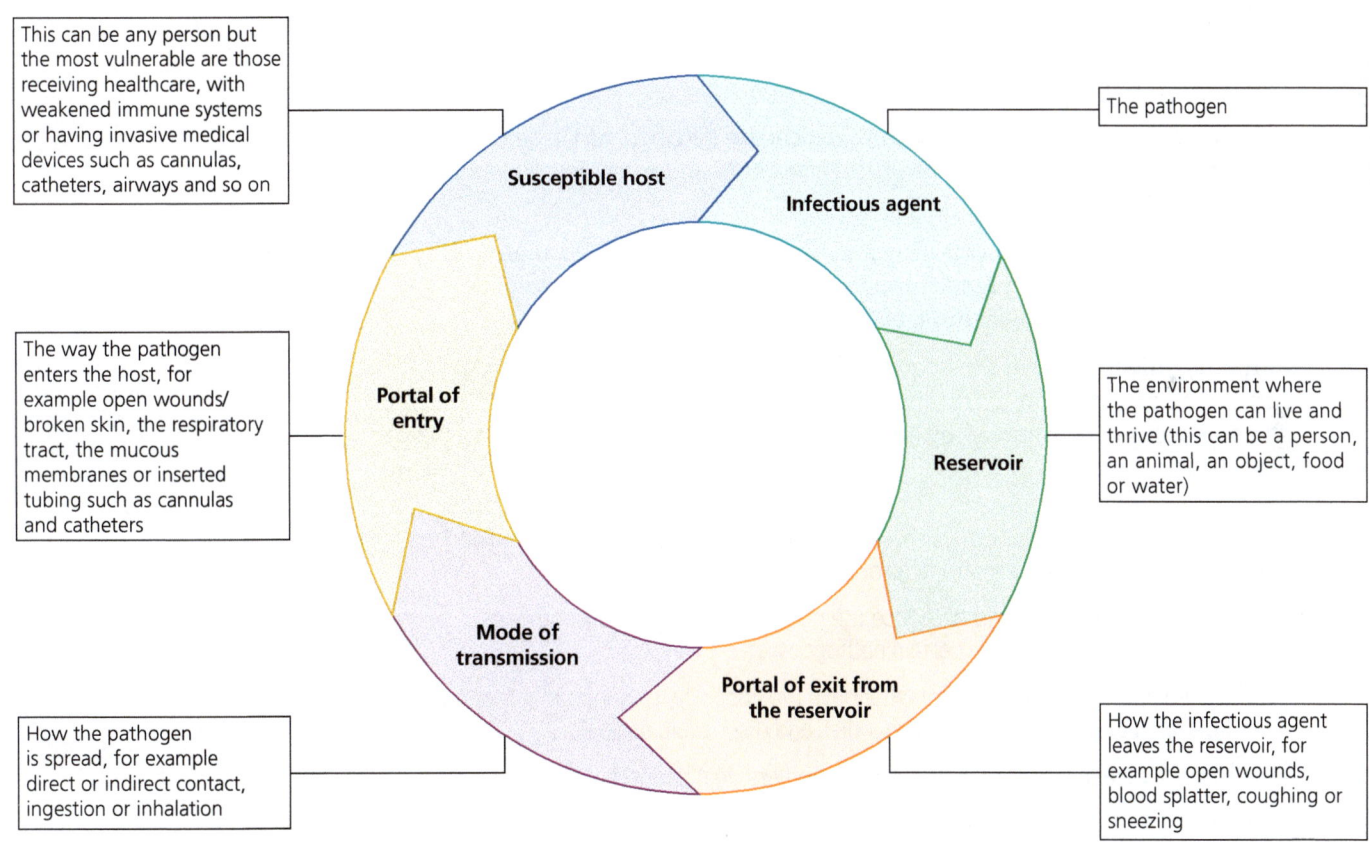

Figure 10.1 The six links of the chain of infection

Techniques for infection control

There are multiple techniques for infection control, as shown in Table 10.1.

Table 10.1 Techniques for infection control

Technique	Example
Use of personal protective equipment (PPE)	PPE acts as a physical barrier. For example, wearing gloves prevents pathogens from exiting through any broken skin or wounds on the worker.
Use of cleaning and disinfection agents	Disinfectants are chemicals that can eliminate some but not all microorganisms *when used correctly*. It is important to follow the manufacturer's instructions to ensure appropriate dilutions that will be effective.
Effective handwashing techniques	It is important to follow the '5 moments for hand hygiene' introduced by the WHO.
Good personal hygiene and uniform requirements	Hair should be tied up and nails kept short; uniform should be clean.
Safe disposal of sharps	To minimise risk of transmission of infection and sharps injury, used sharps (for example hypodermic needles) must be disposed of: + at the point of use + by the person generating the waste + with needles and syringes as one unit + with any safety mechanisms deployed + into a dedicated sharps bin
Appropriate waste segregation and disposal	All healthcare waste must be appropriately segregated and disposed of. To this end, waste is classified using a colour-coded system.

Importance in stopping the spread of infection

It is vital to prevent infections within healthcare settings, as these cause harm to both individuals and healthcare workers and may also pose a risk to the public at large.

For example, norovirus (a vomiting and diarrhoeal infection) is highly transmissible and will spread through a hospital or care home quickly without adequate handwashing, use of PPE and isolation measures.

Similarly, infections that are acquired in the community may spread to healthcare settings through staff, visitors and patients. For example, Group A streptococcus can be spread by an asymptomatic person not practising proper respiratory etiquette.

Cleaning A process used to physically remove contamination, for example blood or faeces, that does not necessarily destroy microorganisms.

Disinfection A process used to reduce the number of viable microorganisms (although it may not inactivate certain pathogens).

Sharps Equipment and instruments that have the capability of puncturing the skin, for example lancet devices, hypodermic needles and disposable scalpels.

Isolation Separating infected individuals from others, to prevent the spread of infection.

Respiratory etiquette Covering the mouth and nose when coughing and sneezing; disposing of used tissues; and washing hands after touching the nose or mouth.

Typical mistake

Infection can be spread from workers to service users, between service users, from service users to workers, between workers, and between service users/workers and family/visitors. Infection control protects everyone within a healthcare environment, not just the individuals receiving care and treatment.

Check your understanding and progress at www.hoddereducation.co.uk/myrevisionnotes

> **Revision activity**
>
> 1 Create a concept map for the chain of infection. Ensure you include:
>   + the six links in the chain
>   + an explanation of what each link means
>   + a list of ways to break each link in the chain.
> 2 Create a set of flashcards to help you remember the key terms involved in infection control and prevention techniques.
> 3 Check the colour-coded classifications for healthcare waste on the internet. Create colour-coded flashcards for the different categories of clinical waste.

> **Now test yourself** TESTED
>
> 1 Summarise what is meant by the 'chain of infection'.
> 2 How does using PPE break the chain of infection?
> 3 How does cleaning the healthcare environment break the chain of infection?
> 4 How can a sharps injury or infection from sharps be avoided?
> 5 Why should waste be segregated and colour coded?

A10.2 The importance of good handwashing techniques and personal hygiene and how to practise this in relation to infection control

REVISED

Importance of good handwashing techniques and personal hygiene

Maintaining good handwashing techniques and personal hygiene helps to prevent the spread of infection, and as a result illness and disease.

Washing hands removes physical contamination with dirt or blood which may contain microorganisms. Alcohol-based hand gels are effective at removing microorganisms where there is no visible contamination to be removed. In both cases, the risk of infection and illness being passed from person to person through cross-contamination is reduced.

Effective handwashing and good personal hygiene also form part of the legal requirements for infection prevention and control, for example as found in the:
+ Control of Substances Hazardous to Health Regulations 2002
+ Health and Safety at Work etc. Act 1974
+ Reporting of Injuries, Diseases and Dangerous Occurrences Regulations 2013.

How to practise good handwashing techniques

It is essential to follow workplace guidance on handwashing techniques.

The Ayliffe handwashing technique/5 moments/12-point technique

Ayliffe (a microbiologist in the 1970s) worked out that we did not remove microorganisms from our hands with casual handwashing. He developed a 6-step technique that ensures all parts of the hands and wrists are decontaminated.

This 6-step technique is incorporated into the full 12-point guidance for handwashing used by the WHO, NHS and UK Health Security Agency (UKHSA), as shown in Figure 10.2.

> **Revision activity**
>
> Research the proper technique to use when decontaminating the hands with alcohol-based hand gel. Create your own infographic that illustrates the steps required and provides an explanation of when this is the recommended method of decontaminating the hands.

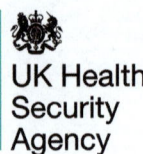

Best Practice: How to hand wash step by step images

Steps 3-8 should take at least 15 seconds.

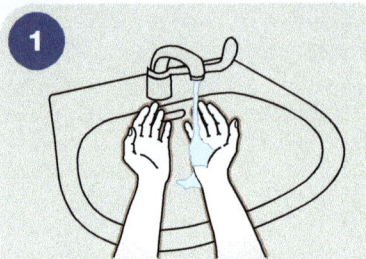

1 Wet hands with water.

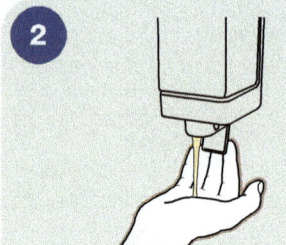

2 Apply enough soap to cover all hand surfaces.

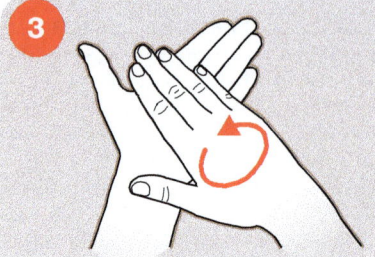

3 Rub hands palm to palm.

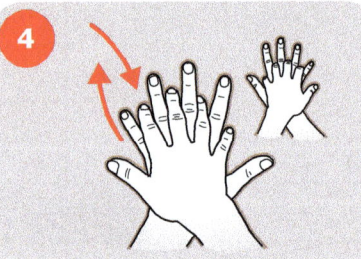

4 Right palm over the back of the other hand with interlaced fingers and vice versa.

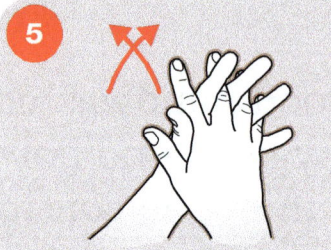

5 Palm to palm with fingers interlaced.

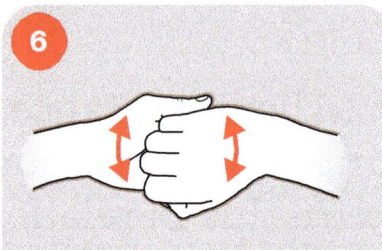

6 Backs of fingers to opposing palms with fingers interlocked.

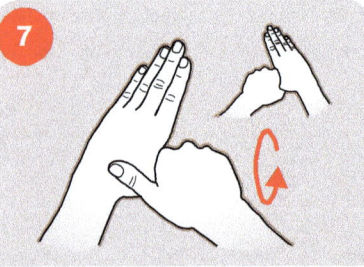

7 Rotational rubbing of left thumb clasped in right palm and vice versa.

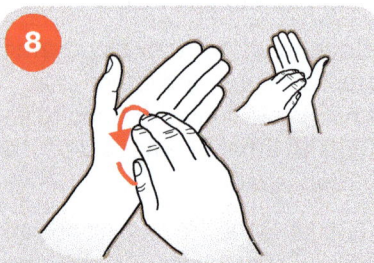

8 Rotational rubbing, backwards and forwards with clasped fingers of right hand in left palm and vice versa.

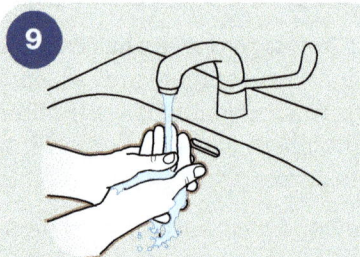

9 Rinse hands with water.

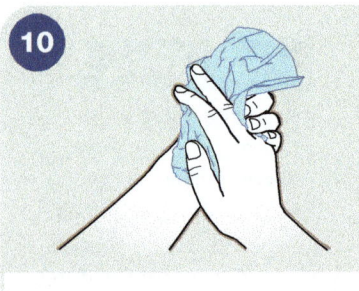

10 Dry thoroughly with towel.

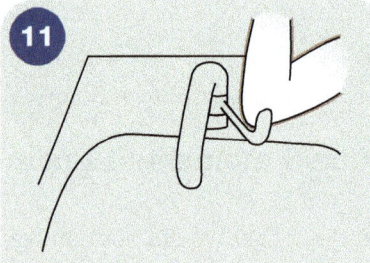

11 Use elbow to turn off tap.

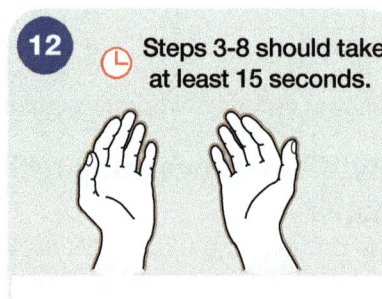

12 Steps 3-8 should take at least 15 seconds.

... and your hands are safe*.

*Any skin complaints should be referred to local occupational health or GP.

Adapted from the World Health Organization/Health Protection Scotland
© Crown copyright 2022

Figure 10.2 UKHSA 12-point handwashing technique with soap and water

Check your understanding and progress at www.hoddereducation.co.uk/myrevisionnotes

In all other circumstances, it is appropriate to use alcohol-based hand gel when giving care.

It is important to know when you should attend to your hand hygiene when giving care. The WHO's '5 moments for hand hygiene' (as used by the NHS) provides guidance on this, shown in Table 10.2.

Table 10.2 The WHO's 5 moments for hand hygiene

Moment	When	Why
Before touching a patient	Clean your hands before touching a patient.	To protect the patient from pathogens on your hands
Before clean/aseptic technique	Clean your hands immediately before performing a clean/aseptic procedure.	To protect the patient from pathogens entering their body
After body fluid exposure risk	Clean your hands immediately after body fluid exposure risk and after removing gloves.	To protect yourself and the healthcare environment from pathogens from the patient
After touching a patient	Clean your hands after touching a patient and their immediate surroundings, when you leave their side.	To protect yourself and the healthcare environment from pathogens from the patient
After touching patient surroundings	Clean your hands after touching any object or furniture in a patient's immediate environment, even if you did not touch the patient, as you leave.	To protect yourself and the healthcare environment from pathogens from the patient

Source: Adapted from the WHO's poster, www.who.int/publications/m/item/five-moments-for-hand-hygiene

How to practise good personal hygiene

Good personal hygiene prevents the body from becoming a reservoir of infection and a method of transmission of infection. Figure 10.3 shows what practising good personal hygiene includes.

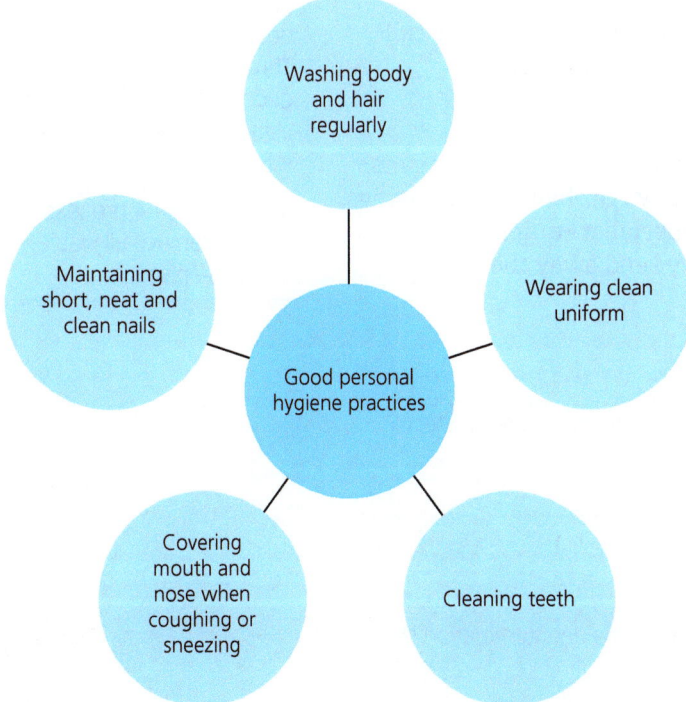

Figure 10.3 How to practise good personal hygiene

> **Revision activity**
>
> Create a method to help you remember the WHO's 5 moments for hand hygiene. For example, can you create an acronym, a mnemonic or a phrase to help you remember each of the five moments?

My Revision Notes: Health T Level

> **Now test yourself** TESTED
>
> 1 Why is it important to maintain good hand hygiene?
> 2 Why is it important to maintain good personal hygiene?
> 3 List **three** ways you can maintain good personal hygiene.

A10.3 The scientific principles of cleaning, disinfection, sterilisation and decontamination

REVISED

The principles

Decontamination

Decontamination is the overarching process used to describe cleaning, disinfection and sterilisation. The healthcare environment and equipment must be decontaminated according to the organisation's policies and procedures.

Cleaning

- Physically reduces the presence of microorganisms that may be present on surfaces and instruments through the removal of visible foreign material.
- Minimises the risk of transfer of microorganisms from one surface or object to another, or from surface to hand or hand to hand.
- Cleaning uses detergent (soap) and water and should be the first step in the decontamination process.

Disinfection

- Disinfection is achieved by using either a specific chemical disinfectant or a physical process such as heat.
- It reduces nonvisible pathogenic microorganisms by destroying the cell wall of the microorganism or interfering with cell metabolism.

Sterilisation

- Sterilisation is the complete elimination (removal) of all microorganisms.
- It is a specialist procedure, usually carried out in larger healthcare settings, such as a hospital, by a specialist team using specialist equipment.
- Smaller settings, for example GP surgeries, may send away their equipment for sterilisation as required.

> **Decontamination** A process to remove or destroy contamination. Three processes of decontamination are used: cleaning, disinfection and sterilisation.
>
> **Sterilisation** A process used to remove all viable microorganisms.

> **Revision activity**
>
> Draw a table or create a spider diagram to show which equipment requires either cleaning, disinfecting or sterilising, based on its use/purpose.

> **Now test yourself** TESTED
>
> 1 What is meant by decontamination?
> 2 The GP reception area is muddy on a wet day. What type of decontamination is most appropriate?
> 3 A patient has been sick on the floor. Why should disinfectant be used?
> 4 Why must instruments used in surgery be sterilised?

A10.4 The differences in procedures for cleaning, disinfection and sterilisation

REVISED

Cleaning

Cleaning procedures are those which result in a surface being visibly clean. There is a universal colour code used by the cleaning industry to prevent cross-contamination between cleaning areas.

It is vital that the correct colour-coded mops and mop buckets, brushes and dustpans, and cleaning gloves are used. The colour coding is shown in Table 10.3.

Table 10.3 The different colour coding used by the cleaning industry

Colour	Area of use
Red	Where the risk of cross-contamination is high, for example toilets
Green	Where the risk of cross-contamination is medium, for example kitchens
Blue	Where the risk of cross-contamination is low, for example general areas
Yellow	Generally used in clinical settings and isolation areas, for example cleaning equipment in hospital

Other tools used for cleaning include:
+ vacuum cleaners
+ floor scrubbers
+ cleaning agents (some of these may eliminate microorganisms).

Disinfection

Disinfection is the use of an agent known to destroy pathogenic microorganisms, for example sodium hypochlorite (commonly referred to as bleach).

Disinfection should be carried out when surfaces and objects have already been cleaned (that is, all visible dirt and contaminants have been removed).

Sterilisation

Sterilisation can be achieved through a variety of methods, depending on the equipment or instrument being sterilised. These methods are shown in Table 10.4.

Table 10.4 Methods of sterilisation

Method	Example
Application of chemical(s)	This is a common method for sterilising metal surgical instruments.
Application of high pressure	This is used to sterilise biomedical devices and implants. (As it does not involve moisture or high temperatures, it does very little damage and does not interact with drugs.)
Application of heat	Dry heat sterilisation is used for items that may be damaged by moist heat.
Application of both high pressure and heat	An autoclave machine (see Figure 10.4) is a common method for sterilising metal surgical instruments.
Irradiation	This is used to sterilise already-packaged, single-use medical devices such as gloves and syringes.
Filtration	This removes microorganisms rather than killing them. It is used to remove microorganisms from heat-sensitive solutions, such as liquid antibiotics and vaccines.

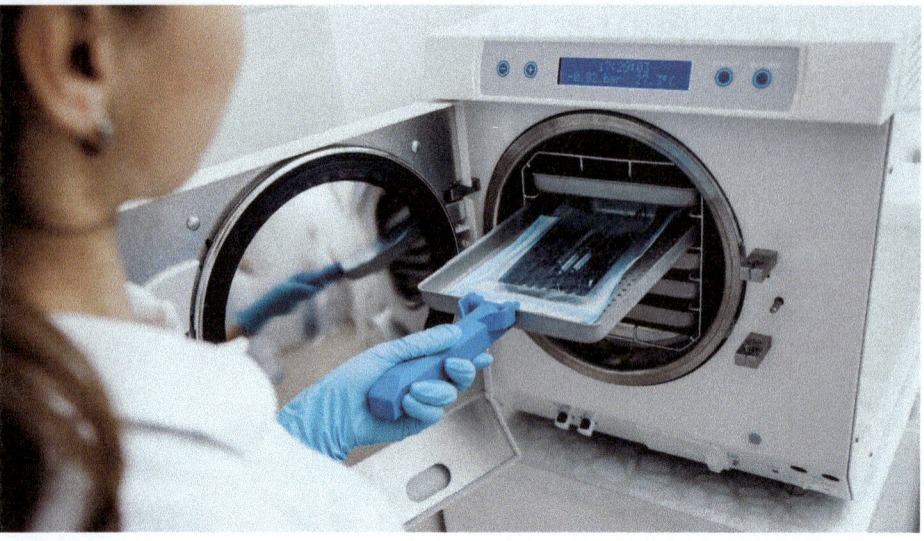

Figure 10.4 An autoclave machine uses steam under pressure to kill harmful microorganisms

> **Now test yourself**   TESTED
>
> 1 What is the difference between cleaning, disinfection and sterilisation?
> 2 When is cleaning sufficient?
> 3 What is the purpose of colour coding cleaning tools?
> 4 What is an autoclave machine?

A10.5 The meaning of impact of antimicrobial resistance, including how this can potentially impact infection control and the ways in which to reduce microbial resistance

REVISED

Antimicrobial resistance

Antimicrobial resistance is the ability of a microorganism to survive exposure to antimicrobial agents, for example antibiotics and disinfectant chemicals.

This resistance is a normal process; bacteria mutate to survive and that includes mutations to become resistant to antibiotics.

However, antimicrobial resistance is accelerated by our actions, specifically by poor infection prevention and control measures and the overuse of antibiotics.

If we take antibiotics when we do not need them, or we do not finish a course of antibiotics, there is more chance that bacteria can mutate to develop a resistance to the antibiotic and then multiply, so there are even more resistant bacteria.

> **Antimicrobial** A substance that kills microorganisms or stops their growth.
>
> **Antimicrobial stewardship** The effort to measure and improve how antibiotics are prescribed by clinicians and used by patients. Improving antibiotic prescribing and use is critical in continuing to treat infections effectively.

The impact of antimicrobial resistance

Antimicrobial resistance has reduced the overall effectiveness of antibiotics. In some cases, it has reduced the number of antibiotics that continue to work against certain bacteria. This can mean that some infections are very difficult to treat effectively.

Overuse of antibiotics has also led to the emergence of new strains of microorganisms and an increase in so-called super bugs, for example MRSA and *Clostridium difficile* (*C. diff*).

Check your understanding and progress at www.hoddereducation.co.uk/myrevisionnotes

Reducing antimicrobial resistance

Antimicrobial stewardship describes a co-ordinated program in the healthcare sector to promote appropriate use of antimicrobials, for example antibiotics.

Stewardship requires different things of different professionals and services within the sector, however what they all have in common is responsible use of antimicrobials and education of end-users.

For example, in the case of antibiotics, doctors must ensure they make a correct diagnosis, when necessary select the right antibiotic, dose and duration, and inform the patient about how to take the antibiotic responsibly.

> **Typical mistake**
>
> Remember, antibiotics have no use in the treatment of viral infections and diseases. Antiviral drugs are a type of medication used specifically for treating viral infections.

> **Now test yourself**   TESTED
>
> 1 Write your own definition of antimicrobial resistance.
> 2 Why is it important to finish a course of antibiotics?
> 3 What does antimicrobial stewardship mean?

> **Exam practice**
>
> 1 Adele is working as a healthcare assistant in a residential nursing home. She has been asked to clean up after a patient has soiled the bed.
>
>   Identify **three** infection-control techniques Adele will need to use in this situation. [3]
>
> 2 Oliver is a new healthcare assistant on a surgical ward. On his first day, he is issued with a uniform and advised how to launder it. He is asked to tie back his long hair.
>
>   Explain why Oliver has been asked to implement these two measures. [4]
>
> 3 Kylie has been asked to clean and disinfect the floor in the ward bathroom.
>
>   a Identify which colour-coded mop should be used in this situation. [1]
>   b Explain the purpose of disinfection. [2]
>
> 4 Dr Frith is a GP. Her patient is a 6-year-old child with a heavy cold. The mother of the patient insists that she needs antibiotics for her cold virus. Dr Frith tells the patient's mother that this is not a responsible use of antibiotics.
>
>   Explain why this is not a responsible use of antibiotics. [4]

A11 Safeguarding

A11.1 The meaning of safeguarding in the health sector and the importance of the key principles of safeguarding

REVISED

Meaning of safeguarding in the health sector

Safeguarding is the protection of the health, wellbeing and rights of individuals. It provides individuals and groups with protection from harm, abuse and neglect. Safeguarding is a key responsibility in the health sector, and workers at all levels must be aware of their role in fulfilling safeguarding legislation, policies and procedures.

The key principles of safeguarding in the health sector

The key principles of safeguarding in the health sector are shown in Figure 11.1.

> **Making links**
>
> A1.1 covers the purpose of safeguarding policies and procedures in the health and science sectors.

> **Making links**
>
> The key principles of safeguarding are detailed further in A8.2. You should refer to Table 8.1 while reviewing this section.

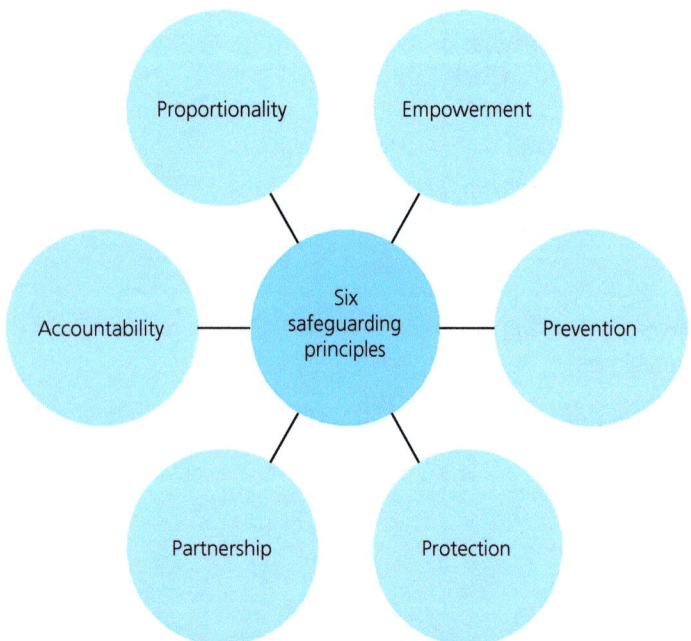

Figure 11.1 The key principles of safeguarding in the health sector

Why safeguarding is important

Safeguarding exists to provide individuals with protection from abuse, harm and neglect. It is a statutory as well as a moral responsibility.

> **Now test yourself** TESTED
>
> 1. Why is safeguarding important?
> 2. Why is empowerment a key principle of safeguarding?
> 3. Who needs to work in partnership to achieve safeguarding?
> 4. What does accountability mean?

> **Revision activity**
>
> Create a set of seven flashcards to help you remember the definition of safeguarding and the six key principles of safeguarding. Use Figure 11.1 along with section A8.2 to help you.

Check your understanding and progress at www.hoddereducation.co.uk/myrevisionnotes

A11.2 How legislation, policies and procedures support the safeguarding of individuals

Mental Capacity Act 2005 plus Amendment (2019)

The Mental Capacity Act (MCA) 2005 empowers and supports people to make their own decisions where at all possible, providing a decision-making framework.

In all safeguarding activities, regard must be given to the provisions of the MCA. This is particularly the case when individuals may have some limit to their capacity, for example due to mental ill health, a learning disability, a brain injury or their level of consciousness.

Safeguards such as Deprivation of Liberty Standards (DoLS) and Liberty Protection Safeguards (LPS) are used to protect individuals who lack capacity to consent to their care arrangements.

> **Making links**
>
> A8.1 explores the purpose of the Mental Capacity Act (MCA) 2005. A8.8 explores the application of the MCA, Liberty Protection Safeguards (LPS) and the deprivation of liberty.

Care Act 2014

The Care Act 2014 provides the legal framework for how local authorities should protect adults at risk from abuse and neglect. It establishes the duties of the local authority to:
+ lead a multi-agency safeguarding system in their locality
+ make necessary safeguarding enquiries, or request that others do so
+ establish safeguarding adults boards (SABs)
+ carry out safeguarding adults reviews (SARs)
+ arrange independent advocates.

> **Making links**
>
> The key principles of the Care Act 2014 are covered in A8.2.

Health and Care Act 2022

The Health and Care Act 2022 established:
+ integrated care systems (ICSs)
+ integrated care boards (ICBs)
+ integrated care partnership (ICP) structures.

ICSs bring together NHS, local authority and non-profit-sector bodies to take on responsibility for delivering health services in an area or 'system'. Their aim is to deliver better, more integrated care for patients, which includes more effective safeguarding actions and processes.

Safeguarding Vulnerable Groups Act 2006

The Safeguarding Vulnerable Groups Act 2006 aims to prevent people that are deemed unsafe or unsuitable for working with adults at risk and children from gaining access to those groups through work.

Under this Act, settings that provide care and treatment for adults at risk and children must use the Disclosure and Barring Service (DBS) to make safer recruitment decisions. Anyone recruited to provide health or personal care should be subject to a DBS check.

Mental Health Act 2007

The Mental Health Act 2007 sets out when someone can be detained and treated for a mental health condition, with the express purpose of reducing threats to the health and safety of the public and the detained individual.

This ensures individuals who pose a risk to themselves are protected from harm, the public are protected from harm and only those individuals who meet the threshold for detention can be detained, thus protecting individuals from unnecessary detention and associated harm.

Equality Act 2010

The Equality Act 2010 provides legal protection for individuals with protected characteristics from discrimination within society.

Discrimination can include reduced access to services, poorer treatment within services and wilful harm, therefore this Act provides legal safeguards from harm.

Human Rights Act 1998

The Human Rights Act 1998 sets out the fundamental rights and freedoms that individuals are entitled to, such as the right to life, prohibition of torture and inhuman treatment, and the right to liberty and freedom.

Upholding these rights promotes safeguarding, as legal protections are given against harm and abuse.

Domestic Abuse Act 2021

The Domestic Abuse Act 2021 provides a framework designed to support organisations to identify and respond to domestic abuse and promote best practice.

It includes a duty on local authorities in England to provide support to victims of domestic abuse and their children in refuges and other forms of safe accommodation.

Through this provision, survivors of domestic abuse and their children are protected from further harm and empowered to live safer lives.

NICE guidance and quality standards

There are six published National Institute for Health and Care Excellence (NICE) guidelines and four published NICE quality standards relating to safeguarding of adults, children and young people with different conditions in a variety of settings (for example schools, care homes and support services across health and social care).

In each case, the guidelines and standards are underpinned by the key principles of safeguarding, aim to protect individuals from harm, abuse and neglect, and make it clear that safeguarding is everyone's responsibility.

NHS England guide

The NHS England pocket guide *Safeguarding Adults* defines guidance in relation to safeguarding requirements to comply with legislation and regulations within health and social care services and settings. The NHS has also produced an app to enable professionals to have 24-hour access to its guide on safeguarding.

The app includes sections on:
+ raising concerns
+ the context of NHS safeguarding
+ types of abuse, exploitation and neglect
+ multi-agency safeguarding arrangements
+ safeguarding commissioning and assurance in the NHS
+ contacts.

> **Making links**
> Discrimination and protected characteristics are covered in A1.1.

> **National Institute for Health and Care Excellence (NICE)** An organisation that uses the best available evidence to compile guidelines and quality standards for health and social care provision. These guidelines make recommendations for best practice and what care the public should expect to receive.

> **Revision activity**
> Create a concept map on how to safeguard individuals in relation to legislation, policy and procedure. Split your map into areas based on the legislation and guidance referenced in this section and make notes in each area, stating how the Act or guidance informs safeguarding and what safeguarding principles are being used.

> **Now test yourself** — TESTED
> 1. List **three** pieces of legislation that support safeguarding of individuals.
> 2. The Care Act 2014 puts a duty on which authority to do what?
> 3. What is DBS and how does it relate to safeguarding?

Check your understanding and progress at www.hoddereducation.co.uk/myrevisionnotes

A11.3 Factors that may contribute to an individual being vulnerable to harm or abuse and the vulnerable groups that require protection

Factors that can contribute to abuse

There are a number of factors that can contribute to an individual being vulnerable to abuse. These are detailed in Table 11.1.

Table 11.1 Factors that can contribute to abuse

Factor	Explanation
Age	Very young and elderly people are vulnerable as they have a physical size difference. Infants and children will also lack understanding of abuse and tend to trust adults without question.
Health issues	Individuals may lack physical power in a relationship because of their illness, which can mean they can be overpowered and abused. Health issues may result in dependence on others in meeting daily activities and for treatment and recovery.
Being physically dependent on others	This carries a risk of the caregiver exploiting this dependence and being abusive, or omitting to care for the individual appropriately, resulting in neglect.
Lack of mental capacity	Individuals may not understand whether something is abusive or may be easier to coerce or convince that abuse is acceptable. These individuals might also find it challenging to speak up about and report abuse.
Previous history of abuse	Individuals may be more vulnerable to recurrent abuse because they may see abusive acts as inevitable or part of life. They may also feel powerless to stop it.
Social isolation	Individuals who do not have support networks may be easier to coerce into abusive situations. These individuals may also find it harder to report abuse as they are isolated.
Drug/alcohol misuse	Individuals may have periods where they lack mental capacity. They may also experience low levels of consciousness, which makes them vulnerable to abuse.
Finance	Individuals may be abused for financial gain, or they may be financially dependent on their abuser.
Religion	Abuse may be motivated by a perceived religious belief or due to discrimination.

Vulnerable groups

Although anyone can be a victim of abuse, members of certain groups are more vulnerable to it. These groups are shown in Figure 11.2.

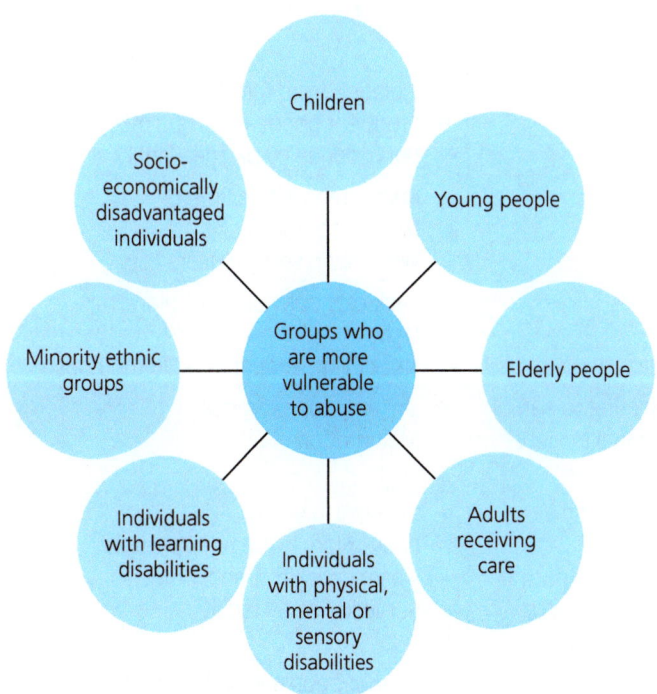

Figure 11.2 Groups who are more vulnerable to abuse

Revision activity

Add another column to Table 11.1 and add in the relevant vulnerable groups (as shown in Figure 11.2) for each factor. For example, for 'age' add children, young people and elderly people.

Now test yourself

1. Why does being physically dependent on someone else increase vulnerability to abuse?
2. How does mental capacity relate to vulnerability to abuse?
3. Why are adults receiving care in their own homes more vulnerable to abuse?

A11.4 A range of different types of abuse and harm

REVISED

A11.5 The types and possible signs of abuse or harm that may be identified in individuals using healthcare

REVISED

Table 11.2 outlines the main types of abuse or harm with examples or explanations, and the possible signs of abuse or harm that healthcare workers may observe in individuals using healthcare.

> **Typical mistake**
>
> An individual may be experiencing more than one type of abuse at once. It is important to know that many of the signs of abuse overlap. Healthcare workers must use their observation skills, their knowledge of individuals and what is normal behaviour for them, their knowledge of an individual's situation and their own knowledge of types and signs of abuse to inform any conclusions they may reach.

Gaslighting Making an individual question their perception of reality.

Table 11.2 Types and possible signs of abuse or harm that may be identified in individuals using healthcare

Type of abuse/harm	Examples/explanation	Possible signs
Physical abuse	+ Female genital mutilation + Hitting + Burns	+ Bruising + Unexplained bleeding
Modern-day slavery	+ Illegal exploitation of individuals for work using threats and violence	+ Reluctance to interact or to talk to others/make eye contact + Workers that look unkempt or malnourished
Sexual abuse	+ Forcing someone to take part in or watch sexual activities	+ Unwanted pregnancy + Sexually transmitted infections + Sexual promiscuity
Emotional abuse	+ Belittling (making someone feel unimportant) + Bullying + Verbal abuse + Gaslighting	+ Depression + Low self-esteem
Coercion/control	+ Assaults + Threats and intimidation + Humiliation	+ Isolation from friends + Frequent phone calls/text messages + Surveillance by partner/family
Organisational/institutional abuse	+ Regimented mealtimes + Removing personal choices	+ Restricted visiting times + Patient complaints + Withdrawn service users
Financial abuse	+ Withholding or taking of money	+ Lack of money and/or belongings + Debt + Not having enough food in the house
Neglect	+ Self-neglect, for example neglecting to eat, or neglecting one's health or personal hygiene + Neglect by others	+ Unkempt appearance + Malnutrition
Domestic abuse	+ Abuse that takes place in the home by a family member + Abuse from an intimate partner or ex-partner + Forced marriage (a marriage where one or both people do not or cannot consent)	+ Physical injuries + Fear of family member/partner + Absence from school or work + Surveillance by family
Professional abuse	+ Abuse by someone in a position of power over the victim or a position of trust	+ Fear of people in authority positions + Low self-esteem

Check your understanding and progress at www.hoddereducation.co.uk/myrevisionnotes

Type of abuse/harm	Examples/explanation	Possible signs
Honour-based abuse	+ Acts of physical, sexual, financial or emotional abuse committed to protect or defend the honour of an individual or family	+ Signs as for the relevant types of abuse
Discriminatory abuse	+ Unequal treatment of an individual based on a protected characteristic, for example race	+ Signs as for the relevant types of abuse
Child sexual exploitation or child criminal exploitation (sexual, labour or forced criminality)	+ Using children for sexual or criminal gain + Child labour	+ Absence from home or school + New and/or older friends + New possessions/unexplained gifts

> **Now test yourself** TESTED
>
> 1 List **two** examples of emotional abuse.
> 2 List **two** signs of financial abuse.
> 3 Summarise the meaning of honour-based abuse in your own words.

> **Exam tip**
>
> It is important to remain objective and to use professional, clear language when responding to questions around abuse.

A11.6 What action to take if abuse is suspected or disclosed

REVISED

It is important to take appropriate action if abuse is suspected or disclosed.

Communicate with the individual

+ Although respecting confidentiality is most important, this must be balanced with assessing risk.
+ It can be appropriate to break confidentiality if an individual is at risk of harm or poses a risk to someone else.
+ It is important to ensure a record of any disclosure is recorded word for word and with impartiality, for example by using a safeguarding disclosure form or a safeguarding incident report form.

> **Exam tip**
>
> Ensure you can clearly describe the process that must be followed when responding to concerns or suspicions of abuse. The same principles will be followed irrespective of the context.

Reporting

+ Everyone in an organisation must know the procedure to follow for reporting concerns or disclosures of abuse.
+ As everyone has a responsibility for safeguarding, understanding the next point of escalation – the report line – is necessary if suspected abuse is not investigated after the first report.
+ It is important to report instances of abuse, however individuals should not intervene unless there is an immediate or imminent threat to safety.

Ability to challenge authority

Healthcare workers require courage to challenge authority, for example when suspicions or disclosures of abuse are not being investigated, or if institutional or professional abuse is occurring.

Preserving evidence

When there is evidence of abuse, it is important to preserve that evidence for the investigations that will follow. This includes:
+ documentation of facts, for example in medical notes or on safeguarding disclosure or safeguarding incident forms
+ observation charts, for example of vital signs, as well as body maps showing the location of injuries
+ clinical photography, for example of bruises.

> **Disclosure** The process in which an individual shares or starts to share information about abuse or neglect.
>
> **Impartiality** Not taking sides and remaining objective.
>
> **Escalation** Taking your concern further or to a more senior person.
>
> **Report line** The direction of communication and responsibility within an organisation. Also known as the chain of command.

> **Now test yourself** TESTED
>
> 1 What should you remember when communicating with an individual who discloses abuse?
> 2 Why do you need to know the report line for safeguarding in an organisation?
> 3 Why does safeguarding require courage?
> 4 Summarise what preserving evidence means in safeguarding.

> **Typical mistake**
>
> All concerns of safeguarding must be reported. Objective, neutral and clear language should always be used when making reports. It is never the responsibility of a healthcare assistant to investigate allegations of abuse.

A11.7 Action that can be taken by individuals and organisations to reduce the chances of abuse

REVISED

It is important to be proactive to reduce the chances of abuse. Table 11.3 lists actions and how they can reduce the chances of abuse.

> **Making links**
>
> A6.9 covers the responsibilities that organisations and individual staff members have in terms of whistleblowing and escalating issues.

Table 11.3 Action that can be taken to reduce the chances of abuse

Action	How it reduces the chances of abuse
Raising awareness and educating others	National campaigns and television adverts, for example by the NSPCC, raise awareness of abuse among the public. This means that individuals know what abuse looks like, so they are more likely to detect and report it or take action to stop it.
Staff training	Staff will complete up-to-date training courses on the types and signs of abuse, so they are more likely to detect and report it or take action to stop it. They are more aware of their own responsibilities and the procedures that must be followed.
Creating a whistleblowing policy	This enables staff to escalate concerns of abuse, harm, neglect and safeguarding failures. It is important that everyone feels empowered to use it.
Creating a complaints policy	This enables individuals and their families to escalate concerns of abuse, harm, neglect and safeguarding failures.
Creating risk management procedures	Organisations will have procedures to identify at-risk individuals and minimise risks of harm and abuse. It is important that everyone knows how to use the procedures.
Carrying out a risk assessment for each individual	Organisations will have procedures to identify at-risk individuals so that specific procedures can be put in place to minimise risks of harm and abuse for that individual. This recognises that every case is different and not all solutions work for all people.
Working with person-centred values	Staff will treat individuals with dignity and respect, reducing risk of abuse. Individuals themselves will feel worthy and empowered and stand up to abuse and neglect. This is underpinned by the initiative Making Safeguarding Personal, which places people and their desired outcomes at the centre of all safeguarding activities.
Multi-agency working	This requires the appropriate sharing of relevant information. It reduces the chance of omissions and gaps in service provision that can result in harm and abuse going undetected.
Implementing holistic approaches	This ensures care and treatment go beyond focusing on physical health and acknowledges emotional, social and spiritual health, which can be compromised by harm and abuse.
Promoting and facilitating access to advocacy	This enables vulnerable individuals to have a voice to report their concerns and empowers individuals to have more control over their lives.

> **Now test yourself**
>
> 1 List **three** actions to reduce the chances of abuse.
>
> TESTED

A11.8 The meaning of patient safety and clinical effectiveness, including why they are important

REVISED

Patient safety

This is the avoidance of accidental or unintended injury or harm during a period of receiving healthcare. This encompasses:
+ safety of the physical environment, for example through fire safety procedures
+ ensuring unauthorised persons do not have access to healthcare settings, by having 24-hour security, security doors and alarms
+ procedures to make clinical care as safe as possible, for example the WHO Surgical Safety Checklist used prior to surgery
+ the use of reporting systems for critical incidents and near misses, so there is continuous learning and improvement
+ audits of practice to ensure safety standards are met.

Clinical effectiveness

This is the application of healthcare, taking into consideration the individual's wishes, the healthcare professional's experience, and evidence-based research in the approach. This requires:
+ a competent workforce
+ the use of evidence-based best practice guidelines, such as those from NICE
+ person-centred care practices and values.

Importance of patient safety and clinical effectiveness

Patient safety and clinical effectiveness are important because they:
+ raise the standard of care
+ improve the patient's experience and quality of care
+ avoid negative outcomes for the provision of care.

> **Making links**
>
> This area of safeguarding is closely linked to what you have learned about health and safety and relevant legislation, regulations and best practice in A3 and A4.

> **Exam tip**
>
> The WHO Surgical Safety Checklist is a good example of how patient safety is maintained. It is a tool used to confirm that critical safety measures are performed before, during and after an operation. You can see the checklist here: www.who.int/teams/integrated-health-services/patient-safety/research/safe-surgery/tool-and-resources

> **Now test yourself** TESTED
>
> 1 Write **one** sentence summarising patient safety.
> 2 What is clinical effectiveness?
> 3 Why is patient safety important?

A11.9 What is meant by radicalisation, identifying signs of radicalisation and the purpose of the Prevent strategy (2011)

REVISED

Radicalisation is the action or process of someone supporting terrorism, or adopting radical extremist beliefs connected with terrorism or terrorist groups.

Identifying signs of radicalisation

The signs of an individual being radicalised include:
+ detachment from family and friends
+ raised levels of anger
+ failing to discuss or avoiding discussing their own or alternative views
+ increased interest in privacy or secretive behaviours.

> **Making links**
>
> The key definition for the term *radicalisation* is in A6.9.

The purpose of the Prevent strategy

The Prevent strategy was published by the UK Government in 2006 and reviewed in 2011.

The specific purpose of Prevent is to work with communities to support vulnerable people at risk of becoming radicalised, therefore safeguarding those individuals from abuse and harm.

The strategy places a duty on specified authorities, which includes the health sector, to have 'due regard to the need to prevent people from being drawn into terrorism'.

The key areas of focus are:
+ awareness of the risks of radicalisation in their area and organisation
+ ensuring staff understand the risk of radicalisation, the importance of Prevent and the measures available to stop radicalisation
+ working in partnership with other agencies as required, including the sharing of information.

> **Now test yourself** TESTED
> 1 What does the term *radicalisation* mean?
> 2 List **three** possible signs of a person undergoing radicalisation.
> 3 What is the Prevent strategy?

> **Exam tip**
> The recognised signs of radicalisation are deliberately broad because the specifics of how these signs present will be different for every individual and their circumstances. This is why person-centred approaches are so important. If we try to get to know people in our care, find out about their usual patterns of behaviour and have open and honest conversations with them and their carers, it is easier to detect a change that could be a cause for concern.

A11.10 The importance of positive behaviour, including a range of positive behaviours expected of a health professional

REVISED

Managing work stress and presenting a positive, professional and caring face to service users and their families is key to positive behaviour. Being positive can help to overcome challenges.

The range of positive behaviours expected of a health professional

+ Taking a people-first approach, for example not making assumptions about individuals and groups but instead acknowledging and accepting diversity and encouraging choice.
+ Demonstrating effective, practised clinical competence in carrying out roles and responsibilities, for example communicating effectively, sharing best practice and working co-operatively.
+ Maintaining safety, for example observing and reporting on an individual's condition and escalating any issues where necessary as soon as possible.
+ Encouraging professionalism and trust in others, for example by modelling positive behaviours and being open and honest and acting with integrity.
+ Promoting individual choice, dignity, inclusion, independence, individuality, identity, privacy and confidentiality of information.

The importance of positive behaviour

Positive behaviour is important for several reasons:
+ It is key to safeguarding individuals and protecting them from harm, abuse and neglect.
+ Taking a positive approach improves the quality of service provision, which in turn leads to positive outcomes.
+ Failing to comply with behavioural standards could result in noncompliance with the contract of employment, which may lead to a warning or dismissal.
+ Failing to comply with behavioural standards could result in deregistration for registered professionals.

> **Exam tip**
> When writing a response to an extended-response exam question on positive professional behaviours, you can demonstrate the breadth of your knowledge by discussing interrelationships between different areas of the specification as appropriate. Taking a people-first approach is a positive behaviour underpinned by legislation, for example the Equality Act 2010 (A11.2), the NHS Core Values (A8.5) and the professional values of the 6Cs (A8.15).

Check your understanding and progress at www.hoddereducation.co.uk/myrevisionnotes

> **Now test yourself** TESTED
>
> 1 List **three** examples of positive behaviour in the healthcare sector.
> 2 List **three** reasons why positive behaviour is important in the healthcare sector.

A11.11 The types of support for managing positive behaviour

REVISED

There are many ways that positive behaviour is supported. The types of support are shown in Table 11.4.

Table 11.4 The types of support for managing positive behaviour

Behavioural frameworks	+ All workplaces will have guidance on how they expect employees to behave. + This may be built into the contract of employment as well as in a separate code of conduct or behaviour guideline. + Professionally registered staff will also have a code of conduct to adhere to established by their regulator, for example nurses must follow the Nursing and Midwifery Council (NMC) Code.
Workplace policies	+ All workplaces have policies that are underpinned by legal obligations. + For example, whistleblowing policies will outline when concerns about poor behaviour should be escalated and how to do this. Another example is social media policies, setting out what employees should or should not do when using social media.
Performance management	+ Employees should have regular work performance appraisals that lead to the creation of a personal development plan, so they can improve their performance. + If an employee has gaps in their knowledge or behaviour, a performance improvement plan can be created, pinpointing not only what they need to improve but also how they can be supported to do this.

> **Revision activity**
>
> Make a list of workplace policies. For each policy, indicate how it links to positive (professional) behaviours and state which legislation it is underpinned by.

> **Now test yourself** TESTED
>
> 1 Give **one** example of a behavioural framework.
> 2 Give **one** example of a workplace policy that supports positive behaviour.

A11.12 What is meant by a conflict of interest and how to deal with this while practising healthcare

REVISED

What is meant by a conflict of interest

A conflict of interest is a situation that arises where the interests of a person of trust (such as a healthcare professional) or an organisation are in direct conflict with the interests of a patient.

An example would be when a patient is hoping to have planned surgery but it is cancelled because there are insufficient staff and resources to carry it out safely or because a higher-priority emergency case arises.

It can also refer to situations where the person of trust may benefit in some way from the patient or has a pre-existing relationship with the patient.

For example, the patient and person of trust may be related or be close friends. These are situations where it may be difficult to remain objective and not allow personal beliefs or feelings to interfere with the professional relationship.

How to deal with conflicts of interest

+ Be open and honest and act with integrity, for example explain why a conflict has arisen and listen carefully to the other person.
+ Follow workplace guidelines on conflict of interest, as well as those relating to patient rights and complaints policies.
+ Declare any personal conflicts, for example that you have a personal relationship with an individual.

> **Typical mistake**
>
> It is sometimes presumed that a conflict of interest results from a disagreement or argument. This is not the case. Make sure you are clear on the definition and that you can apply it to different contexts.

Now test yourself   TESTED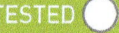

1 Write your own definition of 'conflict of interest'.
2 Give an example of a conflict of interest.

Exam practice

1 Mo is learning about safeguarding. He has read that any action taken to safeguard must be proportionate. He is not sure what this means.
   Explain the concept of proportionality in safeguarding. [2]

2 Rufus is a nursing associate and he wants to update his knowledge regarding safeguarding in the context of domestic violence abuse.
   Describe **two** sources of information that Rufus could consult on safeguarding best practice. [4]

3 a Identify **two** groups that are more vulnerable to abuse. [2]
   b Explain why each of the two groups identified in **a)** are more vulnerable to abuse. [4]

4 Raj is working in A&E. He calls a patient into triage who has a suspected broken arm. She is accompanied by her partner whom she appears to be frightened of. Raj asks the woman to provide a urine sample. Her partner insists on going to the bathroom with her.
   Explain what types of abuse Raj may suspect in this case. [4]

5 Pantelis is a healthcare assistant. A person on the ward where he is working has made a disclosure of abuse to him.
   Outline what action should be taken if abuse is disclosed. [4]

6 State **two** reasons why all hospital staff receive Prevent training. [2]

7 Johann has been struggling at work. He is finding it difficult to communicate with his colleagues in the health centre.
   Describe how performance management can be used to support Johann. [3]

8 Abraham is a healthcare assistant in a busy acute admissions ward in the hospital. He is assigned a new patient and is surprised to see that the patient is a relative.
   a Identify why this is a problem. [1]
   b Outline what Abraham should do in this situation. [3]

Check your understanding and progress at www.hoddereducation.co.uk/myrevisionnotes

B1 Core science concepts

Cells

B1.1 The three principles of cell theory

REVISED

Classical cell theory has three principles:
1. All livings things are made up of cells.
   + Unicellular organisms are made up of single cells (for example bacteria).
   + Multicellular organisms are made up of more than one cell (for example humans).
2. The cell is the basic unit of structure and function of all living things.
   + Cells contain multiple components known as organelles (see B1.3).
3. Cells are created by pre-existing cells.
   + This happens through the process of cell division known as mitosis.

> **Structure** An arrangement of organised elements in a part or system.
>
> **Function** The role of a part or system; what it does.
>
> **Mitosis** A process of cell reproduction in which one cell gives rise to two genetically identical daughter cells.

B1.2 The different types of cells that make up living organisms

REVISED

There are two types of cells: prokaryotes and eukaryotes. Table 12.1 summarises the similarities and differences between them.

Table 12.1 Prokaryotic and eukaryotic cells

Prokaryotic cells	Eukaryotic cells
Small, simple cells	Larger, more complex cells
Unicellular	Unicellular or multicellular
Contain membranes, cytoplasm and DNA	Contain membranes, cytoplasm and DNA
No membrane-bound organelles	Membrane-bound organelles such as mitochondria
DNA is free in cytoplasm, not associated with proteins, or found as plasmids	DNA is contained in the nucleus, associated with histone proteins
For example, bacteria	All animal and plant cells, as well as yeasts, other fungi and algae

> **Typical mistake**
>
> A prokaryote is an organism consisting of a single prokaryotic cell. In other words, prokaryotes, such as bacteria, are *always* unicellular. A eukaryote is an organism consisting of one or more eukaryotic cells. Eukaryotes can be multicellular *or* unicellular, for example humans (multicellular) or yeast (unicellular).

> **Revision activity**
>
> Draw up a list of organisms (living things). Identify whether each organism is
> + unicellular or multicellular
> + prokaryotic or eukaryotic.

> **Now test yourself** TESTED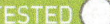
>
> 1. What is the difference between structure and function in biology?
> 2. Explain what is meant by the phrase 'Cells are created by pre-existing cells.'
> 3. a) Give an example of **one** prokaryotic cell and **one** eukaryotic cell.
>   b) Describe **two** differences between prokaryotic cells and eukaryotic cells.

My Revision Notes: Health T Level

B1.3 The structure and function of the organelles found within eukaryotic cells

REVISED

The structure of an animal cell is shown in Figure 12.1, with more information about the structure and function of each organelle given in Table 12.2.

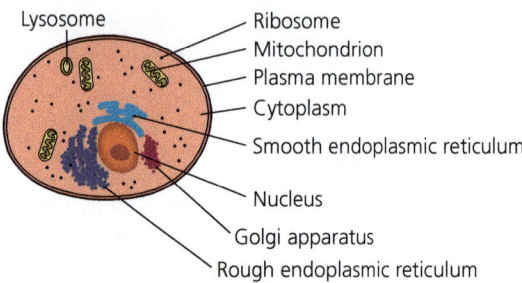

Figure 12.1 Structure of an animal cell

> **Phospholipid bilayer** A two-layer arrangement of phosphate and lipid molecules that form cell membranes.
>
> **DNA (deoxyribonucleic acid)** A double-stranded molecule containing the genetic information responsible for the development and function of an organism.

Table 12.2 Organelles found in eukaryotic cells

Organelle	Structure	Function
Cell-surface membrane (plasma membrane)	**Phospholipid bilayer** with peripheral (surface) proteins and integral (embedded) proteins. Membrane structure is known as the fluid mosaic model.	Controls entry and exit of substances and is the site of antigens.
Nucleus	Enclosed by a double membrane (nuclear envelope) containing pores (openings). Contains **DNA** and histone proteins. DNA combined with histones forms a complex called chromatin. Chromatin is coiled to form chromosomes.	Contains the cell's hereditary information and controls its growth and reproduction.
Mitochondria (singular: mitochondrion)	Enclosed by a double membrane; the inner membrane is folded to form cristae.	The site of aerobic respiration and so adenosine triphosphate (ATP) production. ATP is the energy store of a cell.

Check your understanding and progress at www.hoddereducation.co.uk/myrevisionnotes

Organelle	Structure	Function
Ribosomes	Can be found floating free in the cytoplasm or attached to the rough ER. Made of proteins and RNA.	Bring together amino acids to make particular proteins in the process of protein synthesis (translation).
Rough endoplasmic reticulum (ER)	A system of membrane-enclosed, flattened sacs, with ribosomes attached to the surface.	The attached ribosomes make proteins which are packaged and transported by the rough ER to the Golgi apparatus.
Smooth endoplasmic reticulum (ER)	A system of membrane-enclosed, flattened sacs *without* ribosomes.	Synthesises, stores and transports lipids and some carbohydrates.
Golgi apparatus and Golgi vesicles	Enclosed by a membrane and consisting of flattened sacs known as cisternae.	Modifies proteins, by adding carbohydrates or lipids, which are then transported by the vesicles to other destinations in the cell.
Centrioles	Consist of microtubules arranged in a cylindrical shape.	Form the spindle fibres that separate the chromosomes during mitosis.
Lysosomes	Enclosed by a membrane and contain digestive enzymes.	Break down excess or worn-out cell parts. May be used to destroy invading viruses and bacteria (pathogens).

> **Making links**
> The fluid mosaic model is covered in B1.11.

> **RNA (ribonucleic acid)** A single-stranded molecule that turns genetic information into proteins.

> **Now test yourself** — TESTED
> 1. Describe the structure of the nucleus.
> 2. How do the rough and the smooth endoplasmic reticulum differ in structure?
> 3. Explain the function of lysosomes.

> **Revision activity**
> Draw an animal cell and label the organelles.

B1.4 The structure and function of specialised cells in complex multicellular organisms

REVISED

In multicellular organisms, eukaryotic cells become specialised to perform specific functions. Groups of specialised cells form tissues, which co-operate to form organs and organ systems. This ensures the organism as a whole works together.

In humans, specialisation of embryonic stem cells occurs rapidly to support the development of the foetus. Embryonic stem cells can develop into any cell type.

> **Stem cells** Unspecialised cells that can give rise to other stem cells or differentiate into specialised cells.

All stem cells that develop after the embryonic stem cells have differentiated are known as adult stem cells and are found in specific locations of the body, such as bone marrow. These adult stem cells can only differentiate into a limited number of cell types, for example blood cells.

Specialisation occurs due to cell differentiation. This is controlled by which genes are expressed (switched on).

Specialised cells have different components and adaptations which allow them to carry out specific functions (Table 12.3).

> **Flagellum (plural, flagella)** A slender, thread-like structure that is used to move cells, such as sperm cells.

Table 12.3 Examples of specialised cells

Specialised cell	Structure	Function
Erythrocytes (red blood cells) *View from above — Cell is full of haemoglobin pigment which absorbs oxygen — No nucleus – more room for haemoglobin. Side view — Biconcave shape gives greater surface area for oxygen absorption*	No nucleus so they can carry a large amount of haemoglobin. Small and flexible to fit through blood vessels. Have a biconcave shape (flattened disc) to maximise surface area for oxygen absorption. Very thin cell membrane to allow efficient diffusion.	Transport of oxygen.
Sperm cells *Middle piece, Neck, Head — Acrosome contains enzymes used to penetrate the egg cell — Reduced cytoplasm to reduce mass for swimming — Spiral mitochondria to provide energy for swimming — 'Tail' provides propulsion*	Haploid nucleus in the head of the sperm cell contains genetic material for fertilisation. The head of the cell contains an acrosome with enzymes to break down the female egg cell to allow penetration. Have a flagellum (tail) for propulsion. Full of mitochondria to supply energy for movement.	Fertilise the female egg/ovum.
Ova (singular ovum) *Nucleus, Egg cytoplasm, Follicle cell, First polar body, Gel layer*	Haploid nucleus contains the genetic information; an ovum is much larger than a sperm cell.	Forms the zygote when fertilised by a sperm cell.

Specialised cell	Structure	Function
Neurones (nerve cells) Dendrites — Cell body — Node of Ranvier — Axon — Myelin sheath — Axon terminals	The axon is long and thin to carry messages quickly over long distances. Branched connections (dendrons and dendrites) at each end to join other nerve cells and so transmit/receive electrical impulses. Covered in a myelin sheath which insulates the cell and allows quick, efficient transmission of electrical impulses.	Receive information from cells and transmit this information to other cells.
Squamous epithelial cells Nucleus — Basement membrane	Relatively unspecialised flattened cells.	Make up the layer of epithelium of exchange surfaces such as the lungs, gut and kidney.
Striated muscle cells	Long cells with multiple nuclei that make up skeletal muscles; often referred to as muscle fibres. Striated relates to their striped appearance.	Contract to cause movement of the body.

Making links

Exchange surfaces are covered in B2: see B2.9 for the lungs, B2.12 for the gut and B2.20 for the kidney.

Now test yourself

TESTED

1. How are embryonic and adult stem cells different?
2. What are specialised cells?
3. Describe the specialised structure and function of sperm cells.

Revision activity

Draw and label a sperm cell. Annotate the drawing to explain how the structure of each part of the cell is adapted for its function.

B1 Core science concepts

My Revision Notes: Health T Level

B1.5 The role of a light microscope and how to calculate magnification

REVISED

A light microscope consists of:
+ a light source
+ a stage, where the specimen (usually on a glass microscope slide) is placed
+ an objective lens, usually low-, medium or high-power.
+ an eyepiece lens.

Samples must be very thin to allow light to pass through. This usually means cutting sections with a sharp blade or a microtome. The section is placed on a slide and covered with a thin cover slip. Stains are often used to make the cells more visible. Permanent mounts can be made by fixing the tissue with a preservative before cutting sections.

The magnification of a microscope is calculated using the equation:

$$\text{magnification} = \frac{\text{size of image}}{\text{size of object}}$$

Now test yourself

TESTED

1. You are given a photograph of a bacterial cell. You measure the length of the cell in the magnified image and it is 90 mm. The actual length of the cell is 3.6 μm. Use the equation above to calculate the magnification of the image (1 mm = 1000 μm).

Exam practice

1. Which of the following best describes a prokaryotic organism? [1]
   A A living thing comprised of multiple, complex cells.
   B A living thing comprised of a single, complex cell.
   C A living thing comprised of a single, basic cell.
   D A living thing comprised of both single and multiple cells.
2. State **one** function of mitochondria. [1]
3. Explain why multicellular organisms require specialised cells. [2]

Exam tip

You may not have to remember the equation for magnification – you will probably be given it in the exam – as well as the conversion between mm and μm. You do need to understand how to use the equation.

Make sure you work in the same units, so in the question on the left convert 90 mm into μm or 3.6 μm into mm before you do the division. Magnification values are typically 10×, 100×, 200× etc.

If your answer is less than 1, such as 0.1×, then you have done the calculation the wrong way round (divided the size of the object by the size of the image). Always check your work!

Cell cycle

B1.6 The function of mitosis in nuclear division within cells

REVISED

Mitosis produces two daughter nuclei that have the same number of chromosomes as the parent cell and each other. Each of the daughter cells has an exact copy of the DNA of the parent cell.

This means the daughter cells are genetically identical. This is important in growth of the organism, as well as in producing new cells to replace damaged or worn-out cells (repair and replacement).

Revision activity

Make a list of some of the cell types that are important in:
+ growth of an organism
+ repair and replacement.

Daughter cells may not be identical to the parent cell, but they will be genetically identical. Think about why this is.

B1.7 The purpose of each stage of the cell cycle

REVISED

The cell cycle is shown in Figure 12.2.

The cell cycle consists of:
+ interphase (DNA replication)
+ mitosis (nuclear division).

DNA carries the genetic information and is contained in the chromosomes. Therefore, when the DNA replicates, the chromosomes replicate. Once the chromosomes have replicated, the process of nuclear division can begin. This is why interphase always precedes mitosis.

The stages of mitosis are illustrated in Table 12.4. The diagrams for each stage show how the nucleus appears when viewed under a light microscope. During interphase, even when the DNA has replicated, the chromosomes are too long and thin to be seen with the light microscope.

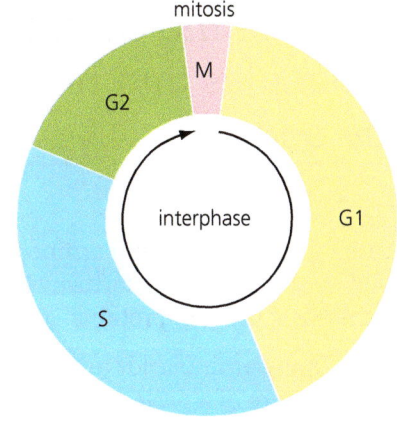

Figure 12.2 The cell cycle

Table 12.4 The stages of mitosis

	Prophase	Chromosomes become visible as two chromatids. The nuclear envelope (see B1.3) disappears.
	Metaphase	The chromosomes line up on the equator at the centre of the cell.
	Anaphase	The chromatids are pulled apart to opposite poles of the cell. At the end of anaphase, we use the term *chromosome*, rather than *chromatid*.
	Telophase	The two sets of chromosomes collect at opposite poles of the cell. The nuclear envelope reforms around each set. Two daughter nuclei are produced.

Following mitosis, the cytoplasm divides to form two daughter cells in a process known as cytokinesis.

Cell cycle The cycle of division, growth and further division that all dividing cells go through.

Chromatids Sometimes called sister chromatids. The two identical copies of a chromosome formed as a result of DNA replication. The term *chromatid* is a shorter way of saying 'one of a pair of identical chromosomes'.

Cytokinesis When the cytoplasm divides to form two daughter cells after nuclear division.

Now test yourself
TESTED
1 What is meant by mitosis?
2 Why does interphase always precede mitosis in the cell cycle?

Exam practice
1. Describe two features of mitosis that ensure the production of genetically identical cells. [2]
2. Explain the difference between nuclear division and cell division. [2]
3. There are stages in the cell cycle where DNA is checked for damage or errors. If any are found, the cycle stops and the cell does not undergo mitosis. Suggest and explain an advantage of this process. [2]

Revision activity
The diagrams in Table 12.4 show the stages of mitosis in a cell with one pair of chromosomes. Draw diagrams to show the stages of mitosis in a cell with three pairs of chromosomes. Make each pair a different length.

Annotate your diagram to show how the different stages ensure mitosis produces two genetically identical daughter cells.

Large molecules

B1.8 The molecular structures of the large molecules and how they are used within the body

REVISED

Proteins

Proteins are formed from amino acids. These are joined together in a condensation reaction, forming a peptide bond. You can think of amino acids as the basic units of proteins.

When many amino acids are joined by peptide bonds, a polypeptide is formed. The structure of a protein is described in relation to the polypeptide chain:
+ The primary structure is the sequence of amino acids in a polypeptide chain.
+ The secondary structure is the way the polypeptide chain is folded.
+ The tertiary structure is the three-dimensional shape of a protein.
+ The quaternary structure is the formation of a functional protein from two or more polypeptide chains.

This is summarised in Figure 12.3.

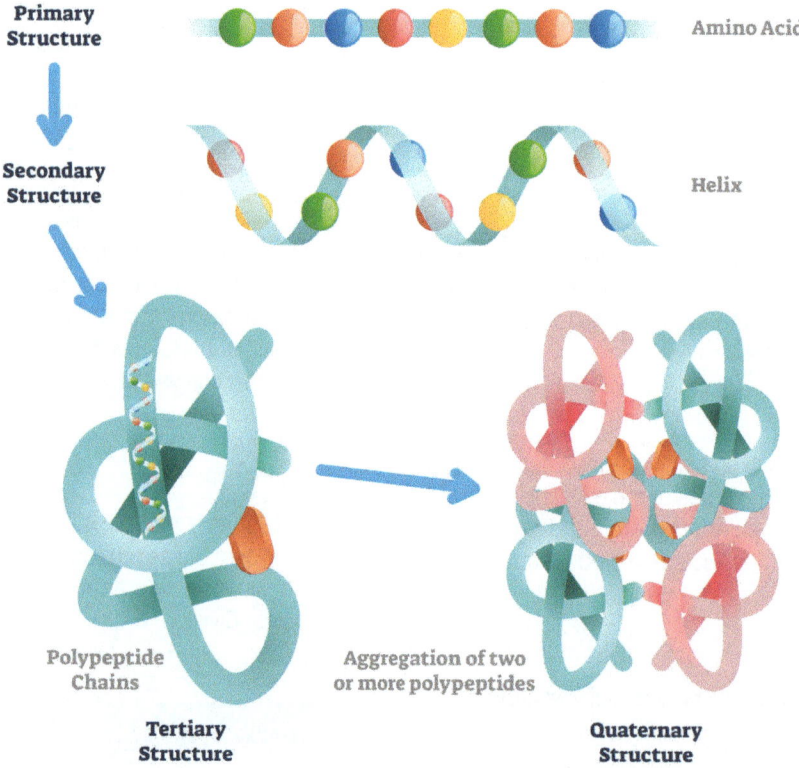

Figure 12.3 The four levels of structure in proteins; not all proteins have quaternary structure

Proteins are used within the body for growth and repair, for example:
+ proteins in muscles, ligaments and tendons
+ enzymes that take part in all cellular processes
+ proteins in skin, nails, hair and bones.

Carbohydrates

Carbohydrates are made up of monosaccharides, which contain carbon, hydrogen and oxygen. Monosaccharides are the most basic carbohydrate.

Condensation reaction
A reaction between two small molecules to produce a larger molecule and water. A number of large biological molecules are formed by condensation reactions.

Monosaccharide
The most basic carbohydrate. Glucose is a monosaccharide.

When combined in pairs, monosaccharides form disaccharides in a condensation reaction. The bond between the monosaccharides is known as a glycosidic bond. This is shown in Figure 12.4.

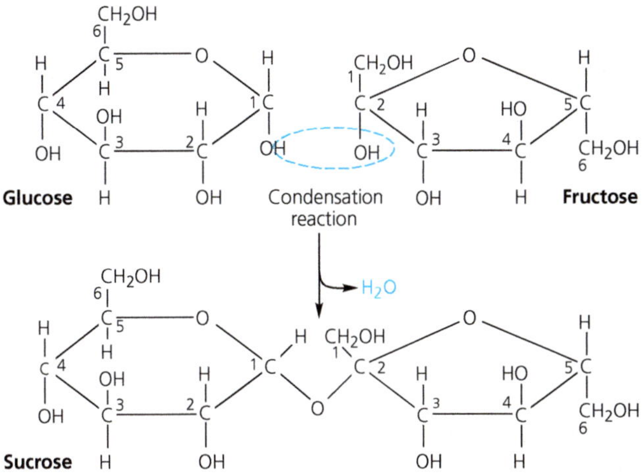

> **Disaccharides** Made up of two monosaccharides joined by a glycosidic bond.
>
> **Polysaccharide** A long polymer molecule made up of many monosaccharide units joined by glycosidic bonds.

Figure 12.4 A condensation reaction between two monosaccharides (glucose and fructose) forms a disaccharide (sucrose) containing a glycosidic bond

Carbohydrates are a source of energy:
+ Glucose is used in respiration.
+ Glycogen is a polysaccharide stored in liver and muscle cells. It contains thousands of glucose units joined by glycosidic bonds.

Lipids

Triglycerides are formed in a condensation reaction between one molecule of glycerol and three fatty acid molecules (Figure 12.5).

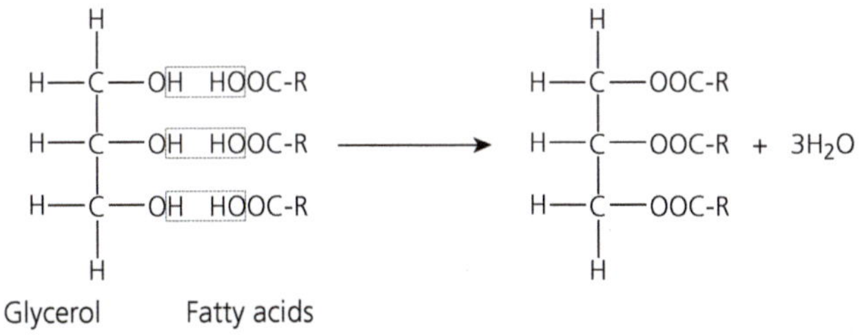

Figure 12.5 Formation of a triglyceride from one glycerol and three fatty acids; R represents a long carbon chain; the R groups can be the same or different

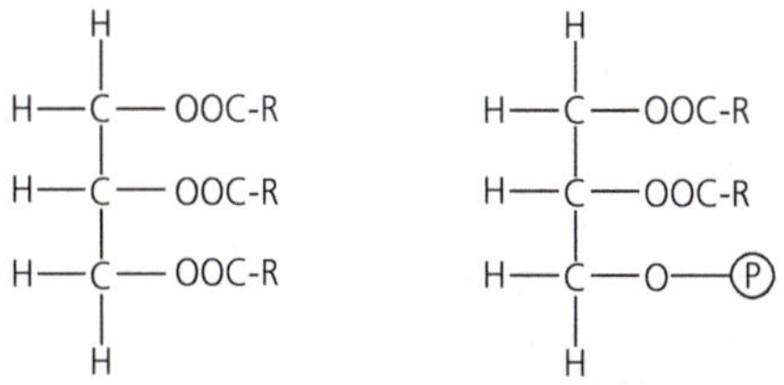

Figure 12.6 Comparing the general structures of a triglyceride (left) and a phospholipid (right). The P in a circle represents the phosphate group

Phospholipids are formed when one of the fatty acids of a triglyceride is substituted by a phosphate-containing group (Figure 12.6).

Fatty acid molecules are hydrophobic (they repel water), while glycerol molecules are hydrophilic (they attract water). A phospholipid is made up of two parts: a hydrophilic head and a hydrophobic tail. As a result, the molecules can come together to form a bilayer that is the basis of the fluid mosaic model of membrane structure and is important for all membrane functions.

> **Making links**
>
> The fluid mosaic model is covered in more detail in B1.11.

Lipids are also used within the body:
+ for thermal insulation
+ for physical protection
+ as an energy source.

> **Now test yourself**
>
> 1 Describe the four levels of protein structure.
> 2 Describe a disaccharide.
> 3 What is the difference between a triglyceride and a phospholipid?
>
> TESTED

Exam practice

1. Name the type of reaction that forms polypeptides, polysaccharides and triglycerides. [1]
2. Explain why glycogen stored in muscle cells is a good source of energy. [2]
3. Explain how phospholipids are able to form bilayers. [3]

Enzymes

B1.9 The properties and functions of enzymes that are determined by their tertiary structure

REVISED

Enzymes are biological catalysts; they speed up cellular reactions. Like all proteins, their properties and functions are determined by their tertiary structure.

Properties

The shape of the active site matches the shape of the substrate(s) – we say it is complementary – so an enzyme will be specific for a particular substrate (Figure 12.7).

The substrate binds to the active site because of bonds between parts of the substrate and amino acids in the active site of the enzyme.

All chemical reactions get faster as temperature increases, including enzyme-catalysed reactions. But because enzymes are proteins, their tertiary structure starts to change as temperature increases. Above a certain temperature, the substrate no longer binds properly, so the rate of the reaction decreases. Eventually, the enzyme loses its structure and no longer works. This is shown in Figure 12.8.

Active site The part of the enzyme where the substrate binds. Its shape is complementary to that of the substrate.

Substrate The substance on which an enzyme acts to form the products.

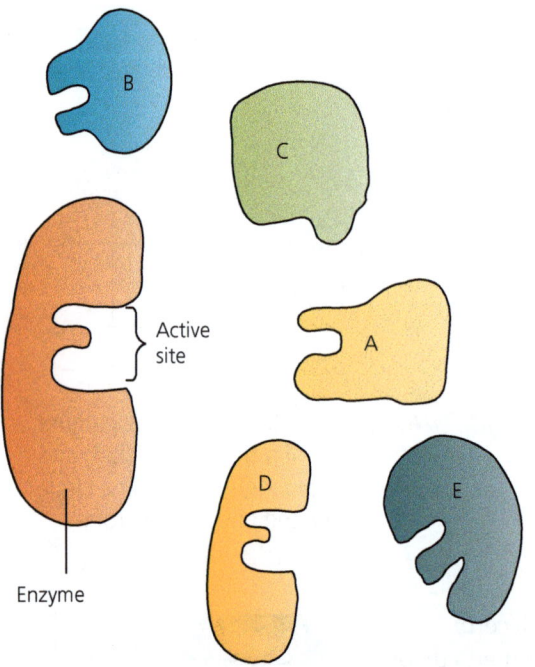

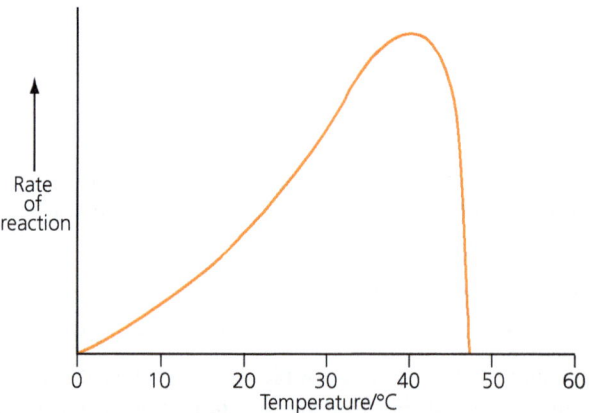

Figure 12.7 The active site of this enzyme is only complementary to the shape of substrate molecule A, the other substrates cannot bind

Figure 12.8 The effect of heat on the rate of an enzyme-catalysed reaction

The role of enzymes

Enzymes play an essential part in all metabolic reactions in cells and in the digestion of foods.

+ Protease enzymes, such as trypsin, break proteins down into smaller polypeptides. Other proteases convert polypeptides into dipeptides and/or amino acids.
+ Carbohydrase enzymes, such as amylase, break down long-chain polysaccharides into disaccharides. (Amylase converts starch into maltose.) Other carbohydrases convert disaccharides (such as maltose) into monosaccharides (such as glucose).
+ Lipase enzymes convert triglycerides into fatty acids and glycerol.

Check your understanding and progress at www.hoddereducation.co.uk/myrevisionnotes

> **Exam practice**
>
> 1. Explain what would happen to an enzyme that was stored on a shelf above a radiator. [3]
> 2. Changes in acidity can affect the bonds that maintain the tertiary structure of enzymes. Explain why salivary amylase no longer works in the stomach, which is highly acidic. [2]
> 3. Thrombolytics are 'clot busting' enzymes that are used to treat heart attack. They act by breaking down the fibrin proteins that form clots. Explain why these drugs do not damage other blood proteins. [2]

> **Now test yourself**
>
> 1 Explain the terms *substrate* and *active site*.
> 2 Explain the shape of the curve in Figure 12.8.
>
> TESTED

Exchange and transport mechanisms

B1.10 How the surface area to volume ratio and additional factors affect the rate of exchange and give rise to specialised systems

REVISED

All organisms exchange substances with their surroundings, to take in oxygen and nutrients or get rid of waste products. For efficient exchange, the surface area of an exchange surface must be large in comparison to the volume. We say it must have a large surface area to volume ratio. This is calculated by dividing the surface area by the volume.

If the surface area is small compared to the volume, then additional exchange and transport mechanisms, such as lungs, will be needed to maximise the rate of exchange.

The rate of exchange depends on:
+ diffusion distance, so exchange surfaces are usually thin; the alveoli in the lungs are only one cell thick
+ temperature, as the rate of diffusion increases with temperature
+ metabolic rate; as this increases, the demand for glucose (absorbed in the gut) and oxygen (absorbed in the lungs) increases.

> **Diffusion** The movement of a substance from a high concentration to a low concentration.

> **Now test yourself**
>
> 1 A cube has sides of 2 cm. Calculate its surface area to volume ratio.
>
> TESTED

B1.11 The structure of the cell-surface membrane and mechanisms of cellular exchange and transport

REVISED

The fluid mosaic model

The cell-surface membrane consists of a phospholipid bilayer that acts as a barrier to diffusion of polar substances (such as water, glucose and ions such as Na^+ and Cl^-). The proteins, lipids and carbohydrates that are found in the membrane vary in shape, size and location, creating a mosaic pattern, so the way we describe the structure of the cell-surface membrane is known as the fluid mosaic model (Figure 12.9). The membrane is described as fluid as components can move throughout it.

> **Fluid mosaic model** A model of the structure of the cell-surface membrane and how its components are arranged like tiles in a mosaic.

> **Making links**
>
> The fluid mosaic model was covered briefly in B1.3 and B1.8. Exchange and transport mechanisms are important in the way cells work.

My Revision Notes: Health T Level

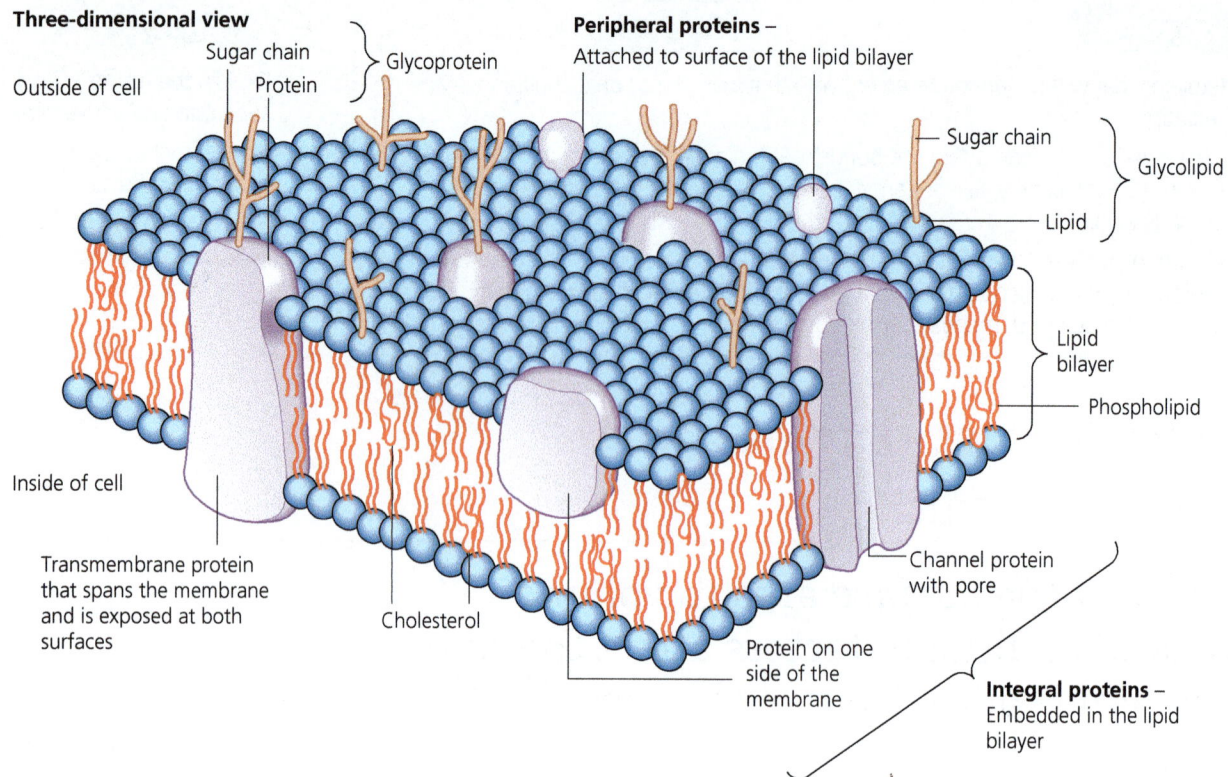

Figure 12.9 The fluid mosaic model of the cell-surface membrane

Mechanisms: passive, active and co-transport

Passive transport

Passive means without using energy from ATP, so substances always diffuse from high to low concentration, i.e. down a concentration gradient.

The cell-surface membrane is described as being partially permeable.
+ Small, non-polar molecules (such as oxygen or carbon dioxide) can move through the phospholipid bilayer by simple diffusion.
+ Polar substances (such as water, glucose or ions (for example Na^+)) cannot diffuse through the phospholipid bilayer and are transported by facilitated diffusion. This involves channel proteins or carrier proteins (Figure 12.10).

Facilitated diffusion of water is known as osmosis. This means that water diffuses from a high concentration of water molecules to a low concentration of water molecules.

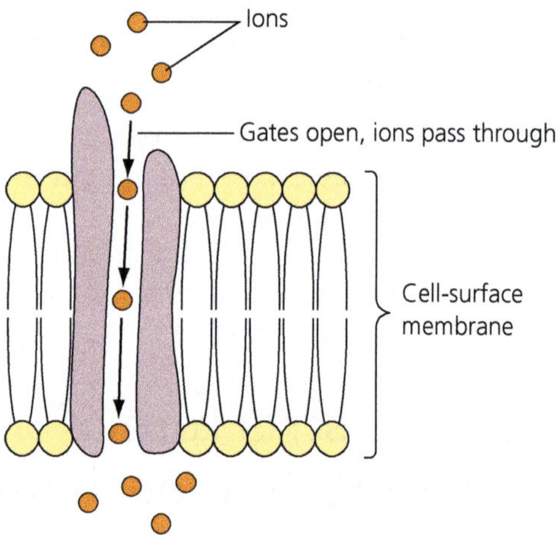

Figure 12.10 Channel proteins help diffusion of ions

Active transport

In facilitated diffusion, substances always move from a high concentration to a low concentration. In active transport, carrier proteins use energy from ATP to move substances from a low concentration to a high concentration.

Co-transport mechanisms

Co-transport is a type of facilitated diffusion using carrier proteins that will only transport one substance together with another substance. Epithelial cells in the lining of the small intestine have carrier proteins that only allow movement of glucose when it is together with sodium ions. Active transport of sodium ions out of the epithelial cells into the blood sets up a concentration gradient of sodium ions that drives the uptake of glucose from the intestine. Movement of glucose from the epithelial cells into the blood requires facilitated diffusion. This is illustrated in Figure 12.11.

Check your understanding and progress at www.hoddereducation.co.uk/myrevisionnotes

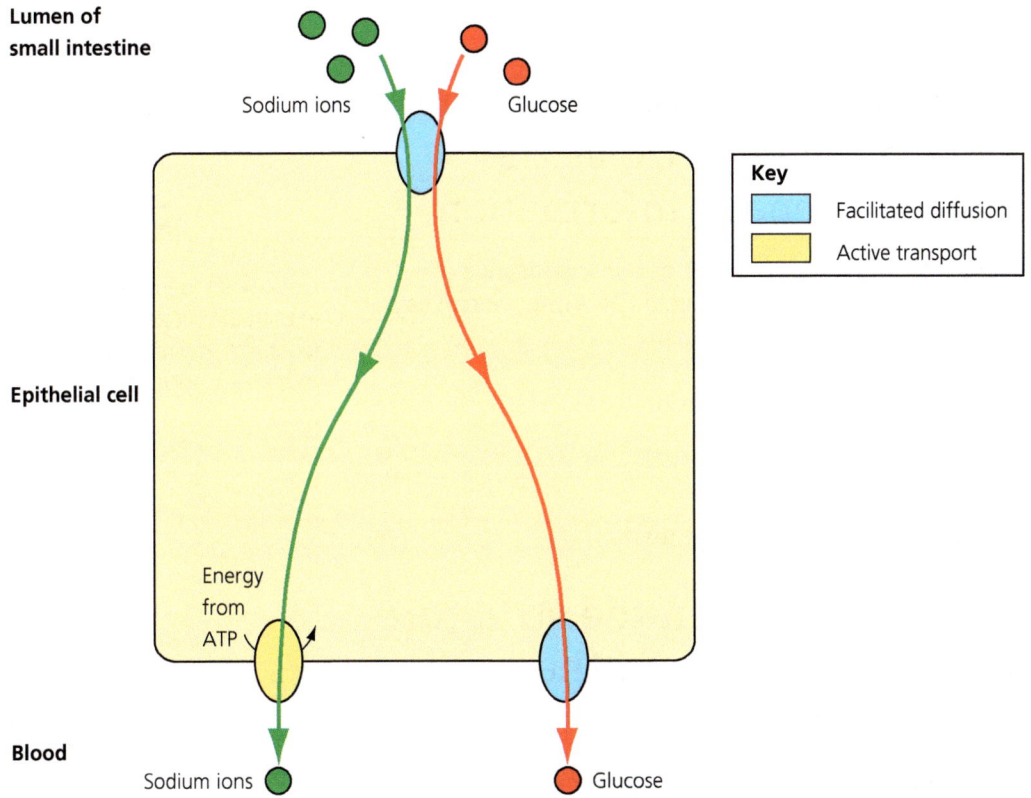

Figure 12.11 Uptake of glucose from the small intestine

Now test yourself

TESTED

1. For each of the following, state whether they would move across the cell-surface membrane by simple diffusion, facilitated diffusion or active transport:
   a. calcium ions from high to low concentration
   b. potassium ions from low to high concentration
   c. oxygen from high to low concentration.
2. What is the name given to the movement of water across the cell-surface membrane from a high concentration of water molecules to a low concentration of water molecules?

Exam practice

1. Cubes are often used to model the effect of surface area to volume ratio on the rate of exchange.
   a. Cube A has sides of 5 cm and a total volume of 125 cm³. Calculate the surface area to volume ratio for Cube A. [2]
   b. Cube B has a surface area to volume ratio of 5 : 1. Explain which cube, A or B, would have the greatest rate of exchange. [2]
2. In which one of the following processes can carbon dioxide, a small, non-polar molecule, pass through the cell-surface membrane? [1]
   A Active transport
   B Diffusion
   C Facilitated diffusion
   D Osmosis
3. A yellow dye, which is a polar molecule, is used to study uptake of substances by cells in culture solution. At the start of the experiment, the cells are colourless and the solution is deep yellow. After 60 minutes, the cells are all stained yellow and the solution is colourless. Explain the results of the experiment. [3]

My Revision Notes: Health T Level

Genetics

B1.12 The purpose of deoxyribonucleic acid (DNA) and ribonucleic acid (RNA) as the carrying molecules of genetic information

REVISED

Genes are passed from parent to offspring and control the appearance of those offspring. Genes consist of deoxyribonucleic acid (DNA), so we can say that DNA holds the genetic information of an organism.
+ Genes control production of proteins.
+ RNA (ribonucleic acid) transfers genetic information from DNA to the ribosomes, where proteins are synthesised.
+ The sequence of bases in DNA determines the sequence of amino acids in the protein.
+ Proteins determine the characteristics of an organism.

Gene A sequence of bases in DNA that codes for (contains the information to make) a polypeptide (protein).

B1.13 The relationship between the structure of DNA and RNA and their role in the mechanism of inheritance

REVISED

DNA and RNA are made up of nucleotides. These small molecules, or monomers, are formed from:
+ pentose (5-carbon sugar)
+ a nitrogen-containing organic base
+ a phosphate group.

The general structure of a DNA nucleotide is shown in Figure 12.12 and a comparison of DNA and RNA nucleotides is given in Table 12.5.

Table 12.5 Similarities and differences between DNA and RNA nucleotides

Component	DNA nucleotide	RNA nucleotide
Pentose sugar	Deoxyribose	Ribose
Organic base	Adenine (A), cytosine (C), guanine (G) or thymine (T)	Adenine (A), cytosine (C), guanine (G) or uracil (U)
Other	Phosphate group	Phosphate group

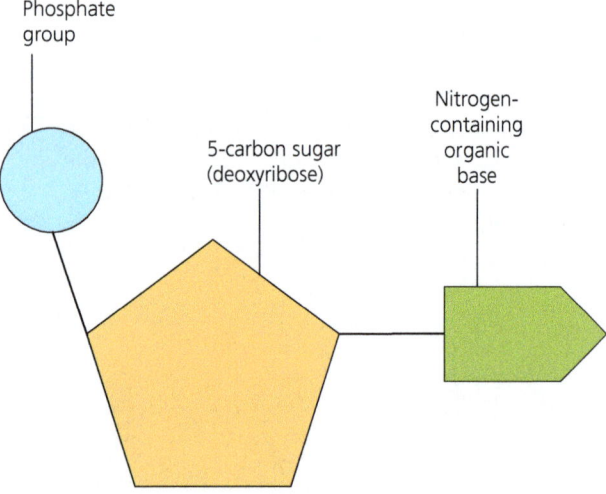

Figure 12.12 General structure of a DNA nucleotide

The nucleotides are joined together in long chains by phosphodiester bonds between the pentose sugars. These bonds are formed in condensation reactions.

Check your understanding and progress at www.hoddereducation.co.uk/myrevisionnotes

A DNA molecule is a double helix with two polynucleotide chains (often called a sugar–phosphate backbone) held together by hydrogen bonds between specific complementary base pairs: A always pairs with T; G always pairs with C.

An RNA molecule is a relatively short, single-stranded polynucleotide chain. A comparison between DNA and RNA molecules is given in Figure 12.13.

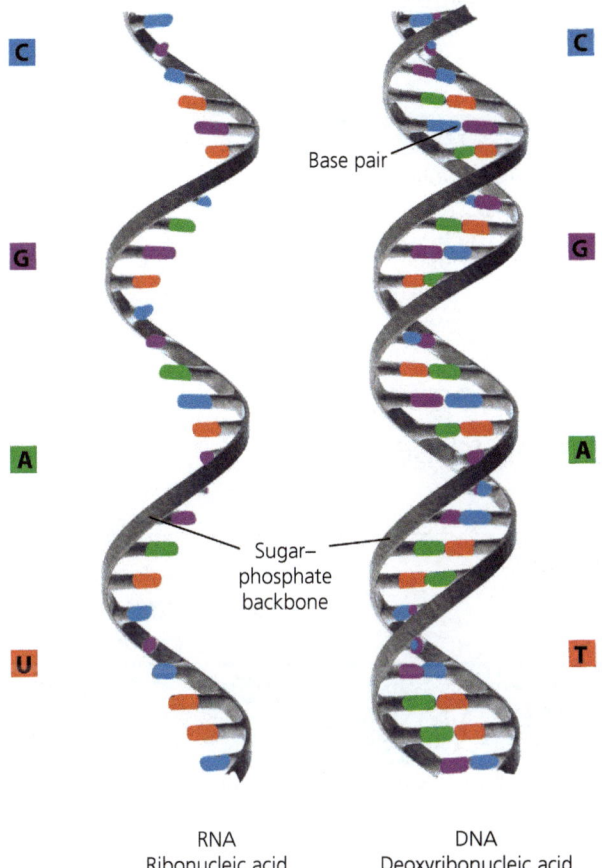

Figure 12.13 The structure of RNA and DNA

> **Now test yourself** TESTED
>
> 1 What is a gene?
> 2 What are the three components of a nucleotide?
> 3 Describe **two** similarities and **two** differences between DNA and RNA nucleotides.

> **Exam practice**
>
> 1 Which of the following is correct? [1]
>   A DNA contains the genetic information, which is transferred to proteins that use it to make RNA.
>   B DNA contains ribose, RNA contains deoxyribose.
>   C RNA contains C, G, A and U.
>   D RNA molecules contain a double helix.
> 2 A mutation is when one base in a gene is changed for another base. Explain why mutations may change the characteristics of an organism. [4]

Immunology

B1.14 The characteristics of key microorganisms

REVISED

You need to know the characteristics of the four types of microorganism shown in Table 12.6.

Table 12.6 Characteristics of some microorganisms

Type of microorganism	Average size of microorganism	Type of cell
Bacterium	0.5–5 µm	Prokaryotic
Fungus	5–50 µm	Eukaryotic
Protist	1 µm–2 mm	Eukaryotic
Virus	20–350 nm	N/A

B1.15 The definition and types of pathogen, including common types of condition/disease caused by them

REVISED

You need to be familiar with the pathogens given in Table 12.7.

Pathogens Disease-causing microorganisms.

Table 12.7 Pathogens and some diseases they cause

Pathogen	Example of condition/disease caused	Notes
Bacteria	Chlamydia Gonorrhoea Tuberculosis	Bacterial infections can be treated with antibiotics, but bacteria are becoming more resistant to them.
Viruses	Common cold Mumps Measles	SARS-CoV-2, the coronavirus that causes COVID-19, has become the best-known virus. Viruses must infect body cells in order to replicate (reproduce).
Fungi	Yeast infection (thrush)	Other examples of fungal skin infections include toenail fungus and athlete's foot.
Prions	Creutzfeldt–Jakob disease (CJD)	Prions are non-living, pathogenic proteins. If ingested, a mutant form of a prion protein can cause normal prion proteins to change shape. This causes damage to the nervous system and may lead to death.
Protists	Malaria	Do not confuse the pathogen (*Plasmodium*, a protist) with the *Anopheles* mosquito that carries the pathogen.
Parasites	Toxoplasmosis	This infection is caused by the parasitic protoctist *Toxoplasma gondii*. Many multicellular parasites can also cause infections, particularly in developing countries.

Now test yourself

TESTED

1. A typical light microscope can be used to view objects larger than about 0.5 µm. Which microorganisms could be viewed with a light microscope?
2. Which of the following diseases are caused by eukaryotic pathogens: chlamydia, toxoplasmosis, yeast infection (thrush), malaria, Creutzfeldt–Jakob disease and mumps?
3. Name **one** disease caused by a bacterial pathogen and **one** caused by a viral pathogen.

Making links

Microorganisms are very small and are usually viewed with a light microscope (B1.5). When you come across images (e.g. photomicrographs) of pathogens, use this as an opportunity to practise measuring and calculating magnification.

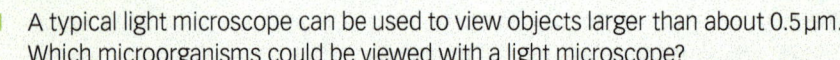
Check your understanding and progress at www.hoddereducation.co.uk/myrevisionnotes

B1.16 The different ways in which pathogens may enter the body

REVISED

If we can understand how pathogens enter the body, we can try to prevent this happening.

Direct transmission

+ There may be physical contact with an infected person (for example shaking hands) or a contaminated surface (for example a door handle).
+ Sharing of needles can allow transmission of blood-borne pathogens such as HIV.
+ Unprotected sexual contact can lead to sexually transmitted infections (STIs) such as chlamydia and gonorrhoea (both caused by bacteria) or genital herpes (caused by a virus).
+ Airborne transmission is where the pathogen is carried by dust or droplets (aerosols) in the air. Some can remain in the air for many hours. COVID-19 and tuberculosis are both spread by inhaling infected droplets.

Some pathogens can cause infection rapidly, while others require much longer exposure.

Indirect transmission

+ This may involve vehicle transmission, for example ingesting infected food or water. Faecal–oral transmission is the result of poor hand hygiene and is a significant cause of food poisoning. Blood from inanimate objects (for example bedding) can also be a source of infection.
+ It can also involve being bitten by an infected vector. Malaria is transmitted when an infected mosquito (the vector) transfers the *Plasmodium* protist in its bite.

> **Typical mistake**
>
> Do not confuse the vector (that transmits the disease) with the pathogen (the disease-causing microorganism).

B1.17 How infectious diseases can spread among populations and communities

REVISED

The greatest contribution to reducing disease has come from what is commonly described as 'public health'. This means understanding the ways in which infectious diseases spread and, therefore, what can be done to prevent or reduce that spread. The three main ways in which infectious diseases can spread are as follows:

+ Inadequate sanitation, for example lack of access to clean water without water-borne diseases. Inadequate sewage disposal can increase the risk of faecal–oral transmission.
+ High population density. Overcrowding in households, along with a lack of social distancing outside the home, can increase the risk of airborne transmission and transmission by physical contact.
+ Lack of accessible health promotion information. Without information, people are less likely to take precautions to prevent the spread of infection. They may also be less likely to take up vaccinations or other health-protection measures.

B1.18 The definition of an antigen and an antibody

REVISED

The immune response is an important part of the body's method of protecting against infection. When an antigen enters the body, it triggers the production of antibodies to counteract it.

> **Making links**
>
> The binding of an antibody to an antigen is specific in a similar way to an enzyme binding to its substrate (B1.9).

> **Typical mistake**
>
> Make sure you do not confuse the terms *antibody* and *antigen*.

Antigen A substance recognised by the immune system as self or non-self and that stimulates an immune response.

Antibodies Blood proteins produced in response to, and counteracting, specific antigens.

B1.19 The link between antigens and the initiation of the body's response to invasion by a foreign substance

REVISED

Antigens are chemical markers (usually proteins or glycoproteins) found on the surface of cells.

The body can recognise self and non-self antigens (see Figure 12.14).

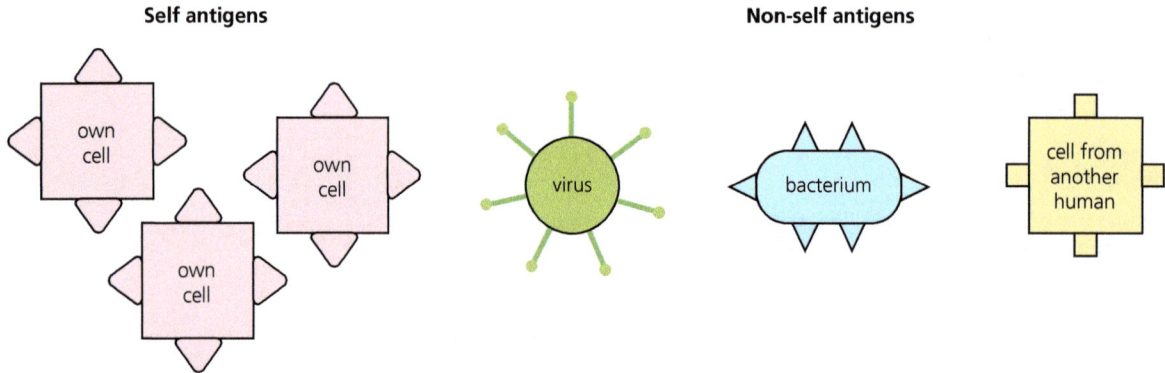

Figure 12.14 We have self antigens on the surface of all our cells

The presence of a non-self antigen in the body is recognised and this leads to the initiation of an immune response. Not all non-self antigens are present on pathogens. They can be on the surface of cells from another human (for example from a blood transfusion or an organ transplant). They can also be present in other substances, such as dust or pollen grains; this is the basis of allergies.

B1.20 The role of non-specific and specific defences to protect the body against invasion from a foreign substance

REVISED

The immune response is not the only way the body protects itself from invasion and is not the first line of defence. Defence mechanisms are summarised in Figure 12.15.

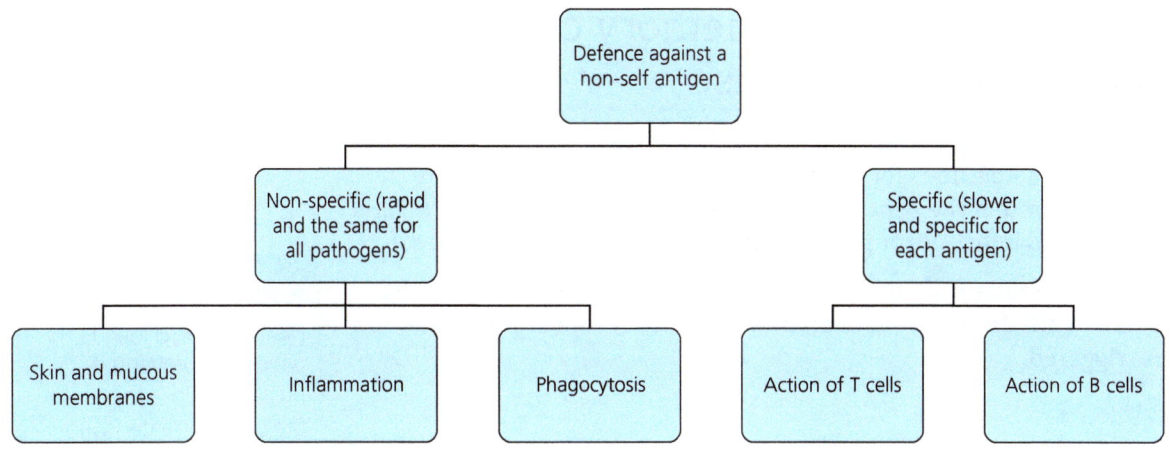

Figure 12.15 Defence mechanisms

Non-specific defences

These are rapid and are not specific for any particular type of pathogen.
+ Physical and chemical barriers help prevent pathogens from entering the body. The skin and mucous membranes (for example in the lungs, gut and reproductive system) act as physical barriers and also produce chemicals that can destroy pathogens.
+ Inflammation is a local response to injury and infection. Blood flow increases and this helps deliver lymphocytes and phagocytes to the site of infection. Chemicals are also released that promote phagocytosis. Swelling can occur as a result of fluid leaking out of blood vessels into the tissues.
+ Phagocytosis involves pathogens being engulfed and digested by phagocytes.

Specific defences

These are slower and are specific for a particular antigen or pathogen. When pathogens enter the body, T cells and B cells are activated by foreign (non-self) antigens on pathogens or other foreign cells.

Activation of T cells leads to the cell-mediated response:
+ Activated T cells bind to non-self antigens on infected cells and destroy them.
+ This removes (kills) bacteria and viruses that replicate inside cells.
+ Activated T cells form memory T cells.

Activation of B cells leads to the antibody-mediated response:
+ Activated B cells produce antibodies.
+ These antibodies are specific to the antigens on the pathogens that led to activation of B cells.
+ Antibodies bind to and neutralise the antigens on the pathogens.
+ Activated B cells form memory B cells.

> **Inflammation** A local response to injury and infection.
>
> **Lymphocytes** Small white blood cells. B lymphocytes, or B cells, are involved in the antibody-mediated response. T lymphocytes, or T cells, are involved in the cell-mediated response.
>
> **Phagocytes** Cells that are produced in the bone marrow and circulate in the blood. Some leave the blood and are present in the tissues. They ingest pathogens.
>
> **Phagocytosis** The process of a phagocyte engulfing and digesting a pathogen or other foreign material.

> **Making links**
>
> The role of memory cells in the secondary immune response is covered in B1.22.

B1.21 The differences between cell-mediated immunity and antibody-mediated immunity

REVISED

There are two parts to the immune response:
+ Cell-mediated response: T cells destroy pathogens but do not produce antibodies. The T cells destroy infected cells and so the pathogens cannot replicate.
+ Antibody-mediated response: B cells produce antibodies against the pathogens. When antibodies bind to antigens on pathogens, they counteract the pathogens and can lead to killing of the pathogens.

B1.22 The role of T and B memory cells in the secondary immune response

REVISED

Activation of T cells and B cells leads to production of memory cells. These remain in the body, sometimes for years, and trigger a stronger and more rapid immune response if they encounter the same antigen in the future. This can prevent a second infection, or prevent infection developing into disease.

Vaccines work by stimulating a primary immune response, which produces T and B memory cells. In the event of an infection, the secondary immune response is triggered.

> **Revision activity**
>
> Defence mechanisms are complicated. It will help if you prepare a wallchart showing how all the different components covered here work together.
>
> Vaccines usually contain some form of antigen from a pathogen and are designed to prevent infection or make it less serious. Incorporate vaccines into your wallchart to show how they stimulate the immune system and can produce long-lasting protection.

> **Making links**
>
> Many bacterial infections cannot be prevented by vaccination. These are usually treated with antibiotics. However, increasing antimicrobial resistance means that many antibiotics are no longer effective; this is covered in A10.5.

> **Now test yourself** TESTED
>
> 1 Briefly describe the role of the following in defence against foreign substances:
>   a macrophages (a type of phagocyte)
>   b B cells
>   c T cells.
> 2 Describe the role of memory cells in the secondary immune response.

B1.23 How the body reacts to injury and trauma

REVISED

The difference between *injury* and *trauma* is how severe it is. The body responds in the same way at first, but trauma is more severe so the response becomes greater.

> **Injury** Damage to the body caused by external force.
>
> **Trauma** An injury that has the potential to cause disability or death.

How the body responds to injury

There are two stages in the body's response to injury:
+ The involuntary inflammatory response is similar to the body's response to infection (see B1.20). It is described as involuntary because it happens automatically and can involve increased blood flow and metabolic rate, redness, pain and swelling.
+ The proliferation phase is where tissue repair takes place. Some key processes are:
  + formation of a blood clot to reduce blood loss and prevent entry of pathogens
  + removal of dead or damaged body cells by phagocytosis
  + growth of new tissue to replace the damaged tissue.

How the body responds to trauma

At first, the involuntary inflammatory response occurs like in injury. However, because trauma involves more serious injury, there can be other responses:
+ loss of organ function; some organs can stop working partially or totally
+ bone structure deformity, damage or loss of structure (for example a fracture)

- haemorrhaging, including bleeding at the site of injury and bruising (bleeding under intact skin)
- multi-organ failure, if the inflammatory response is severe
- ischaemia, a decrease in blood supply to tissues leading to a decrease in supply of nutrients and oxygen; it can, if severe, cause ischaemic shock (known as 'going into shock') which can lead to organ failure and death if not treated correctly

if the trauma or subsequent shock is not fatal, the body goes through a proliferation phase similar to that described above.

> **Making links**
>
> Inflammation is a response to injury or infection. It also plays a part in several chronic diseases, such as rheumatoid arthritis, atopic eczema, Crohn's disease, COPD and endometriosis that are covered in B2.

> **Revision activity**
>
> Make a list of different types of injury that you can think of.
>
> For each, list the effects that they would have on the body and how it might respond.
>
> Now think about what might cause the injuries you have listed to become trauma. How would the body respond differently?

B1.24 The role and considerations of using magnetic resonance imaging (MRI) scanning in the detection and monitoring of trauma and injury

REVISED

MRI scanners use strong magnetic fields and radio waves to generate detailed images of the inside of the body. Unlike X-rays, an MRI scan will show details of soft tissues and is used extensively in diagnosis of soft tissue injuries (for example tendon or ligament damage), as well as to identify the presence of tumours.

The powerful magnetic fields generated in an MRI scanner will strongly attract any metal objects.

To avoid this, a patient medical history will be taken before the MRI scan. This should identify whether the patient has any medical implants containing magnetic metals, such as:
- a pacemaker or ICD used to control irregular heartbeat
- metal plates, wires or screws used for bone fractures
- a contraceptive coil (IUD).

The presence of any of these may not mean the patient cannot have an MRI scan, but special precautions may be needed.

The patient can normally eat, drink and take medication on the day of the scan, but all external metallic objects (like piercings) will have to be removed.

> **Typical mistake**
>
> Do not confuse an MRI scan with a CT scan. They both produce three-dimensional images of the inside of the body, but the CT scan uses X-rays.

> **Revision activity**
>
> Take the list of the types of injury you prepared in B1.23 and, for each, note whether an MRI scan would be useful to help diagnose the nature of the injury.

> **Exam tip**
>
> In questions where you are asked to assess, you need to give reasons. You will not get marks for just saying 'the treatment is inadequate'.

> **Exam practice**
>
> 1 Which of the following is an example of a self antigen? [1]
>   A A protein on the surface of a red blood cell in a blood transfusion
>   B A protein on the surface of the patient's own red blood cells
>   C A protein on the surface of a virus
>   D A protein on the surface of a transplanted kidney
> 2 The tuberculosis bacterium is spread by droplet infection. Large droplets settle quickly and are less likely to be inhaled. Small droplets are most infective but contain only a few bacteria.
>   a Use this information and your own knowledge to suggest the precautions that should be taken to prevent spread of the disease. [3]
>   b Explain why it is recommended not to sleep in the same room as a person infected with tuberculosis. [1]
> 3 A patient presents to a doctor after having stepped on a nail in the garden. The nail has penetrated the skin but there is minimal bleeding. The patient asks for the wound to be cleaned and dressed. Assess the effectiveness of this treatment and suggest what other treatment should be offered. [4]

My Revision Notes: Health T Level

Epidemiology and health promotion

B1.25 What is meant by epidemiology and some specific terminology that is used

Epidemiology is the study and analysis of the distribution and patterns of disease in populations and why diseases occur. This allows us to understand how to prevent and treat disease.

Specific terminology used in epidemiology

+ Incidence is the probability of a medical condition occurring in a population in a specified time period. It is a measure of the rate at which new cases occur.
+ Prevalence is the proportion of a population affected by a medical condition at a specific time. It is usually expressed as a percentage, fraction or number of cases per size of population, for example ten cases per thousand.
+ Morbidity refers to any physical or psychological state that is thought to be outside of normal wellbeing. More simply, it describes illness or ill health.
+ Mortality means death caused by a particular disease.
+ Mortality rate is the rate at which a disease causes death, for example in deaths per year.

> **Typical mistake**
>
> Morbidity and mortality are easily confused. Also, do not assume that morbidity means a reduced lifespan. A person with well-controlled asthma is likely to have a normal lifespan, but a person with advanced lung cancer would have a reduced lifespan.

> **Now test yourself**
>
> 1. Explain the difference between incidence and prevalence of a disease.
> 2. Explain the difference between morbidity and mortality.

B1.26 How epidemiology is used to provide information to plan and evaluate strategies to prevent disease

Epidemiology relies heavily on mathematics and statistics, using a systematic approach to:
+ count the number of cases
+ calculate the rate of increase or decrease in the number of cases
+ compare rates over time or between different groups, for example in different geographical areas or different age groups.

How epidemiology is used

Epidemiology is used for the following purposes:
+ Identifying the cause of a disease, for example identifying that contaminated water causes cholera.
+ Determining the extent of the disease. Measuring incidence and prevalence of a disease helps measure the extent.
+ Identifying trends and patterns. Is the disease increasing or decreasing (trend)? Does it affect one particular group (pattern)? Is it related to factors such as poverty or living conditions (pattern)?
+ Studying the disease progression. Trends and patterns can show how the disease spreads and what action might be needed. Tracking the mortality rate indicates severity of the disease and also the effect of any therapeutics.
+ Planning and evaluating preventative and therapeutic measures. Preventative measures such as vaccination and therapeutic measures such as drug treatment can be implemented and then monitored, so we can evaluate and, if necessary, improve them.
+ Developing public health policy and preventative measures. Prevention is usually more effective than cure.

Check your understanding and progress at www.hoddereducation.co.uk/myrevisionnotes

B1.27 How health promotion helps to prevent the spread of and control disease and disorder

Reduction of morbidity and mortality rates through improved medication has been significant. But improved public health measures have also been important, for example improvements to:
+ nutrition
+ sanitation (clean water, sewage disposal)
+ housing (reduced overcrowding, improved ventilation)
+ access to basic healthcare
+ education and health promotion.

Table 12.8 Some methods of health promotion

Method of health promotion	Notes
Communication	This can be used to raise awareness of issues (for example risk of disease) as well as required behaviours (for example to reduce risk) through a range of media (for example campaigns) that: + deliver a clear message + will reach the target audience + are expressed in language that recipients can relate to + does not cause unnecessary anxiety.
Policy and systems	Government and public policy can change procedures, regulations or laws to enforce behaviours, for example restricting: + access to drugs of abuse + sale of goods such as alcohol or cigarettes + movement of people during epidemics or pandemics.
Education programmes	Ignorance can be deadly. By improving knowledge, individuals can be empowered to adapt their own behaviour.
Health promotion for specific diseases/disorders	Targeted awareness raising and campaigns include: + Change4Life, a social marketing campaign by PHE to reduce childhood obesity by giving parents support to make healthier choices for their families + the annual flu vaccination, promoted through a range of media, including posters in GP surgeries, radio adverts, emails, social media and letters to vulnerable groups.

> **Revision activity**
>
> Search online for more information about the Public Health England health promotion campaigns. Review the health and wellbeing campaigns covered in A9.
>
> Make a list of some of these different types of health promotion and evaluate them.
> + How do they meet the criteria listed here?
> + Were you aware of any of them?
> + Do you think they would influence your behaviour, that of your contemporaries, or that of older or younger generations?

> **Exam tip**
>
> You will often be asked to 'evaluate'. This might be proposed treatment options for a disease or, as in this case, health promotion. When you do, make sure you address both advantages and disadvantages and, if possible, draw a conclusion.

> **Exam practice**
>
> 1. Explain the importance of mathematics and statistics in epidemiology. [3]
> 2. Chlamydia is a sexually transmitted infection (STI). The incidence of chlamydia is increasing in teenagers and young adults. Suggest how health promotion campaigns could reduce the incidence of chlamydia. [4]
> 3. Tuberculosis (TB) is a bacterial disease common in disadvantaged communities and developing countries. TB is transmitted by inhaling infected droplets from another person. Vaccination can prevent spread of TB. Treatment of TB requires long-term treatment (6–9 months) with a combination of antibiotics. Evaluate the use of vaccination, antibiotic treatment and public health measures in the control of TB. [6]

Homeostasis and physiological measurements

B1.28 The principles of homeostasis and how this links to maintaining the functions within the physiological systems which contributes to maintaining a healthy body

REVISED

Homeostasis describes the regulation of the internal environment, meaning physiological parameters such as body temperature as well as the concentration of water, glucose, oxygen and carbon dioxide in the blood.

Principles of homeostasis

Physiological parameters are maintained within a narrow range. This involves negative feedback, receptors and effectors (Figure 12.16).

Feedback systems also involve:
+ the nervous system communicating between receptors and effectors, via a co-ordination centre such as the brain
+ the endocrine system, where hormones are secreted into the blood in response to receptors detecting changes; hormones then act on effectors (target organs) such as the liver, kidney and muscles.

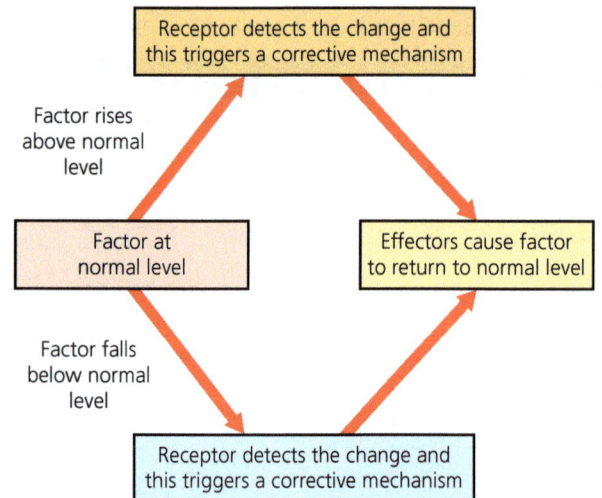

Figure 12.16 Negative feedback involving receptors and effectors

How homeostasis contributes to maintaining a healthy body

Homeostasis maintains the stability and function of physiological systems and cells when there are changes to internal and external conditions that would otherwise prevent enzymes from functioning normally.

> **Homeostasis** The maintenance of an almost constant internal environment despite fluctuations in the external environment.
>
> **Negative feedback** Returns a factor to its normal level when there is movement away from the normal level.
>
> **Receptors** Detect factors such as temperature or blood glucose concentration.
>
> **Effectors** Glands or muscles that make changes to return factors to their normal level.

> **Making links**
>
> Review B1.9, where the effect of temperature on enzyme function is covered. Enzymes also require stable conditions of pH (acidity or alkalinity) to work properly. Homeostasis maintains the pH of the blood within a narrow range so that enzymes function normally.
>
> Cells need a regular supply of glucose for respiration. Homeostasis maintains the blood glucose concentration within a narrow range (B2.15)
>
> If the water content of the body is too high, water will enter cells by osmosis (see B1.11); if it is too low, water will move out of body cells. In either case, the cells will not be able to function properly. The kidney is an important organ that helps maintain the water balance of the body, known as osmoregulation (see B2.15 for the role of glands and hormones and B2.21 for details of the kidney's role in osmoregulation).

B1.29 The normal expected ranges for physiological measurements and the factors which may affect these measurements

REVISED

Normal expected ranges for physiological measurements

Table 12.9 Normal expected ranges for physiological measurements for adults aged 19 to 65

Physiological measurements	Normal expected range
Blood pressure	Systolic 90–120 mmHg; diastolic 60–80 mmHg
Heart rate	60 to 100 beats per minute (bpm)
Respiratory rate (at rest)	12 to 20 breaths per minute (bpm)
Temperature	36–37.5 °C

Factors that contribute to measurements outside of normal parameters

+ Age: blood pressure is lower in children than in adults. In adults, blood pressure increases with age. The normal resting heart rate is higher in children than in adults, but in adults there is little change with age. Respiration rate declines with age, as does lung function.
+ Weight: excess weight can increase blood pressure, which can increase resting heart rate as the heart has to work harder. Being underweight can reduce blood pressure.
+ Exercise: regular running or cycling increases the size of the heart muscle, which means it pumps more blood with every stroke. Therefore, at rest it does not need to beat as fast. A highly trained athlete will have a resting heart rate below the normal range.
+ Sex: men generally have greater body mass, lung capacity and size of left ventricle, all of which can affect normal physiological measurements.
+ Overall health: measurements outside of the normal range are likely to be a sign of poor health or an underlying health condition.

Exam practice

1. Which statement is correct? [1]
   A Effectors detect changes in physiological parameters and stimulate receptors to bring about return to the normal level.
   B Negative feedback ensures body temperature remains constant at all times.
   C Negative feedback works to maintain physiological parameters within a narrow range.
   D Regular exercise leads to an increase in resting heart rate.
2. Hypothermia occurs when body temperature falls below about 34 °C. Body temperature continues to fall and, if not treated, hypothermia can be fatal. Explain why hypothermia represents a failure of normal negative feedback mechanisms. [3]

Classification of diseases and disorders

B1.30 The commonly used classification systems of diseases and disorders

REVISED

Classification systems help to provide a common language for reporting and monitoring health and disease. This makes it easier to share and compare data. Table 12.10 gives an example of ways in which a disease can be classified.

> **Exam tip**
>
> Your understanding of disease classification might be tested in any part of Paper B.

Table 12.10 Example of how angina (chest pain) is a symptom of heart disease which is a type of cardiovascular disease

Type of classification	Basis of classification	Example
Topographical	By bodily region or system	Cardiovascular disease
Anatomical	By organ or tissue	Heart disease
Physiological	By function or effect	Angina

> **Revision activity**
>
> In B2, you will study several chronic diseases. For each of these, try to apply the three classification systems above. Does this help to show connections?

Particles and radiation

B1.31 The types and properties of ionising radiation

REVISED

> **Making links**
>
> Nuclear medicine is the medical specialty that uses radioactive isotopes in diagnosis and treatment of disease. You will see examples of this, particularly the use of radioactive iodine in the treatment of thyroid cancer (see B2.31).

Knowledge of the three types of ionising radiation shown in Table 12.11 helps us to understand their potential uses in healthcare, as well as precautions we need to take when handling or storing radioactive materials.

Ionisation The formation of charged particles from neutral molecules or atoms by adding or removing electrons.

Table 12.11 Summary of the types of ionising radiation

Type	Composition/source	Ionising and penetrating power	Range
Alpha (□)	Two neutrons and two protons (equivalent to a helium nucleus)	High ionising Low penetrating	1–2 cm in air
Beta (□)	High-speed electron ejected from the nucleus as a neutron turns into a proton	Medium ionising Medium penetrating	Approximately 15 cm in air
Gamma (□)	Electromagnetic radiation from the nucleus	Low ionising High penetrating	Many kilometres in air

Check your understanding and progress at www.hoddereducation.co.uk/myrevisionnotes

B1.32 The definition of half-life

REVISED

Half-life is the time taken for half of the unstable nuclei in a sample to undergo radioactive decay.

+ A sample with a short half-life will decay rapidly. It may emit a high level of radiation, which could be dangerous, however it will become safe quite quickly.
+ A sample with a long half-life may emit a relatively low level of radiation, but it could still be dangerous for a very long time.

> **Half-life** The time taken for half of the unstable nuclei in a sample to undergo radioactive decay.
>
> **Radioactive decay** The random process that occurs when an unstable nucleus loses energy by giving out alpha or beta particles or gamma radiation.

Exam practice

1. Radioactive iodine is used in the treatment of thyroid cancer. It emits beta and gamma radiation. Which of the following statements is true? [1]
   - **A** Beta radiation is high-speed electrons and gamma radiation contains protons and neutrons.
   - **B** Alpha radiation contains helium nuclei and gamma radiation is a form of electromagnetic radiation.
   - **C** Beta radiation and gamma radiation are both highly ionising.
   - **D** Gamma radiation has a long half-life.

Units

B1.33 The use of the international system of units (SI)

REVISED

There are seven SI base units and all other units are based on these. You need to know three:
+ mass: kilogram (kg)
+ length: metre (m)
+ time: second (s).

B1.34 How to convert units of measure

REVISED

Length

Metres (m) to millimetres (mm) and millimetres (mm) to micrometres (μm):
+ 1 m = 1000 mm (10^3 mm) so 1 mm = 0.001 m (10^{-3} m)
+ 1 mm = 1000 μm (10^3 μm) so 1 μm = 0.001 mm (10^{-3} mm)

Volume

Litres (L) to millilitres (mL) and millilitres (mL) to microlitres (μL):
+ 1 L = 1000 mL (10^3 mL) so 1 mL = 0.001 L (10^{-3} L)
+ 1 mL = 1000 μL (10^3 μL) so 1 μL = 0.001 mL (10^{-3} mL)

> **Exam tip**
>
> Take care with units, particularly when they contain powers, such as cm^3 (cubic centimetres).

> **Exam tip**
>
> The prefix 'milli' means one thousandth, so you will see that converting milligrams (mg) to grams (g) means dividing by 1000, while converting from grams (g) to milligrams (mg) means multiplying by 1000. You can use the same approach for volume and length.
>
> 1 mg is much less than 1 g, so always check your answer!

> **Exam tip**
>
> You need to be able to convert to and from volumes in mL (millilitres). However, you will often encounter cm³ (cubic centimetres) as an alternative to millilitres, including on the exam papers. Do not be put off by this, they are the same: $1\,mL = 1\,cm^3$.
>
> You will also encounter dm³ (cubic decimetres) as an alternative to L; once again, they are the same: $1\,L = 1\,dm^3$.

Mass

Grams (g) to milligrams (mg) and milligrams (mg) to micrograms (μg):
+ $1\,g = 1000\,mg$ ($10^3\,mg$) so $1\,mg = 0.001\,g$ ($10^{-3}\,g$)
+ $1\,mg = 1000\,μg$ ($10^3\,μg$) so $1\,μg = 0.001\,mg$ ($10^{-3}\,mg$)

Now test yourself — TESTED

Copy and complete the table of conversions.

Convert from	Convert to	Answer
1500 mm	m	
250 μm	mm	
0.00005 m	mm	
0.0035 L	mL	
25 μL	mL	
650 cm³	L	
225 mg	g	
0.03 g	μg	
3.7 μg	g	

B1.35 The importance of using significant figures and science notation

REVISED

Significant figures refer to how accurately we can make measurements. The measurements made by a ruler with 1 mm divisions could result in a calculated answer of 12.7354 mm. However, with 1 mm divisions, we cannot measure to that level of accuracy with this ruler. So we round our answer to 13 mm, which is 2 significant figures. The other digits in the answer are not reliable.

Science notation (also called scientific notation) refers to standard form. This is a method of writing very small or very large numbers in a standard way.

Makes calculations with large or small numbers less cumbersome

Very large numbers, such as 1 500 000, have a lot of zeros at the end (called trailing zeros). You could write 1.5 million instead, which is simpler and shorter. In science and medicine, we use scientific notation where the number is written in standard form. 1.5 million is written as 1.5×10^6.

Very small numbers can have a lot of leading zeros. For example, 0.0000002 would be written as 2×10^{-7} in standard form.

This makes calculations with large or small numbers less cumbersome.

> **Exam tip**
>
> To multiply powers, add the powers: $10^2 \times 10^3 = 10^5$ (the same as $100 \times 1000 = 100\,000$)
>
> To divide powers, subtract the powers: $10^5 \div 10^2 = 10^3$ (the same as $100\,000 \div 100 = 1000$).

Raising numbers to powers

When a number is raised to a power, the power is written as a superscript. 2 to the power of 2 (2 squared) is written 2^2 and is equal to 4 (2×2). Similarly, 2 to the power of 3 (2 cubed) is written 2^3 and is equal to 8 ($2 \times 2 \times 2$).

You will see this in units such as m^2 (square metres) or cm^3 (cubic centimetres).

Science (scientific) notation

Scientific notation allows us to work with all numbers by writing them in standard form. For example: 3 570 000 would be written as 3.57×10^6.

The number before the '×' sign is always between 1 and 10. The number after the '×' sign is a power of 10.

Calculating using standard form

For example, calculate $(4.5 \times 10^3) \times (3.8 \times 10^5)$.

First, multiply 4.5 and 3.8 to give 17.1. Then, multiply the powers $10^3 \times 10^5$ to get 10^8.

That gives 17.1×10^8, but 17.1 is greater than 10, so we must correct this:

$17.1 \times 10^8 = 1.71 \times 10^9$

Reduces the chance of data errors

10^{12} is the same as 1 followed by 12 zeros. It is easy to lose count of the zeros, so working with powers of 10 reduces the chance of data error. Working with numbers in standard form also makes calculations easier and less prone to error.

> **Typical mistakes**
>
> Take care with negative powers, because when you subtract a negative number, you are actually adding the number. For example, $2 - (-3) = 5$ or $-2 - (-4) = 2$
>
> Therefore: $10^2 \div 10^{-3} = 10^5$ ($100 \div 0.001 = 100\,000$)

> **Exam tip**
>
> Numbers less than 1 can also be written in standard form. Therefore, 0.0025 would be written as 2.5×10^{-3}.

> **Typical mistake**
>
> Standard form is not really very useful for numbers between 1 and 10. For example, 5.2 would be written as 5.2×10^0 because $10^0 = 1$, so adding the $\times 10^0$ does not help.

> **Now test yourself** TESTED
>
> 1 Convert the following numbers into standard form (use a scientific calculator).
>   - a 0.00058
>   - b 250 000 000 000
>   - c 135 300
> 2 Evaluate (work out) the following:
>   - a $(2.5 \times 10^3) \times (1.45 \times 10^2)$
>   - b $(7.25 \times 10^2) \times (2.5 \times 10^4)$
>   - c $(1.5 \times 10^{-3}) \times (3.5 \times 10^2)$
>   - d $(4.64 \times 10^3) \div (8.04 \times 10^5)$
>   - e $(5.0 \times 10^3) \times (2.0 \times 10^{-2})$

> **Exam practice**
>
> 1. A new drug is being tested in human volunteers. The recommended dosage is 5 mg per kg per day. Calculate the amount in grams of drug required for treating an 84 kg volunteer for 6 weeks. [3]
> 2. In April 2020, the population of the USA was 331 449 000, and it was estimated that there were 39 000 000 cases of flu during the 2019–20 winter flu season. Calculate the prevalence of flu in cases per 100 000 of population. Give your answer in standard form. [2]

B2 Further science concepts in health

Musculoskeletal system

Musculoskeletal refers to the skeleton and the muscles attached to it. The musculoskeletal system is involved in support of the body and in movement.

B2.1 The structure and function of the musculoskeletal system

REVISED

Structure of the musculoskeletal system

You need to know the anatomical skeletal structure, including the bones as labelled in Figure 13.1.

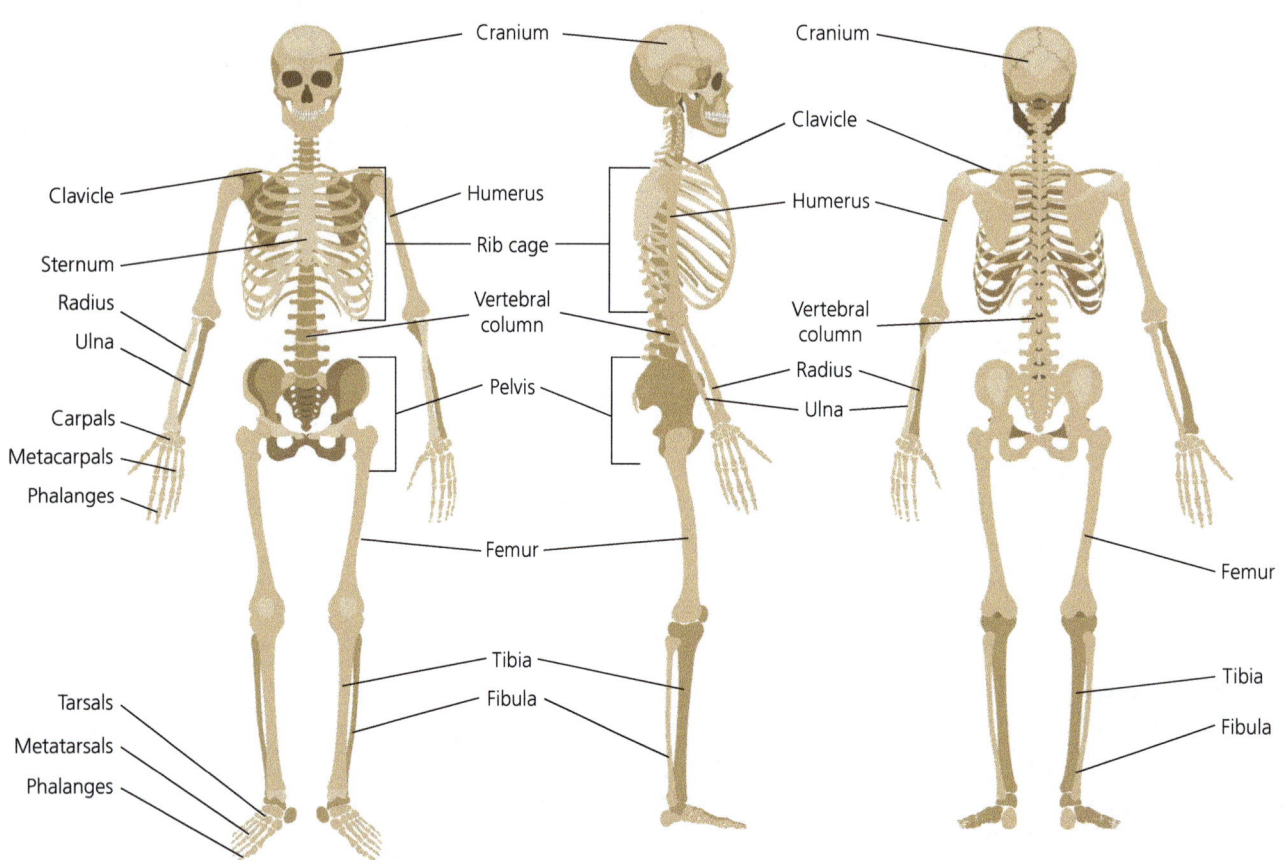

Figure 13.1 The full skeletal structure

You also need to know the types of bones given in Figure 13.2.

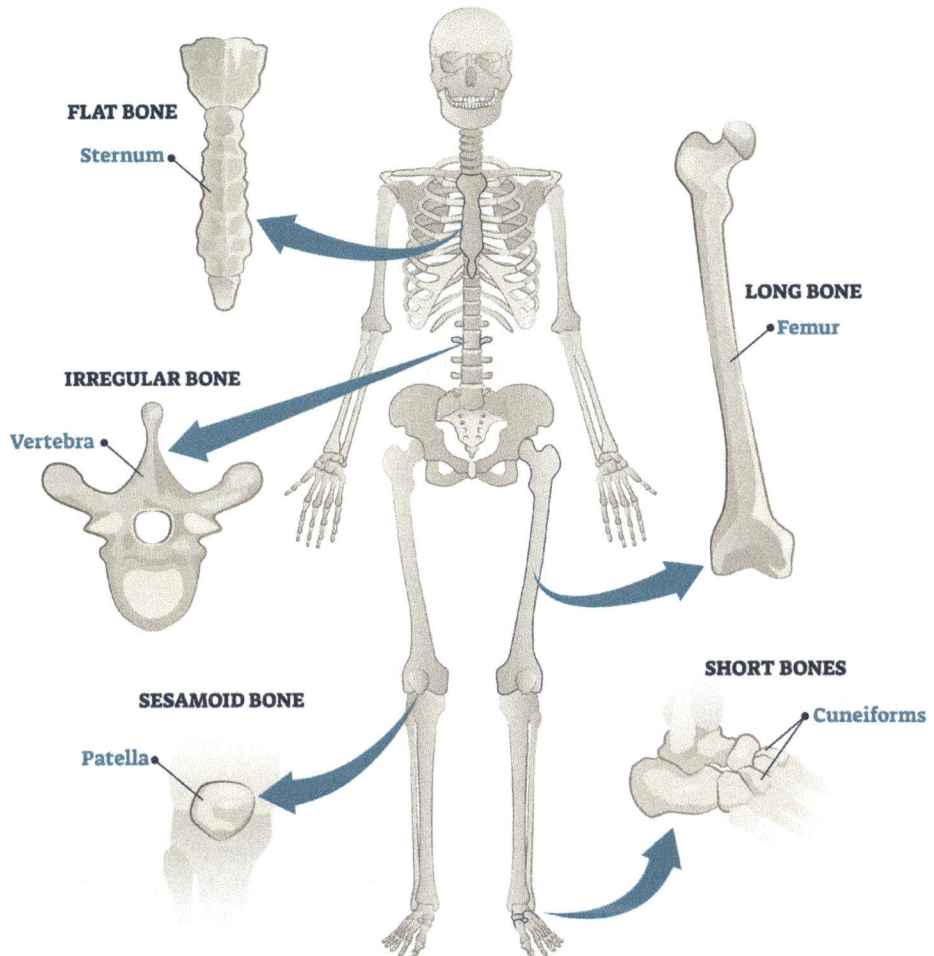

Figure 13.2 The main types of bones in the human skeleton

Joint The area where two or more bones connect.

Cartilage A type of **connective tissue** containing collagen and the elastic protein elastin; it is more flexible than **ligaments and tendons** but not as hard as bone.

Connective tissue Connects, supports or binds tissues or other organs. It consists mostly of the protein collagen.

Ligaments and tendons Both are connective tissues made of collagen. Ligaments join bones together, while tendons attach muscles to bones.

Striated muscle Named for its striped appearance under the microscope, striated muscle is also called skeletal muscle because it is attached to the skeleton and is the main type of muscle involved in movement.

There are three main types of joints:
+ In fibrous joints, the bones are fused together (for example the skull).
+ In cartilaginous joints, the bones are connected by relatively flexible cartilage (for example the rib cage).
+ Synovial joints are the most common. They are flexible and move in a number of ways (for example the hip joint). They all have cartilage providing cushioning between the bones and a synovial capsule containing synovial fluid.

The main type of muscle involved in movement is striated muscle (skeletal muscle). Figure 13.3 shows the arrangement of the individual muscle cells (muscle fibres), while Figure 13.4 shows the striated (striped) appearance of skeletal muscle fibres under a light microscope. The significance of the striations will be explained in the next section.

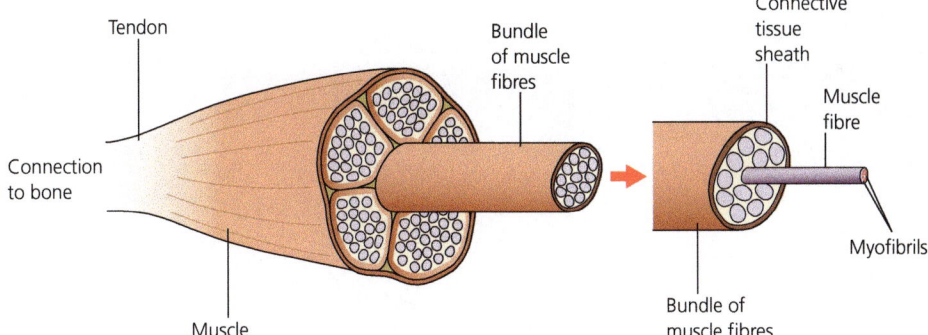

Figure 13.3 The arrangement of muscle fibres in skeletal muscle

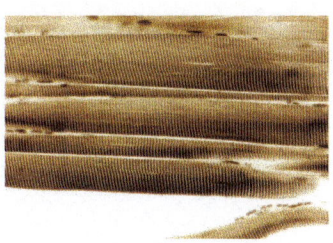

Figure 13.4 Skeletal muscle fibres viewed under a light microscope

My Revision Notes: Health T Level

Functions of relevant components within the musculoskeletal system

The skeleton has a number of functions:
+ It provides support and protection, as well as attachment for muscles/ligaments.
+ It is a source of blood production; bone marrow contains stem cells that produce erythrocytes (red blood cells) and lymphocytes (white blood cells).
+ Bones store minerals in the form of calcium phosphate.

Muscles in the body facilitate movement and are usually arranged in opposing (antagonistic) pairs. Figure 13.5 shows how bones, muscles and joints all work together when the forearm is raised.

Muscles also provide support by helping maintain posture. Even when sitting or standing, our muscles are working.

The sliding filament theory of musculoskeletal function explains how thick (myosin) and thin (actin) filaments slide in and out between each other to bring about contraction and relaxation. Figure 13.6 shows how thick and thin filaments slide across each other when the muscle contracts.

> **Making links**
>
> Stem cells and the production of erythrocytes was covered in B1.4, and the role of lymphocytes in the immune system was covered in B1.20–1.22.

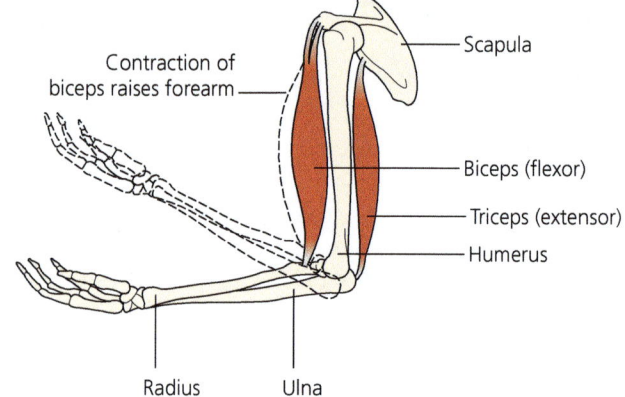

Figure 13.5 The forearm raises when the biceps contracts and the triceps relaxes; the forearm is lowered when the triceps contracts and the biceps relaxes.

Relaxed

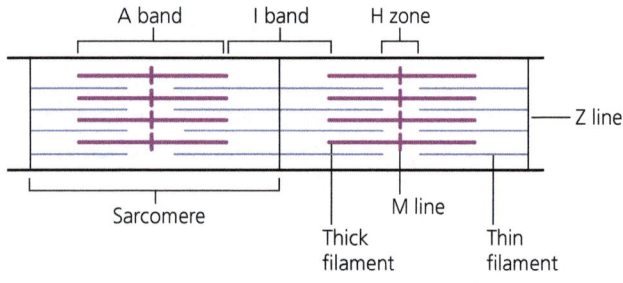

Contracted

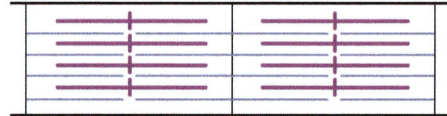

Figure 13.6 The arrangement of thick and thin filaments in a relaxed and contracted myofibril

The sarcomere is the repeating structure in the myofibril. Note how contraction happens because the sarcomeres shorten.

> **Now test yourself**   TESTED
>
> 1 Name the **three** main bones in the arm.
> 2 Name the **three** main bones in the leg.
> 3 Describe the difference between fibrous and cartilaginous joints.
> 4 Name the proteins in:
>   a thick filaments
>   b thin filaments.

Check your understanding and progress at www.hoddereducation.co.uk/myrevisionnotes

B2.2 The process of muscle contraction

The stages of the sliding filament theory for muscle contraction

This is summarised in Figure 13.7.

(a)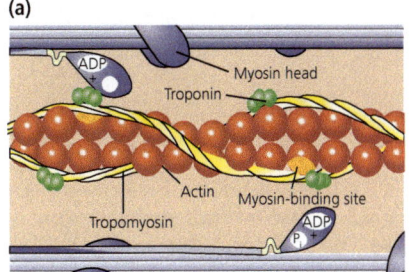
The resting state. The muscle is relaxed.

(b)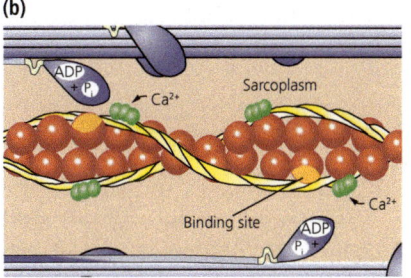
An impulse arrives and calcium ions flood into the myofibril. These ions bind to the troponin, which moves the tropomyosin out of the myosin-binding sites.

(c)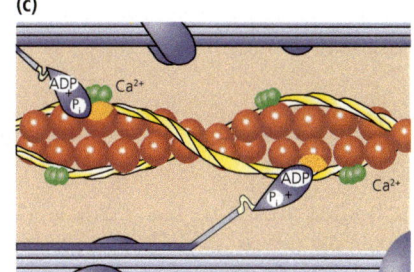
The myosin heads attach to the exposed binding sites.

(d)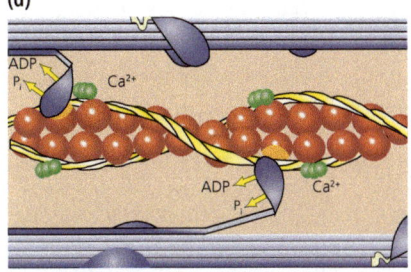
The release of ADP and inorganic phosphate causes the heads to move and pull the actin along.

(e)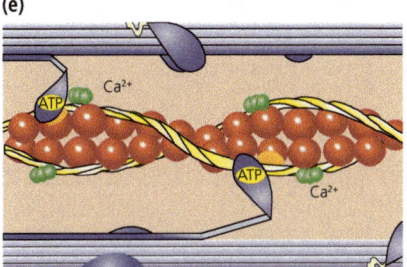
Fresh supplies of ATP enter the myosin heads and this breaks the connection with the binding sites.

(f)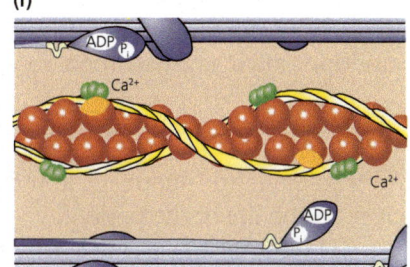
The hydrolysis of ATP to ADP and Pi returns the myosin heads to their starting positions. If calcium ions are still present, each myosin head will then immediately bind to the next myosin-binding site.

Figure 13.7 The stages of the sliding filament theory for muscle contraction

+ Calcium ions bind to troponin; this causes tropomyosin to expose the myosin-binding sites on actin. When adenosine diphosphate (ADP) is bound to the myosin head group, it can form cross-bridges between actin and myosin filaments.
+ When myosin binds, ADP is released and the myosin head bends, pulling the actin towards the centre of the sarcomere.
+ After ADP is released, ATP can bind to the myosin head. This breaks the cross-bridge between the actin and myosin filaments.
+ The myosin head is an ATPase, meaning it can hydrolyse ATP to ADP and P_i, releasing energy that restores the myosin head to its normal position.
+ The cycle is repeated, leading to the shortening of the sarcomere.

Exam tip

Myosin, tropomyosin and troponin all have similar names – try not to get them muddled.

Revision activity

Try to list the stages of muscle contraction from memory. Make sure you do not mix up ADP and ATP, because hydrolysis of ATP releases energy to prepare the myosin head before it binds to actin and then pulls the actin towards the centre of the sarcomere (known as the power stroke).

Now test yourself

1. Describe the function of calcium ions in muscle contraction.
2. State **two** functions of ATP in muscle contraction.

B2.3 The development, impact and management of rheumatoid arthritis

REVISED

Causes of the disease

Rheumatoid arthritis (RA) is an autoimmune disease where the body produces antibodies against antigens in the joints. What triggers this is not clear, but it might have a genetic element.

Impact on systems within the body and on physical and mental health

Antibodies attacking the joints leads to soreness and inflammation, releasing chemicals, particularly TNF-α, that damage nearby bones, cartilage, tendons and ligaments. The joints become stiff and misshapen and can eventually be destroyed.

There is no cure, so patients must learn to live with the disease, as treatment can only relieve symptoms. Pain and stiffness can be much worse on some days (known as a flare-up). This can lead some people to develop depression or emotions such as frustration, fear, anger and resentment.

How common treatments relieve symptoms

Early treatment and support can reduce the risk of joint damage and limit the impact on the life of the patient.
- Anti-rheumatic drugs, such as methotrexate, suppress the immune system.
- Biological treatments include monoclonal antibodies that bind to and inhibit TNF-α.
- Physiotherapy can help strengthen muscles and make joints more flexible.
- If joints become sufficiently damaged, surgery on the affected area can cut or release ligaments and tendons or remove inflamed tissue.

> **Now test yourself** TESTED
> 1. What is meant by an autoimmune disease?
> 2. How do anti-rheumatic drugs help to treat the symptoms of RA?

> **Making links**
> Rheumatoid arthritis (RA) is one of several chronic inflammatory diseases. Others that you will study include COPD (B2.10) and Crohn's disease (B2.13).

> **Autoimmune disease**
> Caused by the immune system attacking the body's own cells and tissues, rather than foreign antigens such as those on pathogens. (See sections B1.20–1.22 for details of the immune system.)

> **Chronic inflammatory diseases** Long-term conditions caused when the body's normal inflammatory response, for example to infection or injury (see B1.23), becomes excessive.

> **Making links**
> TNF-α is also involved in the tissue damage associated with Crohn's disease (B2.13) and the same monoclonal antibodies can be used to treat both diseases.

B2.4 The development, impact and management of muscular dystrophy disease

REVISED

Muscular dystrophies are a group of inherited diseases that cause gradual weakening of the muscles. If this affects the heart or the muscles involved in breathing, it can be life-threatening. The most common form is Duchenne muscular dystrophy (DMD) that usually affects boys in early childhood and often shortens life expectancy.

Causes of the disease

Mutations in the genes for muscle proteins cause changes to the muscle fibres and interfere with the muscles' ability to function.
- Dominant mutations cause disease when inherited from just one parent.
- Recessive mutations must be inherited from both parents to cause disease.
- Sex-linked mutations are more common and more severe in males.

Impact on systems within the body and on physical and mental health

(a) Duchenne muscular dystrophy	(b) Myotonic dystrophy	(c) Limb-girdle muscular dystrophy	(d) Oculopharyngeal muscular dystrophy
• Difficulty walking • Difficulty standing up • Difficulty climbing stairs • Behavioural or learning disabilities • Muscles around the pelvis and thighs appear bulkier	• Muscle stiffness • Cataracts • Excessive sleepiness • Dysphagia (swallowing problems) • Behavioural and learning disabilities • Slow and irregular heartbeat	• Muscle weakness in hips, thighs and arms • Loss of muscle mass • Back pain • Heart palpitations • Irregular heartbeat	• Droopy eyelids • Dysphagia (swallowing problems) • Progressive restriction of eye movement • Limb weakness around shoulders and hips

Figure 13.8 The symptoms of different forms of muscular dystrophy

As with all chronic disabilities, DMD can have a negative impact on a person's mental health. Also, a person with DMD might be concerned about passing on the disease to their children. Genetic testing and genetic counselling can help with this.

How common treatments relieve symptoms

+ Steroids can improve muscle strength and function for six months to 2 years, but side effects mean they cannot be used long-term.
+ Physiotherapy can help maintain muscle strength and flexibility.
+ Low-impact exercise, such as swimming, can also help maintain muscle strength and flexibility.
+ Corrective surgery can be used in severe cases, such as to treat scoliosis (curvature of the spine). Tight joints can be loosened by lengthening or releasing tendons.

> **Making links**
>
> All the chronic diseases that you study are likely to have a negative impact on the patient's mental health. This can be made worse by referring to the diseases as 'incurable', which is why the term 'chronic' is preferred. Nevertheless, knowing that they will have to live with the disease for the rest of their lives can cause many patients to suffer depression.

> **Exam practice**
>
> 1 Arrange the following steps in muscle contraction in the correct order. [3]
>   A Myosin detaches from actin.
>   B Calcium ions bind to troponin.
>   C ATP binds to the myosin head group.
>   D ADP leaves the myosin head group.
>   E The myosin head group returns to its normal position.
>   F ATP is hydrolysed to ADP and P_i.
>   G Tropomyosin moves to expose the binding sites on actin.
>   H Actin is pulled towards the centre of the sarcomere.
>   I The myosin head binds to actin.
> 2 The protein dystrophin connects the muscle filaments to the cell-surface membrane of the muscle fibre. In DMD, mutations in the dystrophin gene lead to deletions in the amino acid sequence of the dystrophin protein.
>   Suggest how this could lead to the symptoms of DMD. [4]

Cardiovascular system

B2.5 The role of the components in performing the functions of the cardiovascular system

REVISED

The cardiovascular system transports:
+ nutrients such as glucose and amino acids to the tissues
+ oxygen from the lungs to the tissues
+ carbon dioxide from the tissues to the lungs.

The components of the cardiovascular system are the heart, blood and blood vessels.

> **Making links**
>
> The cardiovascular system plays an important role in regulating body temperature (B2.15) and transports hormones around the body (B2.14).

Components of the cardiovascular system

Figure 13.9 shows a diagram of the mammalian heart.

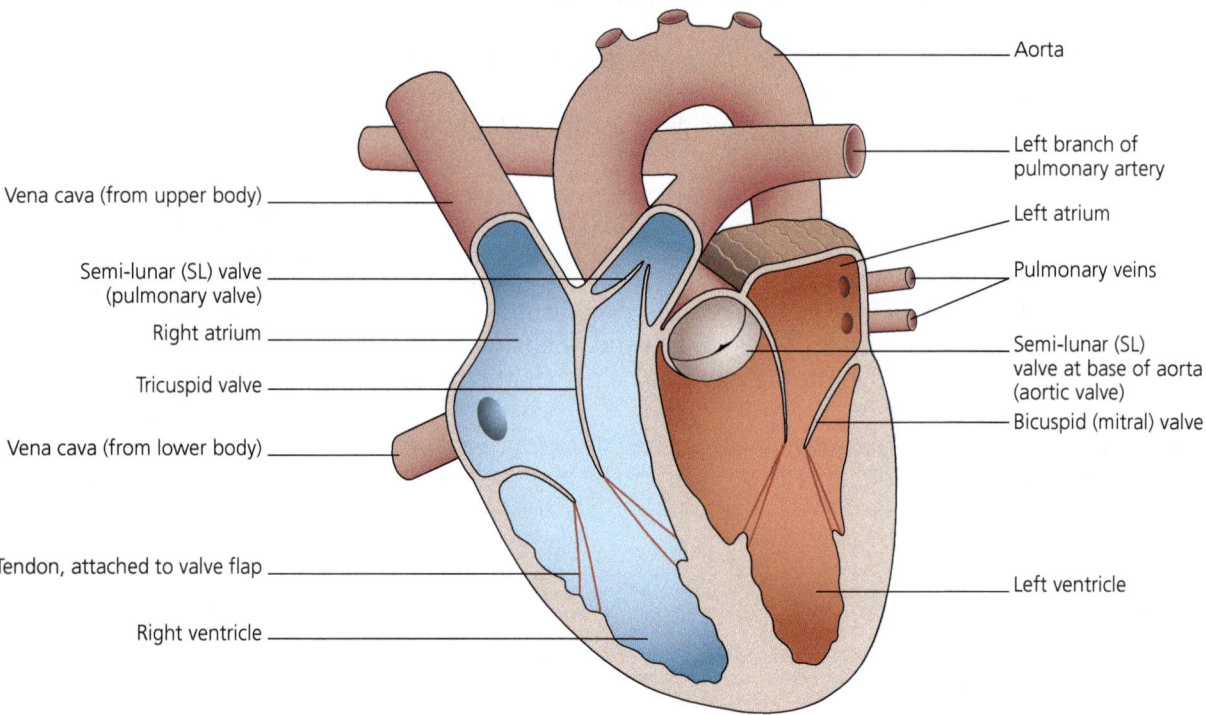

Figure 13.9 Cross-section through the mammalian heart

Note that the pulmonary and aortic valves are also known as semi-lunar (SL) valves, and the tricuspid and mitral (bicuspid) valves are also known as atrioventricular (AV) valves.

Figure 13.10 on the next page shows cross-sections of the three types of blood vessel.

Arteries carry blood away from the heart and have a thick layer of muscle and elastic tissue. Muscle allows constriction (narrowing) and dilation (widening) to regulate blood flow. Elastic tissue allows the artery to expand and withstand the pressure caused by pumping of the heart.

Veins carry blood back to the heart. The blood is at much lower pressure, so the lumen (space for blood) is much wider than in arteries and the walls are much thinner.

Capillaries are the smallest vessels and carry blood throughout the tissues.

> **Exam tip**
>
> Make sure you can identify and label the following components of the heart:
> + atria
> + ventricles
> + aorta
> + vena cava
> + pulmonary artery
> + pulmonary vein
> + tricuspid valve
> + pulmonary valve
> + mitral (bicuspid) valve
> + aortic valve.

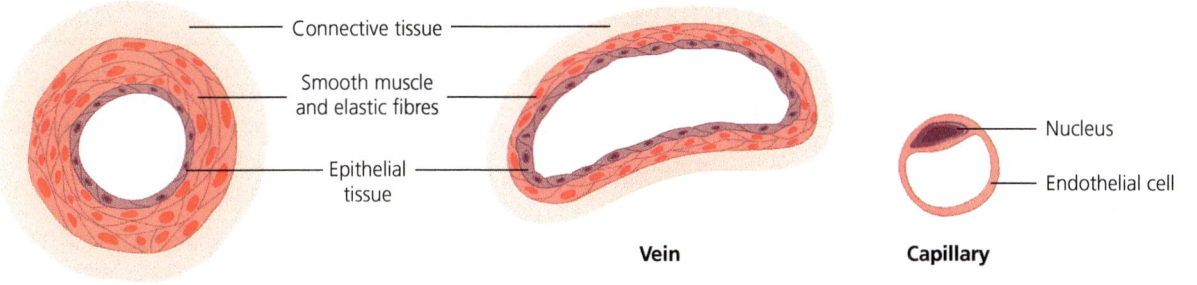

Figure 13.10 Cross-sections of an artery, a vein and a capillary. Capillaries have walls that are a single cell thick or, like this one, consist of single cells wrapped into a tubular shape

Blood is made up of:
+ plasma, the straw-coloured fluid that is left if all cells are removed
+ platelets, the small disc-shaped cell fragments involved in blood clotting
+ erythrocytes, the red blood cells; these have lost most of their organelles (including the nucleus) and contain haemoglobin for transport of oxygen
+ leucocytes or white blood cells; these are involved in protection against infection (B1.20).

The function of the components of the cardiovascular system

Figure 13.11 shows how the cardiovascular system can transport substances around the body. Note how the human cardiovascular system is a double circulation.

> **Revision activity**
>
> Make a list showing the route taken by blood flowing from the heart, to the lungs, back to the heart and around the body, returning again to the heart. Do this for each path shown in Figure 13.11:
> + arms, head, ribs etc.
> + liver, stomach and intestines
> + kidneys
> + legs, abdomen etc.
>
> What is different about the circulation to the liver?

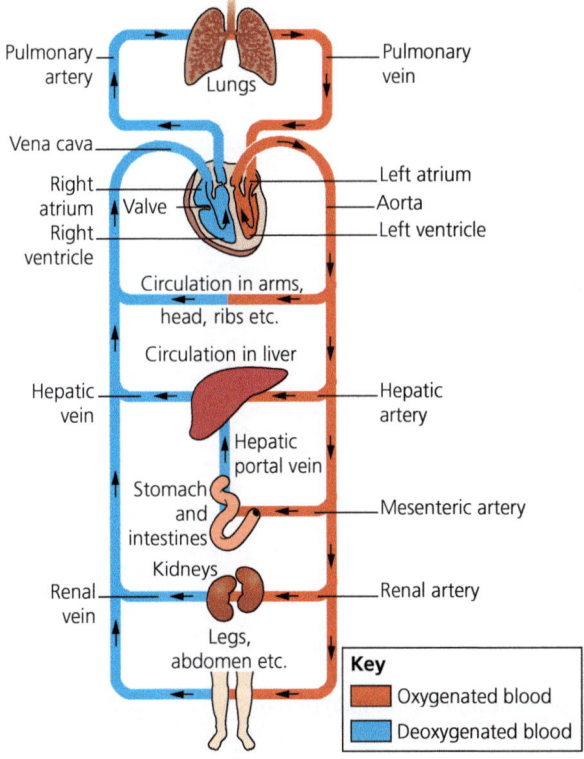

Figure 13.11 The organisation of the human cardiovascular system

> **Now test yourself**   TESTED
>
> 1 Give the names of the **four** valves in the heart.
> 2 Give **two** similarities and **two** differences between arteries and veins.
> 3 Explain why the mammalian circulatory system is described as a double circulatory system.

B2.6 The process of the cardiac cycle

The cardiac cycle describes the pumping of blood by the heart through a series of muscle contractions and relaxations (systole and diastole). The electrical activity of the heart helps control the process and allows us to monitor it. Pressure changes help us to understand how the blood flows through the chambers of the heart.

Figure 13.12 is a simplified diagram of the heart that helps in understanding the flow of blood through the heart.

> **Systole** The contraction of the atrium (atrial systole) or ventricle (ventricular systole).
>
> **Diastole** The relaxation of the atrium (atrial diastole) or ventricle (ventricular diastole).

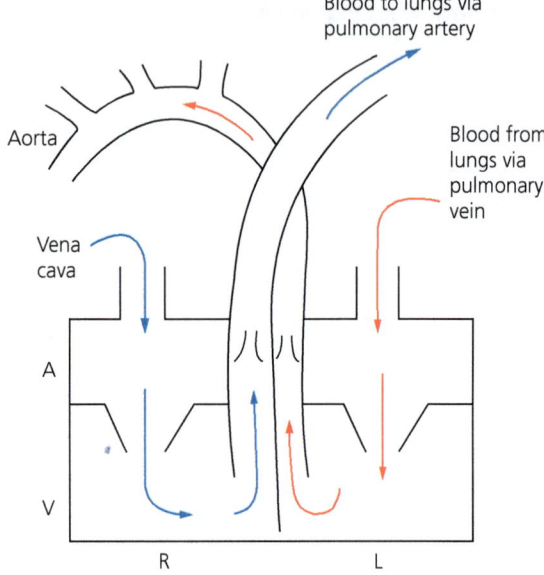

Figure 13.12 Simplified diagram of the heart showing the main chambers, valves and blood vessels, illustrating the route taken by blood through the heart; A = atria, V = ventricles, R = right, L = left

The electrical activity of the heart and how heart rate is controlled and regulated

Figure 13.13 shows how electrical signals produced by the sinoatrial node (SAN) spread out over the surface of the atria and then the ventricles, causing them to contract.

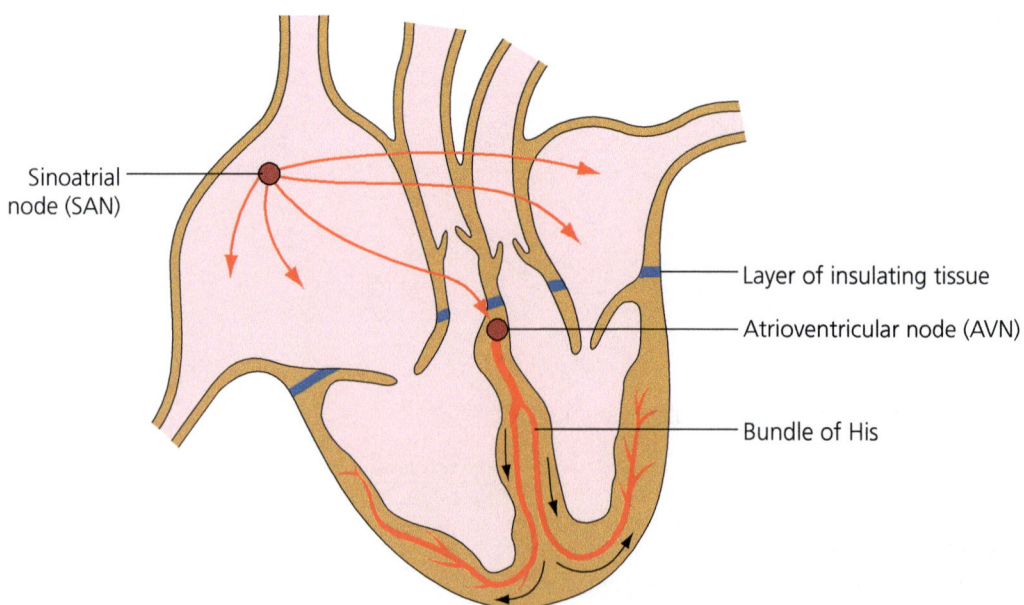

Figure 13.13 Electrical activity in the heart that co-ordinates the heartbeat

Check your understanding and progress at www.hoddereducation.co.uk/myrevisionnotes

This electrical activity can be detected using electrocardiography (ECG) to produce a trace known as an electrocardiogram (also called an ECG), as shown in Figure 13.14.

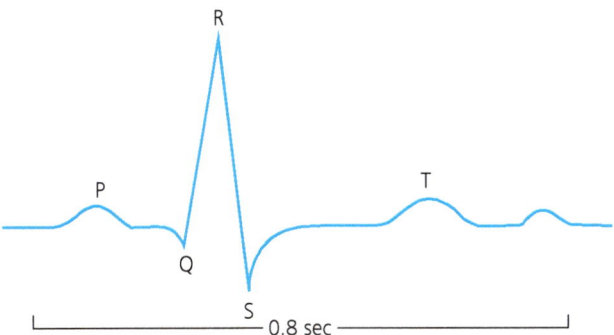

> **Typical mistake**
>
> Do not confuse the terms *electrocardiogram* and *electrocardiograph*. An electrocardiogram is the trace produced by an electrocardiograph, the instrument that measures the electrical activity of the heart. Both terms are abbreviated to ECG.

Figure 13.14 ECG showing one beat of a healthy heart

The graph shows several distinct waves:
+ The P wave is caused by atrial systole.
+ The QRS complex represents ventricular systole.
+ The T wave is caused by ventricular diastole.

Pressure changes in the heart and blood vessels and how this is linked to blood pressure

The chambers of the heart shown in Figure 13.9 consist of muscle and are separated by valves.
+ Muscles contract to push the blood through the heart and out of the heart.
+ Valves prevent backflow, ensuring blood only flows in one direction through the heart.

You can learn the route taken by blood flowing through the heart. However, it is better if you understand how and why this happens. Look at the graph in Figure 13.15. This shows the pressure in the chambers of the left side of the heart and the aorta.

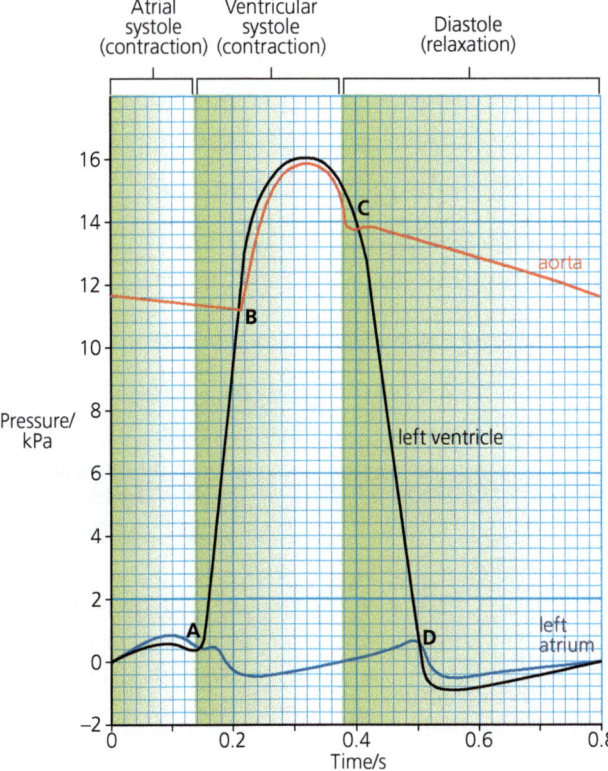

Figure 13.15 A graph showing how pressure changes in the left atrium, left ventricle and aorta during one cardiac cycle

The graph can be interpreted by applying the following principles:
+ Contraction of the atrium or ventricle increases the pressure in that chamber.
+ Blood flows from high to low pressure, pushing open the valve ahead of it.
+ When the pressure in the ventricle is higher than that in the atrium, the bicuspid valve is pushed closed, preventing backflow from ventricle to atrium.
+ The same applies when the pressure in the aorta is higher than that in the ventricle, so the semi-lunar (aortic) valve closes to prevent backflow into the ventricle.

> **Revision activity**
>
> Make a copy of Figure 13.15 and annotate it with a description of how and why blood flows through the heart during a single cardiac cycle.
>
> Pay particular attention to the points marked A, B, C and D. How do the pressure differences at these points ensure blood flows only in the right direction?
>
> How would you expect the graph to be different for the right side of the heart? Think about how far blood must be pumped by the two sides of the heart – Figure 13.12 will help. Does this explain the differences in the thickness of the left and right ventricle walls that you can see in Figure 13.9?

> **Now test yourself** — TESTED
>
> 1 What is meant by systole?
> 2 On an ECG trace, what does the QRS complex represent?
> 3 Explain how the aortic valve prevents backflow of blood.

B2.7 The development, impact and management of coronary heart disease (CHD)

REVISED

Coronary heart disease (CHD) refers to a disease of the coronary arteries. These are the blood vessels that supply the heart muscle with nutrients, such as glucose, and oxygen.

Causes of the disease

Narrowing of coronary arteries will reduce the supply of glucose and oxygen, leading to the symptoms of CHD. Narrowing can be caused by atherosclerosis – a build-up of fatty substances in the wall of the arteries. Thrombosis is when blood clots form in the narrowed arteries. If the clot completely blocks the artery, it causes a heart attack (myocardial infarction).

Risk factors for CHD include:
+ hypertension (high blood pressure), which thickens the walls of the arteries
+ smoking, as it is possible that nicotine in cigarette smoke constricts the arteries, which raises blood pressure
+ excessive consumption of alcohol, which increases blood pressure
+ high cholesterol, which increases the risk of atherosclerosis
+ diabetes, which can increase the risk of atherosclerosis
+ age and sex: the risk of CHD increases with age, as damage to arteries develops slowly; men are more likely than women to get CHD in middle age, although there is little difference between older men and women
+ genetic factors
+ ethnicity: in the UK, people of African–Caribbean, Black African or South Asian background have a greater risk of CHD.

> **Making links**
>
> Shortness of breath is also a symptom of respiratory diseases such as COPD (B2.10).
>
> Smoking is also a risk factor in respiratory diseases such as COPD, as well as several cancers (B2.30).

Check your understanding and progress at www.hoddereducation.co.uk/myrevisionnotes

Impact on systems within the body and on physical and mental health

The symptoms of coronary heart disease depend on the degree and location of the narrowing of the coronary arteries and include:
+ chest pain (angina), as heart muscle becomes starved of blood
+ shortness of breath, as the heart is less able to pump blood around the body
+ pain throughout the body
+ feeling faint
+ feeling sick (nausea).

If CHD is undetected or untreated, it can lead to myocardial infarction (heart attack), when a whole segment of the heart muscle is starved of oxygen (ischaemia) and begins to die. Blockage of one of the larger coronary arteries can be fatal.

CHD can cause a decline in mental health because of the symptoms, concern about the risk of serious heart attack and the need to make lifestyle changes that might be stressful. For example, giving up smoking can have a short-term negative impact on a person's mental health, even though there are long-term benefits.

How common treatments relieve symptoms

There are a number of treatments that can relieve symptoms:
+ Blood-thinning medicines (anticoagulants) can prevent the formation of blood clots. This reduces the risk of thrombosis but can mean that the person may bleed too easily.
+ Statins lower the concentration of cholesterol, which reduces the risk of atherosclerosis.
+ Betablockers oppose the effect of adrenaline acting on the sinoatrial node (see B2.6) and so slow down the heart.
+ Lifestyle changes can include making changes to diet, to reduce body mass or limit intake of saturated fats, stopping smoking and taking regular exercise.
+ Surgical options include:
  + angioplasty, which involves inserting a balloon to widen narrowed arteries or a wire mesh stent that also helps keep the artery open
  + a coronary artery bypass graft to bypass one or more narrowed coronary arteries
  + heart transplant surgery, which can be used in cases where a heart attack is not fatal but causes heart failure; there is a risk of rejection of the transplanted organ, so immunosuppressant drugs must be taken for the rest of the patient's life.

Exam practice

1. Describe the path taken by blood flowing through the left side of the heart. Indicate how pressure differences and the different valves ensure blood only flows in one direction. [6]
2. A patient has presented with chest pain and a history of smoking. They have been diagnosed with coronary heart disease (CHD). An ECG shows no sign of them having had a heart attack. Their doctor has suggested statins and blood-thinning medication (anticoagulants).
   a. Discuss the suitability of these treatments. [4]
   b. Suggest what else the patient could do to reduce their risk of heart attack. [3]

Exam tip

You will often be asked to evaluate or discuss the suitability of different treatment options. Make sure you cover both advantages and disadvantages and also try to draw a conclusion.

Respiratory system

B2.8 The role of the components in performing the functions of the respiratory system

REVISED

Components of the respiratory system

The human respiratory system comprises the following components (see Figure 13.16):

- trachea (windpipe)
- lungs
- bronchi (there are two bronchi; the singular is bronchus)
- bronchioles
- alveoli
- pleural membranes
- ribs
- intercostal muscles
- diaphragm.

> **Alveoli** Small air-filled sacs at the ends of bronchioles. They have a wall consisting of a single layer of epithelial cells. The singular is alveolus.

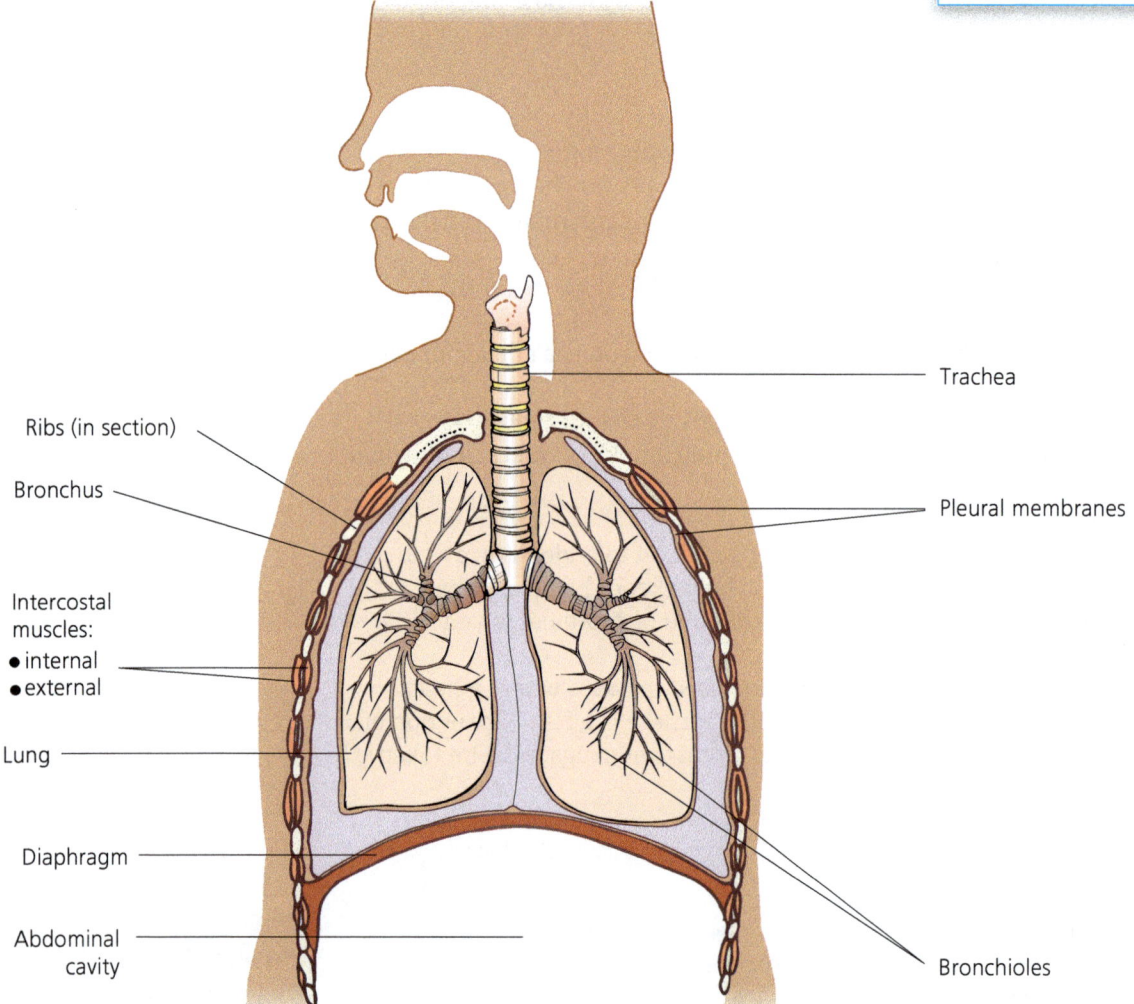

Figure 13.16 The human respiratory system

If you look at Figure 13.16, you will see that the lungs consist of a series of branching tubes:

trachea → two bronchi (one to each lung) → many bronchioles

The bronchioles lead to blind ends called alveoli, which are the site of gas exchange (see B2.9).

> **Revision activity**
>
> Make a copy of Figure 13.16 without the labels. Use this to test your memory – can you label all the structures?

Check your understanding and progress at www.hoddereducation.co.uk/myrevisionnotes

Functions of relevant components within the respiratory system

Inspiration involves:
- contraction of the diaphragm, causing it to move down
- contraction of the external intercostal muscles, causing the rib cage to move up and outward.

This increases the volume of the chest cavity, reducing the pressure below atmospheric pressure (the pressure of the air outside the body). This means that air flows down a pressure gradient into the lungs, causing them to expand.

Expiration at rest involves relaxation of both sets of muscles. This reduces the volume of the chest cavity, so the pressure increases and air is forced out of the lungs. In forced expiration (like blowing out a candle), the internal intercostal muscles also contract, which causes the rib cage to be pulled in and down more forcefully, expelling air more rapidly.

> **Inspiration** Breathing in.
> **Expiration** Breathing out.

> **Now test yourself** TESTED
> 1 Describe the route taken by inhaled air.
> 2 What is the difference between forced expiration and expiration at rest?

B2.9 The role of the alveoli as a specialised exchange surface in the process of gas exchange

REVISED

Like all large mammals, humans have a low surface area to volume ratio. This means that specialised organs are needed for exchange. Gas exchange occurs in the alveoli and they are adapted to maximise the efficiency of this process.

> **Making links**
> B1.10 introduced the concept of the surface area to volume ratio.

How adaptations of the alveoli maximise the rate of diffusion

Figure 13.17 shows the process of gas exchange in an alveolus.

The key features of the alveoli that make a good exchange surface are a:
- large surface area to volume ratio; the surface area is about 75 m² in an adult human
- good blood supply
- short diffusion distance; there are only two layers of cells between the air in the alveoli and the blood.

Two other factors help to maximise the rate of diffusion of gas:
- a film of moisture lining the alveoli allowing oxygen to dissolve before diffusing across the epithelium
- body temperature, as the rate of diffusion increases with increased temperature.

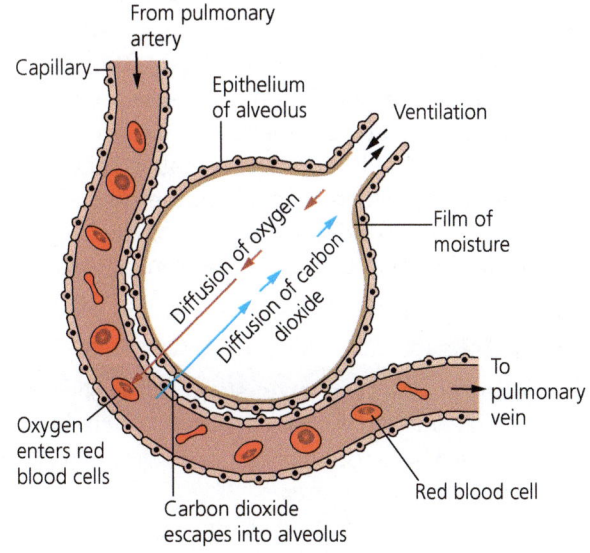

Figure 13.17 Gas exchange in an alveolus

B2.10 The development, impact and management of chronic obstructive pulmonary disease (COPD)

Chronic obstructive pulmonary disease (COPD) describes a group of lung diseases that cause difficulty breathing. These include emphysema and chronic bronchitis.

Causes of the disease

Smoking is responsible for about 90 per cent of cases of COPD. Exposure to some types of dust and chemicals, particularly at work, or other forms of air pollution can increase the risk of COPD.

These harmful substances can damage the epithelia, causing inflammation in the alveoli. Eventually the walls of the alveoli break down, reducing the surface area for gas exchange – this is emphysema.

Inflammation of the bronchioles can lead to chronic bronchitis. The bronchioles are narrowed and produce excessive amounts of mucus, leading to obstruction of the airways.

Impact on systems within the body and on physical and mental health

The main symptoms of COPD include:
+ shortness of breath
+ persistent chesty cough that produces large amounts of phlegm
+ frequent chest infections
+ persistent wheezing.

Without treatment, COPD can restrict daily life and normal activities, which can affect the patient's mental as well as physical health.

How common treatments relieve symptoms

Treatments that relieve symptoms include:
+ lifestyle changes – stopping smoking is the most effective way of preventing the disease from progressing
+ bronchodilator inhalers, like the reliever inhalers used to treat asthma; these relax the muscles in the walls of the bronchi, widening the airways
+ steroid inhalers that help to reduce inflammation of the airways; in severe cases, oral steroids (tablets) can be prescribed, but usually only for a short period because of side effects
+ pulmonary rehabilitation, a specialised course of exercise and education delivered by physiotherapists, nurse specialists and dietitians
+ surgery to remove damaged parts of the lung in severe cases; a last resort is a lung transplant, with a lung from a healthy donor.

> **Making links**
>
> There may be periods when the symptoms of COPD get suddenly worse. This is known as a flare-up. This sudden worsening of symptoms can also be seen in other chronic inflammatory diseases, such as rheumatoid arthritis (B2.3) and Crohn's disease (B2.13).
>
> There is no cure for chronic diseases, although symptoms can be treated. When a person knows that they must live with a disease for the rest of their life, this can cause anxiety, depression or other forms of mental illness. For this reason, you will see that all the chronic diseases that you learn about may have a negative impact on a person's mental health.

> **Exam practice**
>
> 1. A patient presents with a persistent chesty cough. They also wake up at night feeling breathless. They are diagnosed with chronic bronchitis.
>   a. Explain **two** effects this condition will have on their respiratory system and blood oxygen levels. [4]
>   b. What are the **two** most important questions the patient would have been asked when their medical history was taken? [2]
>   c. Outline the first-line treatment options that would be offered to the patient. [3]
>   d. Describe the treatment options for more severe disease. [4]
>   e. Discuss the advantages of pulmonary rehabilitation for the treatment of COPD. [4]

Check your understanding and progress at www.hoddereducation.co.uk/myrevisionnotes

Digestive system

B2.11 The role of the components in performing the functions of the digestive system

REVISED

Components of the digestive system

The digestive system is the group of organs that work together to break down food so that nutrients can be absorbed, and waste got rid of. You need to know the following components:

- mouth
- oesophagus
- stomach
- pancreas
- liver
- duodenum, ileum and colon.

You should also know the associated glands linked to these components, including salivary glands in the mouth, gall bladder and bile duct. These are all illustrated in Figure 13.18.

Figure 13.19 illustrates the layers of the wall of the gastrointestinal tract (GI tract).

> **Gastrointestinal tract (GI tract)** The tube-like structure from mouth to anus that forms a part of the digestive system.

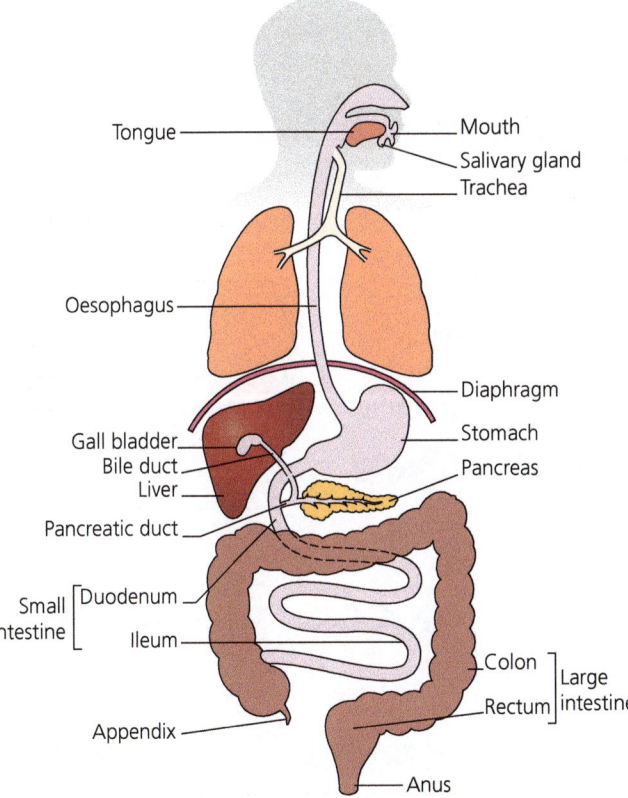

Figure 13.18 The human digestive system

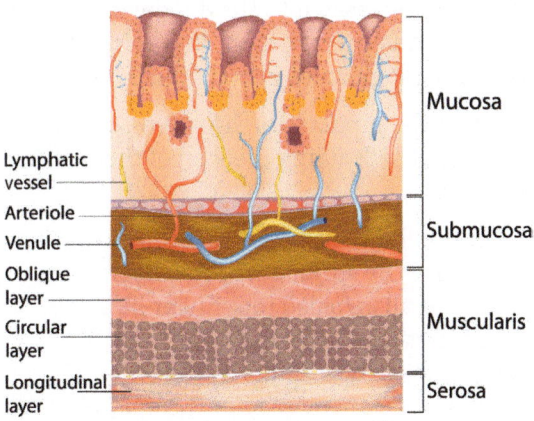

Figure 13.19 The four layers of the wall of the GI tract

> **Revision activity**
>
> Use Figures 13.18 and 13.19 to help you identify and label the components you need to know. Make copies of each and blank out the labels. Now see if you can fill in the blanks.
>
> This is a useful revision method wherever you need to be able to identify structures on diagrams like these.

Function of relevant components within the digestive system

The digestive system breaks down food by physical and chemical digestion, followed by absorption of the products of digestion.

Physical digestion involves breaking food into smaller pieces:
+ Food is chewed in the mouth. Saliva from salivary glands helps lubricate the food and also contains the enzyme salivary amylase.
+ The food is churned in the stomach through contraction of smooth muscle in the stomach wall.
+ Peristalsis (rhythmic movement of the gut wall) moves the food along the length of the GI tract.

Chemical digestion involves enzymes that break down large molecules (proteins, lipids and polysaccharides like starch) into smaller molecules.

Making links

B1.8 covered the formation of proteins and polysaccharides by joining smaller molecules in condensation reactions. Digestion is the reverse of this process.

Table 13.1 A summary of the process of chemical digestion

Enzymes	Location/source	Action
Amylases	Saliva and pancreatic fluid	Digestion of starch
Disaccharidases	Duodenum (for example lactase)	Convert disaccharides into their constituent monosaccharides
Proteases	Pepsin (stomach), trypsin, chymotrypsin and carboxypeptidase (pancreatic fluid)	Convert proteins into smaller fragments: peptides and eventually amino acids
Lipases	Pancreatic fluid	Break down lipids into fatty acids and glycerol

There are two other components of chemical digestion:
+ Hydrochloric acid in the stomach sterilises the food.
+ Bile is produced in the liver, stored in the gall bladder and released into the duodenum via the bile duct and pancreatic duct. Bile helps break down large fat globules into smaller fat droplets.

Absorption of the products of digestion occurs in the epithelial cells lining the wall of the ileum (Figure 13.20).

The wall of the ileum has several features that greatly increase the surface area for absorption:
+ The ileum wall is folded into finger-like projections called villi.
+ These are covered in epithelial cells.
+ The cell-surface membrane of the epithelial cells is folded into microvilli.

Fatty acids are non-polar and so they can diffuse passively through the cell-surface membrane of the epithelial cells.

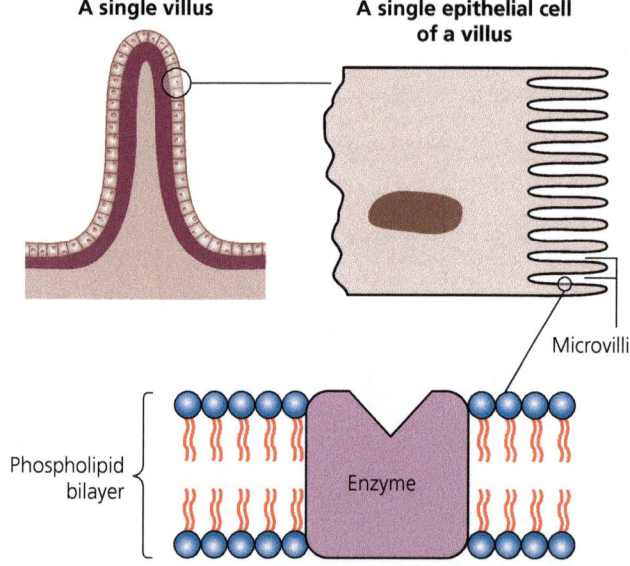

Figure 13.20 The lining of the small intestine showing a villus, microvilli on the surface of an epithelial cell and its cell-surface membrane incorporating an enzyme such as maltase

Now test yourself   TESTED

1. Describe the main function of physical digestion.
2. Name the end products of digestion of:
   a. proteins
   b. polysaccharides.
3. Acidity in the stomach sterilises the food. Suggest one adaptation that stomach enzymes need to be able to work in this environment.

Check your understanding and progress at www.hoddereducation.co.uk/myrevisionnotes

B2.12 The process of cellular transport in the small intestine to absorb glucose and amino acids

REVISED

Apart from fatty acids, all the other products of digestion are polar molecules so they cannot just diffuse through the cell-surface membrane of the epithelial cells. The absorption of glucose and amino acids occurs by a combination of:
+ active transport through the cell-surface membrane
+ co-transport mechanisms
+ facilitated diffusion (passive transport through the cell-surface membrane).

> **Making links**
>
> The process of glucose absorption is covered in B1.11. Amino acids are absorbed by a similar mechanism.

B2.13 The development, impact and management of Crohn's disease

REVISED

Crohn's disease is a type of inflammatory bowel disease that cannot be cured. The lining of the gut is inflamed and damaged.

Causes of the disease

Several factors may play a part:
+ genes
+ the immune system attacks the gut, although Crohn's disease does not seem to be an autoimmune disease
+ smoking
+ a previous gut infection
+ an imbalance in the microbiome (the population of gut bacteria).

The type of diet does not seem to cause Crohn's disease, although some people find certain foods can cause a flare-up (worsening of symptoms).

Impact on systems within the body and on physical and mental health

Crohn's disease most commonly affects the large intestine (colon). Symptoms include:
+ diarrhoea, particularly when it comes on suddenly
+ stomach aches and cramps, particularly in the lower right abdomen
+ blood in the faeces
+ tiredness and weight loss.

In severe cases, inflammation can obstruct the bowel. Patients with Crohn's disease are more likely to develop bowel cancer.

Crohn's disease is linked to a number of mental health disorders, including depression and anxiety.

How common treatments relieve symptoms

+ Steroids, such as prednisolone, reduce inflammation in the gut, but cannot be used for long periods because of side effects.
+ Immunosuppressants can be used if steroids on their own are not effective. They can be used as a long-term treatment.
+ Changes to diet might help control symptoms, although the relationship between food and Crohn's disease is complicated.
+ Biological medicines, such as adalimumab, include monoclonal antibodies that bind to and block TNF-α, a protein that attacks the gut.

> **Making links**
>
> Adalimumab is also a treatment for rheumatoid arthritis (B2.3) and works in a similar way in both diseases. These medicines are given by injection or as a drip into a vein every 2–8 weeks and may be needed for several months or years.

+ Surgery is an option if medicines do not work. In resection of the bowel, a small, inflamed section of the bowel is removed, usually by keyhole surgery. The healthy parts are then stitched back together. Surgery can relieve symptoms and prevent them returning for a time, but they will normally return eventually.

> **Revision activity**
>
> Make a list of the symptoms of Crohn's disease and, for each, think about what effect they would have on the patient's everyday life.
>
> Then do the same with the common treatments. Try to link the type of treatment with the ability of a patient to cope with everyday life. List ways in which this could influence the mental health of the patient and think about ways in which they could be supported.

Exam practice

1 Figure 13.21 shows an epithelial cell in the lining of the ileum.

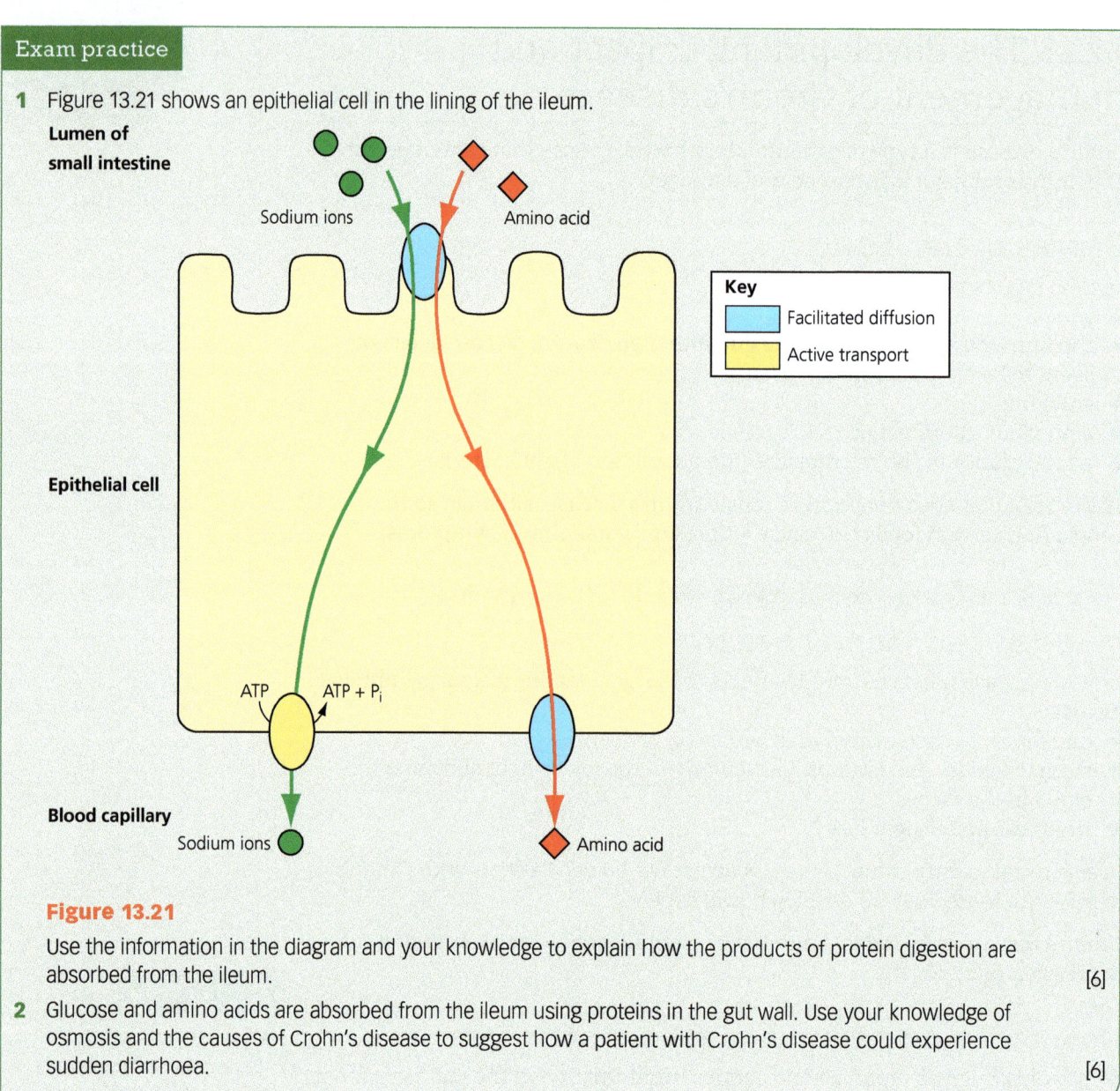

Figure 13.21

Use the information in the diagram and your knowledge to explain how the products of protein digestion are absorbed from the ileum. [6]

2 Glucose and amino acids are absorbed from the ileum using proteins in the gut wall. Use your knowledge of osmosis and the causes of Crohn's disease to suggest how a patient with Crohn's disease could experience sudden diarrhoea. [6]

Endocrine system

B2.14 The role of the components in performing the functions of the endocrine system

REVISED

Endocrine glands secrete hormones into the blood which act as chemical messengers and are transported in the blood around the body to act on specific target cells or organs.

Components of the endocrine system

Figure 13.22 shows the components of the human endocrine system.

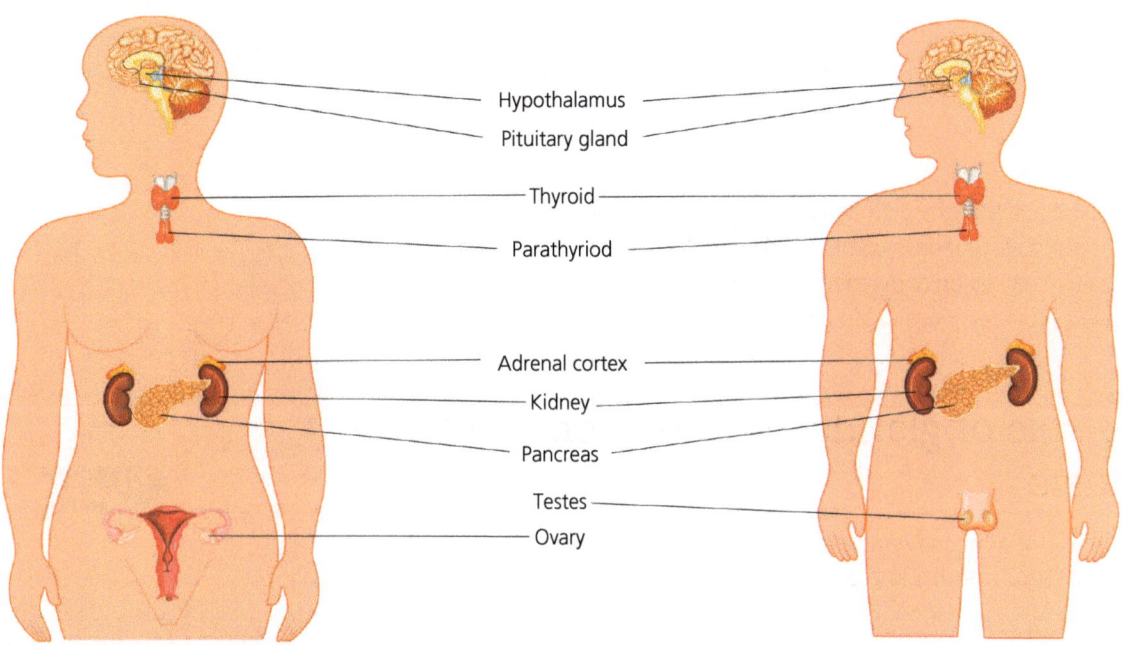

Figure 13.22 The human endocrine system showing the endocrine glands in females (left) and males (right)

> **Revision activity**
>
> Make a copy of Figure 13.22 without the labels and use this to test yourself. You might not be expected to label a diagram, but it is helpful to know where in the body the different glands are located.

Gland A group of cells that make chemicals such as hormones or enzymes.

Endocrine glands These glands release hormones into the blood.

Hormone A chemical messenger released into the blood by an endocrine gland that acts on a target elsewhere in the body.

Functions of relevant components within the endocrine system

Each endocrine gland produces one or more specific hormones that may be stored in the gland and then released into the blood. Table 13.2 shows the activity of common hormones and their specificity in relation to their target cells or organs.

Table 13.2 on the next page shows the production and activity of specific hormones.

Table 13.2 The production and activity of specific hormones

Hormone	Secreted by	Acts on
Thyroxine	Thyroid	Most body cells to regulate metabolic rate
Cortisol	Adrenal cortex	Liver and muscle cells and increases the blood glucose concentration; cortisol is produced in response to stress
Oestrogen	Ovaries	Pituitary and uterus: oestrogen is involved in regulation of the menstrual cycle
Testosterone	Testes	Muscle and bone cells to increase muscle mass and bone density
		Sex organs to stimulate the development of the male sex organs and secondary sexual characteristics; required for production of sperm cells
Gastrin	Stomach	Stomach: gastrin has several actions in digestion involving the stomach and small intestine
Growth hormone (GH)	Pituitary	Most body cells respond to GH, which is responsible for normal growth during infancy and childhood
Follicle stimulating hormone (FSH)	Pituitary	Ovaries: FSH stimulates the growth and development of the egg follicle during the first half of the menstrual cycle

> **Now test yourself** TESTED
>
> 1 Identify the name and site of production of the following hormones:
>   a It stimulates growth and development of the egg follicle.
>   b It is involved in regulation of the menstrual cycle.
>   c It is involved in the response to stress.

B2.15 The role of glands and hormones in homeostasis

REVISED

The regulation of blood glucose concentration involves the pancreas, which produces the hormones insulin and glucagon, as shown in Figure 13.23.

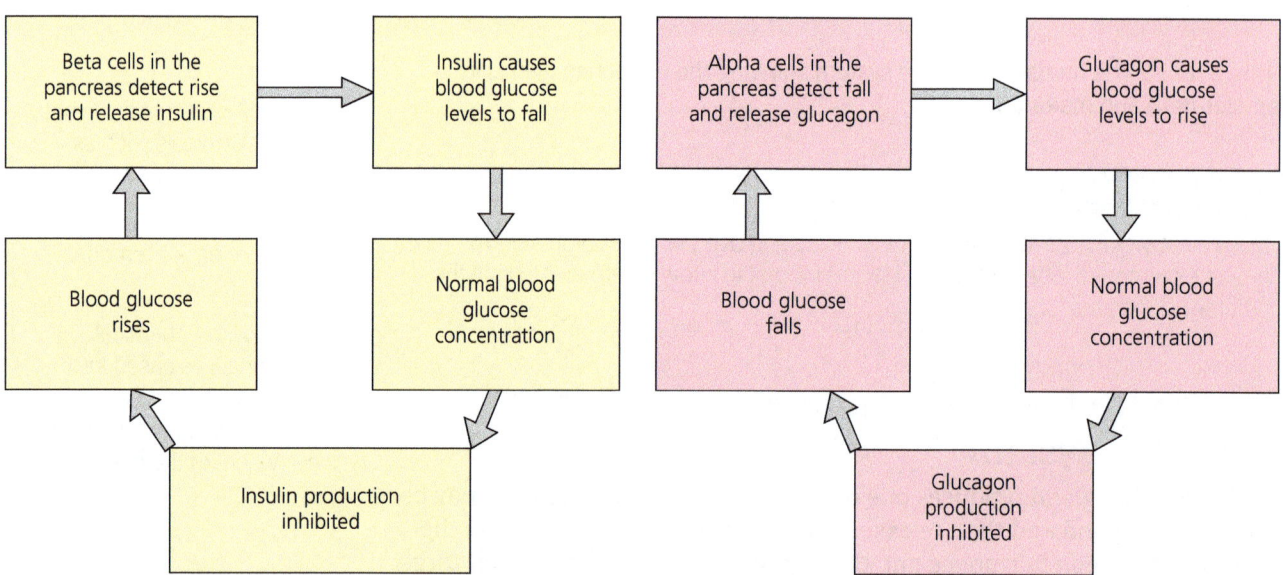

Figure 13.23 Regulation of blood glucose concentration by insulin (left) and glucagon (right); these are both examples of negative feedback

> **Revision activity**
>
> Look back at Figure 12.16 in B1.28. The diagram shows a factor at a normal level and then what happens when the factor rises above or falls below the normal level. Using Figure 13.23 as the basis, produce a similar diagram to show what happens when blood glucose concentration rises above or falls below the normal levels.

Check your understanding and progress at www.hoddereducation.co.uk/myrevisionnotes

The kidneys are involved in osmoregulation – the regulation of the water balance of the body.
+ If there is too little water in the body (low water potential), this leads to dehydration. If there is too much water (high water potential), the body becomes over-hydrated. Both states cause problems for the normal functioning of the body.
+ The hypothalamus controls the amount of water lost in the urine through the kidneys by the action of the hormone ADH. This is shown in Figure 13.24.

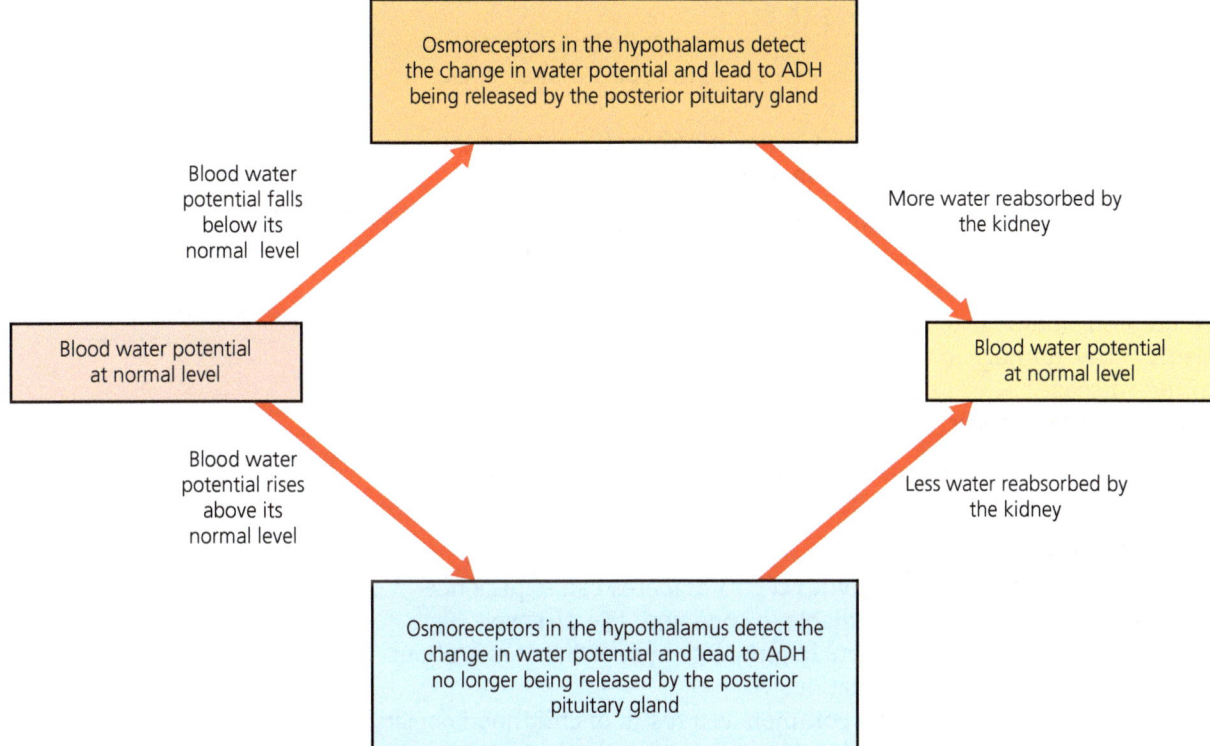

Figure 13.24 Control of the water potential of the blood by ADH

Thermoregulation is the maintenance of the body temperature within a narrow range. This is covered in B2.24. Like osmoregulation, the process is controlled by the hypothalamus. However, the control mechanisms involve nerves rather than hormones.

> **Making links**
>
> The principles of homeostasis and the importance of negative feedback were covered in B1.28.
>
> Osmoregulation involves the renal system; this is covered in more detail in B2.21.
>
> Look at B1.9 on the effect of temperature on the activity of enzymes. This should illustrate the importance of thermoregulation.

B2.16 The development, impact and management of diabetes

REVISED

Diabetes involves a failure in the regulation of blood glucose concentration.

Causes of diabetes

+ Type 1 diabetes is caused by destruction of the beta cells in the pancreas that produce insulin. This means that the body is unable to respond to increases in blood glucose concentration.

+ Type 2 diabetes is caused by insulin resistance – the liver and muscle cells no longer respond to insulin. The mechanism is not clear, but obesity is a major risk factor.
+ Gestational diabetes is similar to type 2 diabetes. Blood glucose concentrations are increased because the pancreas cannot produce enough insulin to meet the extra needs of the body during pregnancy. Hormonal changes in pregnancy may be involved, and obesity is also a risk factor.

Impact on systems within the body and on physical and mental health

Blood glucose concentration rises after a meal. In type 1 diabetes, lack of insulin leads to hyperglycaemia. The excess glucose is excreted by the kidneys, causing glucose to appear in the urine. This can then lead to hypoglycaemia, which can cause coma or even death.

In type 2 diabetes, insulin resistance can also lead to hyperglycaemia. In both types, long-term hyperglycaemia can lead to complications of diabetes as a result of damage to the small blood vessels. These include:
+ retinopathy (damage to the retina)
+ neuropathy (damage to the nerves)
+ kidney disease
+ cardiovascular disease.

This is why it is important to monitor blood glucose concentrations and ensure the disease is well controlled.

Diabetes also affects mental health:
+ Adolescents and young people with type 1 diabetes can experience distress and feelings of being unable to cope with the disease.
+ The incidence of eating disorders in girls with type 1 diabetes is about twice that in the general population.
+ Type 2 diabetes is increasingly common as a result of childhood obesity. The combination of obesity and diabetes can cause mental health issues in young people.

> **Hyperglycaemia** When the blood glucose concentration rises above the normal or optimal level.
>
> **Hypoglycaemia** When the blood glucose concentration falls below the normal or optimal level.

How common treatments relieve symptoms

There is, at present, no cure for diabetes.
+ Type 1 diabetes is treated by replacing the missing insulin, through injection or infusion (using an insulin pump). Patients with type 1 diabetes monitor their blood glucose concentration and adjust their dose of insulin accordingly. An artificial pancreas works by combining a sensor that measures blood glucose concentration with an insulin pump, to try to replicate more closely the normal working of blood glucose regulation.
+ Type 2 and gestational diabetes are treated through lifestyle changes: eating a healthy diet (low in sugar, fat and salt) and keeping active. If this is not sufficient, metformin medication can be used. This increases the sensitivity of the body's cells to insulin. If diet or medication do not work, insulin injections can be used.

> **Exam practice**
>
> 1 An 11-year-old girl is diagnosed with type 1 diabetes. Suggest what advice you could give her to help her avoid the disease having an impact on her mental health. [6]
>
> 2 A 56-year-old man has been diagnosed with type 2 diabetes. He has been offered alternative courses of treatment. He could either:
> + follow a healthy diet, lose weight and take more exercise
> + take metformin tablets.
>
> Evaluate these two options. [6]

Check your understanding and progress at www.hoddereducation.co.uk/myrevisionnotes

Nervous system

B2.17 The role of the components in performing the functions of the nervous system

REVISED

The nervous system controls and co-ordinates our movement and allows us to interact with our environment using receptors and effectors. It also controls many autonomic functions of the body – the ones over which we have no control.

Components of the nervous system

The brain and spinal cord are sometimes called the central nervous system (CNS). The brain is where sensory inputs (hearing, sight, touch etc.) are processed and responses (such as movement) are initiated. In humans, the brain is responsible for conscious thought, memory and learning, as well as emotions. The spinal cord is important in connecting the brain with the nerves in the rest of the body (sometimes called the peripheral nervous system) and particularly important in reflex actions.

Sensory neurones carry nerve impulses that connect receptors to the brain, whereas motor neurones take nerve impulses to the effectors (muscles and glands). These have a similar structure, including:
+ dendrites that make connections with other neurones or receptors
+ a cell body, containing the nucleus
+ an axon which carries the nerve impulse from the cell body
+ a myelin sheath of Schwann cells that insulates the axon
+ nodes of Ranvier, which are small gaps between the Schwann cells
+ axon endings/terminals and synaptic ends (also called synaptic knobs) that make connections with other neurones.

Figure 13.25 shows the structure of a motor neurone.

Relay neurones make connections between other neurones, such as sensory and motor neurones. This is important in the reflex arc (B2.18).

Synapses are the connections between neurones. The nerve impulse is transferred from one neurone to the next via synapses – this is known as synaptic transmission.

> **Making links**
>
> The nervous system plays a part in homeostasis. This is covered in B1.28. The role of the nervous system in temperature regulation is covered in B2.24.
>
> The nervous system is also involved in regulation of heart rate (B2.6).

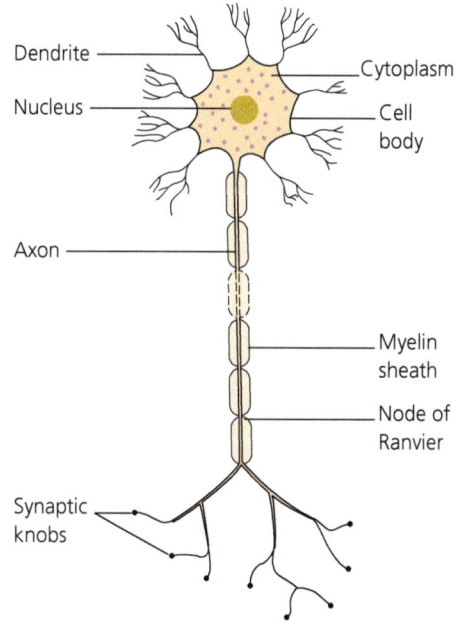

Figure 13.25 The structure of a myelinated motor neurone

Function of the relevant components of the nervous system

Figure 13.26 shows an outline of how signals are transmitted in the nervous system. The process of synaptic transmission is covered in B2.18.

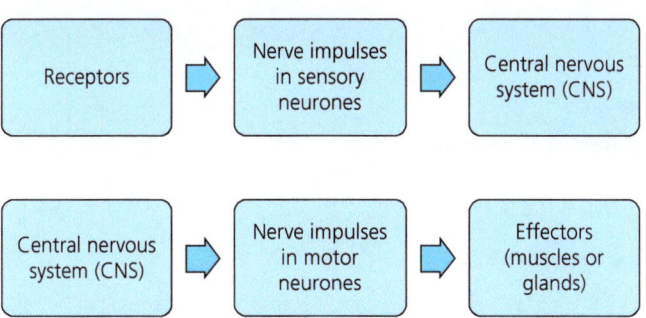

Figure 13.26 How signals from receptors cause effects in the body

> **Revision activity**
>
> An internet search for 'neurone diagram' or 'neurone drawing' will give you a selection of diagrams or drawings of the three main types of neurone: sensory, motor and relay. Find unlabelled diagrams and practise labelling them.

B2.18 The mechanism of nerve impulses via neurones

REVISED

Transmission of action potentials along neurones

Nerve impulses are electrical signals. A rapid depolarisation is followed by a rapid repolarisation. This takes about 1 millisecond and is known as an action potential. A nerve impulse involves propagation (transmission) of the action potential along the neurone towards the axon terminal.

Motor neurones and most sensory neurones are myelinated (surrounded by a myelin sheath). Nerve impulses are propagated faster along myelinated neurones because the action potentials jump from one node of Ranvier to the next (see Figure 13.25).

When the nerve impulse reaches the end of the axon, it must be transmitted to the next neurone. Connections between neurones are known as synapses (Figure 13.27).

> **Depolarisation** The reversal of the resting potential; the inside of the cell is now positive.
>
> **Repolarisation** The return to the resting potential.
>
> **Resting potential** The voltage difference between the inside and outside of a nerve cell. It is usually between −60 mV and −70 mV, i.e. the inside of the cell is more negative than the outside.

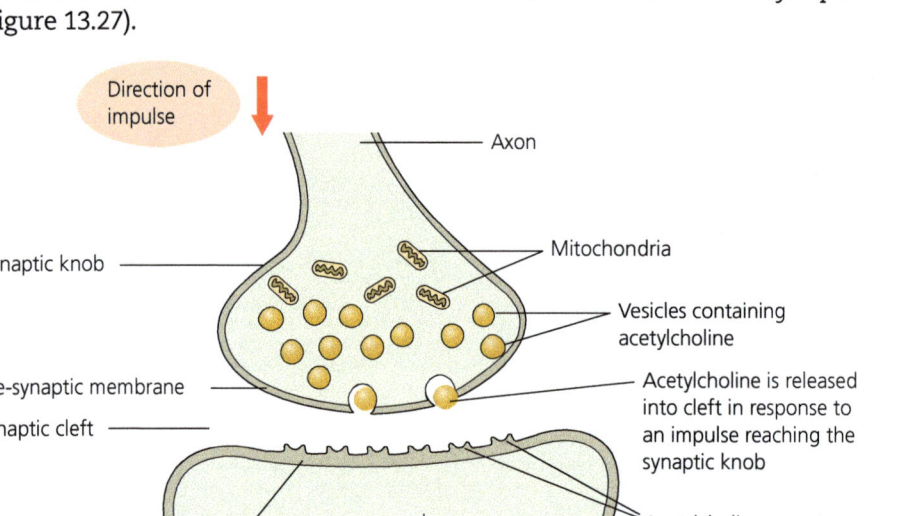

Figure 13.27 The structure of a synapse

When a nerve impulse reaches the synaptic knob, it causes neurotransmitter (usually acetylcholine) to be released. This diffuses across the synaptic cleft and binds to receptors on the membrane of the next neurone (the post-synaptic neurone). If enough neurotransmitter binds, the post-synaptic membrane will be depolarised and a new nerve impulse will be generated in the next neurone.

> **Typical mistake**
>
> An action potential usually takes less than 1 millisecond. Using the term 'speed of nerve impulses' can be misleading. We usually mean the speed or rate at which impulses travel along the neurone, so a better way to describe this is the speed or rate of propagation (of the nerve impulse).

Check your understanding and progress at www.hoddereducation.co.uk/myrevisionnotes

Mechanism of a reflex action

A reflex action is an automatic response to an external stimulus, such as touching a hot surface. This is shown in Figure 13.28.

> **Making links**
>
> Homeostasis was covered in B1.28. If you look back, you will see that there are similarities with the reflex arc. The stimulus (heat) is detected by a receptor that communicates, via the relay and motor neurones, with an effector (the muscle in the arm) to bring about a response (movement away from the source of heat).

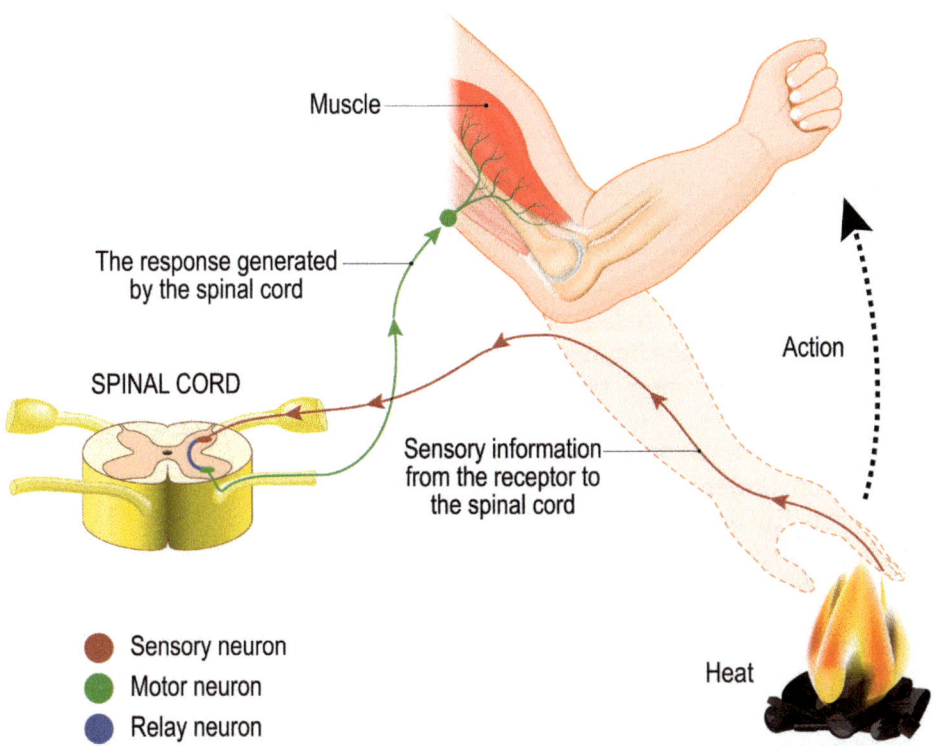

- Sensory neuron
- Motor neuron
- Relay neuron

Figure 13.28 A three neurone reflex arc

> **Now test yourself** — TESTED
>
> 1. Name the three types of neurone.
> 2. Explain the difference between an action potential and a nerve impulse.
> 3. Explain why nerve impulses are propagated faster in myelinated neurones.

B2.19 The development, impact and management of Parkinson's disease

REVISED

Parkinson's disease is a neurodegenerative disease caused by progressive loss of structure or function in the neurones.

Causes of the disease

Parkinson's disease is caused by the loss of neurones in the part of the brain involved in movement. This is thought to be due to a combination of genetic and environmental factors. These neurones release dopamine as their neurotransmitter, and this loss is responsible for many of the symptoms.

Impact on systems within the body and on physical and mental health

The main symptoms of Parkinson's disease are:
+ involuntary shaking of parts of the body (tremor)
+ slow movement
+ stiff and inflexible muscles.

A person with Parkinson's disease can also experience a wide range of other physical and psychological symptoms, including:
+ depression and anxiety
+ balance problems, which may increase the chances of a fall
+ anosmia (loss of sense of smell)
+ insomnia (problems sleeping)
+ memory problems.

How common treatments relieve symptoms

There is no cure for Parkinson's disease. Treatments focus on reducing symptoms and maintaining quality of life.
+ Supportive therapies include physiotherapy and occupational therapy.
+ Levodopa medication helps to replace the lost dopamine. This can cause dramatic improvement at first, but the effects can reduce over time because there are fewer neurones available to take up the medication. Levodopa can also have side effects, such as sickness, tiredness and dizziness.
+ Surgery, called deep brain stimulation, can ease symptoms for patients who have not responded to medication. Under general anaesthetic, electrodes are inserted into the part of the brain responsible for movement. These are attached to a pulse generator that delivers high-frequency electrical impulses. This can lead to improvement of symptoms, but also has risks, such as stroke.

Exam practice

Levodopa is the most common medicine for treatment of Parkinson's disease (PD). Most patients respond well and it is effective at managing symptoms. However, about 75% of patients develop involuntary muscle movement after 10 years of treatment.

The table shows the incidence of side effects of levodopa in a group of patients.

Side effect	Percentage of patients (%)
Nausea	90
Abnormal muscle movement	65
Vomiting	50
Anorexia	35
Abnormal heart rhythm	20

Another group of PD patients was treated with deep brain stimulation (DBS). Of these, about 80% felt that it improved their symptoms, although they had only been receiving treatment for a relatively short time.

The table shows the incidence of side effects in this group of PD patients.

Side effect	Percentage of patients (%)
Electrode leads moving	10
Temporary mental decline	10
Bleeding	10
Deep infection	10
Seizure	8
Superficial infection	2

Use your knowledge and the information provided to evaluate the two treatments for Parkinson's disease. [9 + 3 marks for QWC]

Exam tip

This type of question is marked in bands or levels, and you will be awarded marks for the quality of your written communication (QWC). Some of the marks will be for your knowledge and understanding, but you will also be marked on application of your knowledge and evaluation of the two treatments. When asked to evaluate, you will get more marks if you consider advantages and disadvantages as well as drawing a conclusion.

Renal system

B2.20 The role of the components in performing the functions of the renal system

REVISED

Components of the renal system

The renal system (Figure 13.29) has two main functions:
+ excretion – the removal of nitrogenous waste in the form of urea
+ osmoregulation – the maintenance of the water balance of the body.

The kidneys (left and right) are supplied with blood by the renal arteries, and blood leaves by the renal veins. Urine is formed in the kidneys and transported via the ureter to the bladder, where it is stored prior to urination via the urethra.

The nephron is the main functional unit of the kidney and each kidney contains about 1 million nephrons. Figure 13.30 shows the structure of the nephron.

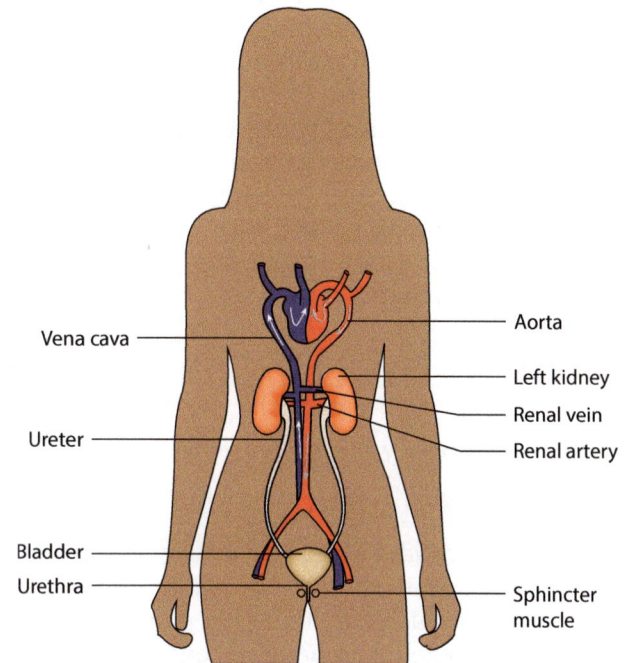

Figure 13.29 The renal system

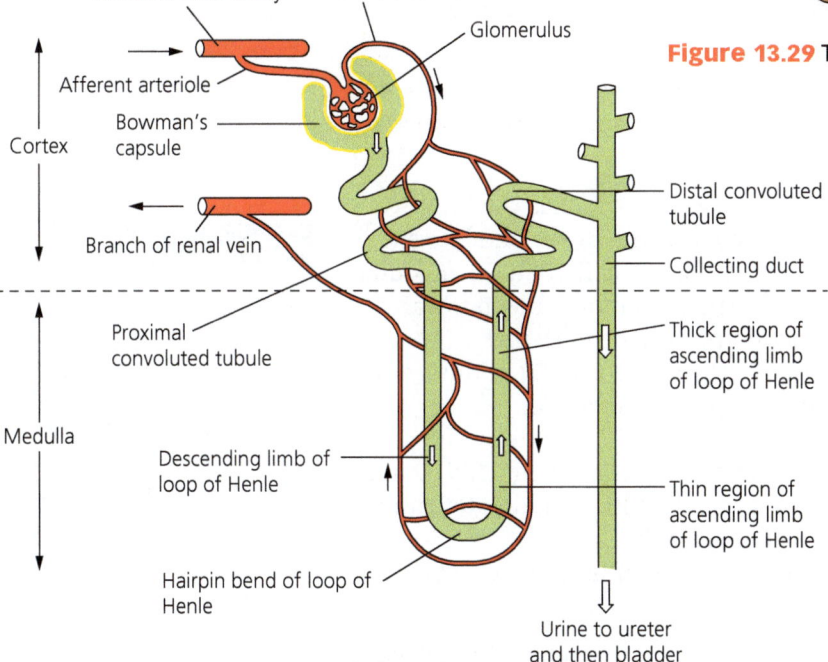

Figure 13.30 One nephron and associated blood vessels. The flow of blood is shown with black arrows and the flow of filtrate and urine with white arrows

Functions of the renal system

The renal system removes waste products, particularly urea, and produces urine. Urea is removed from the blood by the process of ultrafiltration.
+ Blood enters the space surrounded by Bowman's capsule via an arteriole (a branch of the renal artery) that divides into a knot or tangle of capillaries known as the glomerulus.

> **Revision activity**
>
> You are expected to know the following components of the renal system:
> + kidney
> + nephron (Bowman's capsule, glomerulus, proximal convoluted tubule, loop of Henle, distal convoluted tubule)
> + ureter
> + bladder
> + urethra.
>
> Make sure you can identify them on a diagram. The nephron is quite complicated, so make copies of Figure 13.30, remove the labels and use that to help you learn the names and locations.

- High pressure in the glomerulus forces fluid out into Bowman's capsule forming the filtrate. This contains water, small molecules (for example glucose and amino acids), mineral ions (for example sodium, potassium and chloride) as well as urea. Only erythrocytes (red blood cells) and large proteins cannot pass into the filtrate.

The filtrate then moves along the length of the nephron, where it undergoes several changes before becoming urine.
- Substances such as glucose and amino acids are required by the body and are reabsorbed into the blood along the length of the proximal convoluted tubule (PCT).
- Mineral ions (sodium, potassium and chloride) may also be reabsorbed. This depends on whether there is an excess of any of them in the blood. Some of this reabsorption happens in the PCT, but most of it takes place in the distal convoluted tubule (DCT).
- Water is also reabsorbed, depending on the water balance of the body. This is covered in B2.21.

> **Now test yourself**
> 1 Describe the route taken by urea after it is produced in the liver.
> 2 Name the process that takes place in the glomerulus.
> 3 Name **two** components of the blood that do not enter the filtrate in Bowman's capsule.
>
> TESTED

B2.21 The mechanism of osmoregulation

REVISED

The process of water reabsorption within the nephron via osmosis and the role of water potential

When water moves by osmosis, we say that it moves from a high water potential to a low water potential (or down a water potential gradient). Adding solute will reduce the water potential of a solution, so pure water has a high water potential, whereas a concentrated solution has a low water potential.

> **Water potential** A measure of the relative tendency of water to move from one place to another by osmosis.

Some reabsorption of water occurs in the PCT. As solutes such as glucose and amino acids are reabsorbed, they reduce the water potential of the epithelial cells, so water moves into these cells by osmosis.

Most water reabsorption occurs in the collecting duct, which is the final part of the nephron before the urine moves towards the ureter and into the bladder. This happens because the water potential of the fluid in the medulla surrounding the collecting duct decreases as the fluid moves down towards the ureter. This is brought about by the action of the loop of Henle:
- As the filtrate moves up the loop of Henle (towards the DCT), sodium and chloride ions are pumped out into the surrounding medulla.
- From the medulla, they enter the descending limb.
- The filtrate is flowing in opposite directions in the two limbs. This means that the concentration of solutes increases as the filtrate moves towards the hairpin bend at the bottom of the loop of Henle.
- As a result, the concentration of solutes in the medulla is highest at the bottom of the loop of Henle.

> **Making links**
>
> The hypothalamus co-ordinates the process of osmoregulation. This, together with the function of the posterior pituitary releasing ADH, was covered in B2.15. The collecting duct is the site of action of ADH.

This means that the water potential in the medulla surrounding the collecting duct decreases as the urine moves down towards the ureter. Therefore, there will always be a water potential gradient ensuring water can move by osmosis out of the collecting duct into the medulla. How much water is reabsorbed in this way is part of the process of osmoregulation.

Osmoregulation as a homeostatic mechanism

ADH makes the walls of the collecting duct more permeable to water. This means that more water can be reabsorbed by osmosis and so a smaller volume of more concentrated urine is produced. When less ADH is released from the posterior pituitary, the walls of the collecting duct become less permeable to water. Less water is reabsorbed and so a larger volume of more dilute urine is produced.

> **Now test yourself**
> 1 Name the **two** main parts of the nephron where water is reabsorbed.
> 2 Describe the effect of ADH on the walls of the collecting duct.
>
> TESTED

Check your understanding and progress at www.hoddereducation.co.uk/myrevisionnotes

B2.22 The development, impact and management of chronic kidney disease (CKD)

REVISED

Chronic kidney disease (CKD) involves gradual loss of kidney function over months or even years.

Causes of the disease

CKD is caused by other conditions that put strain on the kidneys, most commonly:
+ diabetes (see B2.16)
+ hypertension
+ kidney inflammation.

Impact on systems within the body and on physical and mental health

In the early stages, CKD may not cause symptoms. As it worsens, failures in normal functioning of the kidney can cause:
+ water retention, leading to oedema (swelling) of ankles, feet and hands; in extreme cases, this can cause pulmonary oedema that can be life threatening
+ tiredness and shortness of breath
+ blood in the urine.

In CKD the kidney no longer produces vitamin D and lack of this vitamin can cause disorders of bone metabolism.

Like other chronic diseases, CKD can affect a person's mental health.

How common treatments relieve symptoms or cure the disease

There is no cure for CKD, other than kidney transplant. Other treatments relieve symptoms:
+ Lifestyle changes, such as weight loss and a low-salt, low-protein diet, can slow down progression.
+ Renal dialysis replicates some of the function of the kidney, particularly removal of harmful urea from the blood:
  + A haemodialysis machine requires the patient to be connected via a tube inserted in a vein. This can be carried out in a dialysis centre or at home.
  + Peritoneal dialysis (CAPD) uses a bag of dialysis fluid attached to a catheter leading into the patient's abdomen. This allows the patient to move around during the dialysis.
  + Patients on dialysis can enjoy a reasonable quality of life for several years, but about 2 per cent of patients with CKD will progress to kidney failure that requires a kidney transplant.
+ Kidney transplant uses a healthy kidney from a donor, frequently from a living close relative to minimise the risk of rejection of the transplanted organ.

The need for frequent dialysis can lead to depression and anxiety. This can be made worse when a patient is waiting for a transplant.

> **Exam practice**
>
> 1. People with untreated diabetes can have very high blood glucose concentrations. This leads to there being more glucose in the filtrate than can be reabsorbed. Explain, in terms of water potential, why a person with untreated diabetes will produce larger volumes of urine than normal. [3]
> 2. The loop of Henle is described as a countercurrent flow system.
>   a. Suggest why it is called countercurrent flow. [2]
>   b. Explain how the loop of Henle ensures water can be reabsorbed from the filtrate along the length of the collecting duct. [6]
> 3. Describe how the kidney is adapted for:
>   a. removal of urea from the blood [1]
>   b. reabsorption of glucose and amino acids from the filtrate in the PCT. [4]
> 4. Patients with CKD are usually offered dialysis but may require a kidney transplant later. For each treatment, give **two** advantages and **two** disadvantages. [8]

> **Exam tip**
>
> You will often be asked to evaluate the different treatment options for chronic diseases. Make sure you give both advantages and disadvantages. You will also get extra marks if you can draw a conclusion.

Integumentary system

B2.23 The role of the components in performing the functions of the integumentary system

REVISED

Components of the integumentary system

The integumentary system consists of the skin (Figure 13.31) and associated exocrine glands, as well as hair and nails.

> **Exocrine glands** These glands secrete products onto a surface such as the skin or into ducts such as the pancreatic duct.

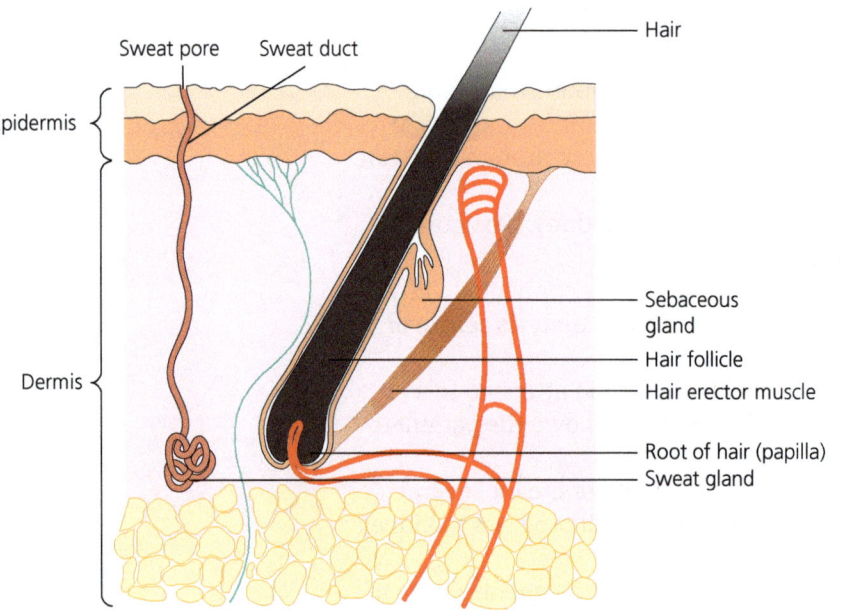

Figure 13.31 Cross-section of human skin

The epidermis is the strong surface layer that consists of squamous (flattened) epithelial cells. Stem cells in the lowest level of the epidermis divide to regenerate the epidermis as epithelial cells are worn away.

The dermis supports the epidermis and helps make the skin elastic. It contains blood vessels, hair follicles and exocrine glands (sweat glands and sebaceous glands).

Hair consists of the fibrous protein keratin and grows outwards from hair follicles. Nails are made of keratin, and keratin also helps waterproof the epidermis.

> **Making links**
>
> Stem cells and the structure of squamous epithelial cells were covered in B1.4.

Check your understanding and progress at www.hoddereducation.co.uk/myrevisionnotes

Functions of relevant components of the integumentary system

- Protection – the skin acts as a physical barrier to infection (see B1.20). Exocrine glands and benign bacteria living on the skin help protect against infection by pathogenic bacteria and fungi.
- Vitamin D is made in the lower layers of the epidermis, in a reaction that depends on sunlight. Lack of sunlight can lead to vitamin D deficiency, so vitamin D is added to some foods such as milk and breakfast cereals.
- Cutaneous sensation depends on mechanoreceptors in the dermis that respond to pressure and vibration. Between them they produce the sense of touch, as well as sensing heat, pain and chemicals such as capsaicin (found in chilli peppers).
- Exocrine glands:
  - The main function of sweat glands is to help reduce body temperature (see B2.24) but sweat contains inorganic ions and urea, so it plays a part in excretion.
  - Sebaceous glands secrete oily sebum that helps lubricate skin and hair. It also keeps the skin slightly acidic, which protects against pathogens.

> **Making links**
>
> Endocrine glands were covered in B2.14. These are glands that release their products (usually hormones) directly into the blood. Exocrine glands release their products onto a surface, such as the skin, or into ducts like the bile duct and pancreatic duct; this was covered in B2.23. Make sure you do not get the two types of gland mixed up.

B2.24 The components and processes involved in temperature regulation

REVISED

Regulation of body temperature is controlled and co-ordinated by the hypothalamus, in the base of the brain (see B2.14). Temperature receptors in the hypothalamus monitor core body temperature, and peripheral temperature receptors, located in the skin, monitor the external temperature.

- Sweat glands release sweat when body temperature rises. Thermal energy is transferred from capillaries close to the surface of the skin to the water in sweat, causing it to evaporate. This cools the skin and reduces body temperature.
- Arterioles regulate the amount of blood flowing near the surface. When they constrict (vasoconstriction), less blood flows near the surface and less heat is lost. When they dilate (vasodilation), more blood flows near the surface and more heat is lost. This is controlled by nerve impulses from the hypothalamus.
- Hair erector muscles (see Figure 13.31) contract to raise the hairs, trapping a thicker layer of air next to the skin. This reduces heat loss when core body temperature falls. When core body temperature rises, these muscles relax and the hair lies flat, allowing for more heat loss. This is controlled by nerve impulses from the hypothalamus.
- Shivering is a reflex action involving small, rapid contractions of skeletal muscles. This generates heat that helps to increase core body temperature.

> **Making links**
>
> The principles of homeostasis were covered in B1.28. Temperature regulation is an important part of homeostasis.

> **Revision activity**
>
> Make a diagram showing the role of receptors, the hypothalamus and effectors in thermoregulation. Add to your diagram what happens when body temperature falls and rises.

B2.25 The development, impact and management of atopic eczema

REVISED

In atopic eczema, the skin becomes dry, itchy, inflamed and cracked. It is common in children, but can improve significantly or disappear completely as some children get older. Adults can develop atopic eczema for the first time.

Causes of the disease

Atopic eczema usually occurs in people with various allergies. These allergies and eczema probably have a common cause. There is a genetic element, as there is usually a family history of eczema or allergies. Food allergies or environmental factors (soaps or detergents), as well as stress or the weather, can act as triggers.

Impact on systems within the body and on physical and mental health

Symptoms range from relatively mild to more serious:
+ Dry, flaky skin affects the hands, insides of elbows, backs of the knees and face and scalp in children.
+ Feet and hands are most affected in adults.
+ In severe cases, the skin can be unbearably itchy. Scratching can damage the skin and increase the risk of infection.

Like other chronic diseases, the lack of a cure and the effect on daily life of having to live with the symptoms can have an impact on patients' mental health. Eczema can affect how a person looks, and so even relatively mild symptoms can cause embarrassment, anger, frustration or depression, particularly if the eczema is prominent, such as on the face.

> **Making links**
>
> People with atopic eczema can have flare-ups where symptoms become more severe. This also happens in other chronic inflammatory conditions, such as rheumatoid arthritis (B2.3) or Crohn's disease (B2.13).

How common treatments relieve symptoms

Table 13.3 Eczema treatments and effects

Treatment	Effect on symptoms
Emollients	Moisturising reduces dry, flaky skin.
Topical corticosteroids, for example hydrocortisone cream	These reduce inflammation, swelling, redness and itching. Side effects can include thinning of the skin.
Dietary changes	These are effective when certain foods are known to trigger symptoms.
Environmental changes	Avoiding pollen, allergens, dust etc. can also help where these are known to trigger symptoms.
Behavioural changes	Avoiding scratching reduces skin damage; avoiding certain fabrics, soaps and detergents can remove these as triggers.

Because symptoms of atopic eczema can vary from mild to severe between patients, or even within a single patient at different times, the most appropriate treatment can vary (see Table 13.3). For example, emollients can be used successfully, but corticosteroids might be required to control more severe flare-ups. In other patients, low-strength corticosteroid cream can be used on a regular basis, with stronger corticosteroid cream being used to control flare-ups. Once under control, the patient can return to a lower-strength corticosteroid.

> **Exam tip**
>
> Exam questions about chronic diseases often suggest a range of different treatments and ask you to evaluate the different options. Make sure you are familiar with the pros and cons of each type of treatment, and remember that for highest marks, you need to consider advantages and disadvantages in your evaluation. Ideally, you should also offer a conclusion.

> **Exam practice**
>
> 1 State the names of the two layers of the skin. [2]
> 2 Describe **two** ways in which sweat glands are involved in homeostasis. [2]
> 3 Describe **two** ways in which the skin helps protect against infection. [2]
> 4 Recent treatments for atopic eczema include creams containing ceramide and probiotics. Ceramide is a lipid normally found in the skin, but levels are reduced in eczema. Probiotic creams contain live bacteria that are normally found on the skin, but which may be reduced or absent in eczema. Evaluate the use of these creams as alternatives to existing treatments. [9 + 3 QWC]

Check your understanding and progress at www.hoddereducation.co.uk/myrevisionnotes

Reproductive system

B2.26 The role of the components in performing the functions of reproductive systems

REVISED

Sexual reproduction involves the production of male and female gametes that are brought together in the process of fertilisation to form a zygote. This develops into the embryo and then the foetus. The components of the male and female reproductive systems are shown in Figure 13.32.

> **Gametes** Gametes (sperm and egg cells in humans) are haploid cells produced by meiosis, a type of cell division that halves the number of chromosomes.
>
> **Fertilisation** Fusion of haploid gametes to produce a diploid zygote with the full number of chromosomes.

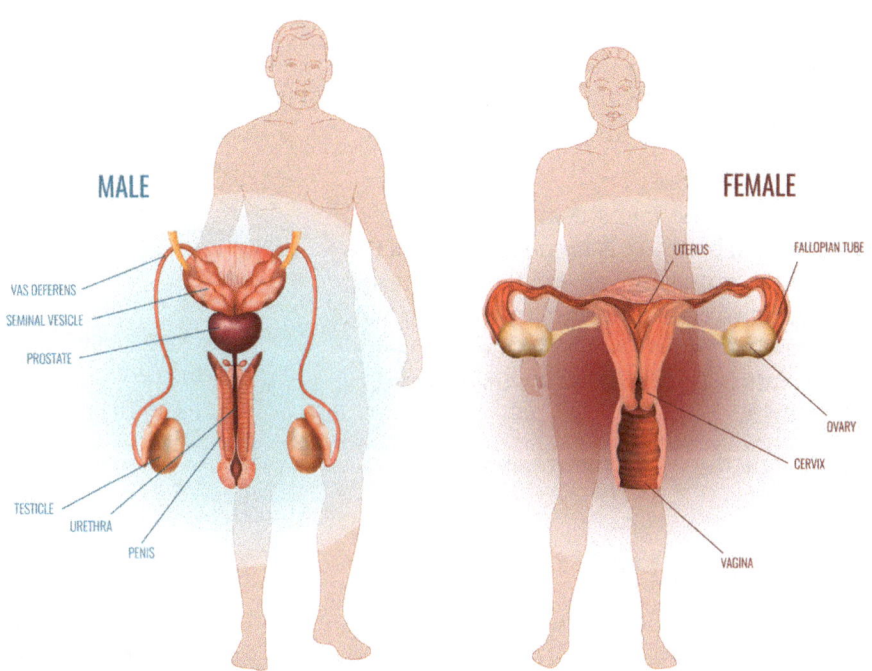

Figure 13.32 The human reproductive system

The components of the female reproductive system

+ Ovaries – the site of production of female gametes (egg cells or ova). There is one ovary on each side.
+ Fallopian tubes – they connect the ovaries with the uterus.
+ Uterus – the organ where the foetus develops following fertilisation.
+ Cervix – a ring of muscle that helps retain the developing foetus within the uterus. A plug of mucus in the cervix acts as a barrier to pathogens while allowing sperm to pass from the vagina into the uterus.
+ Vagina – the elastic, muscular part of the female reproductive system that allows loss of menstrual blood (see B2.27), receives sperm during sexual intercourse and forms the birth canal along which the baby moves during childbirth.

The components of the male reproductive system

+ Penis – erectile tissue that allows insertion of the penis into the vagina during sexual intercourse, and the penis encloses the urethra.
+ Urethra – it transports semen, which is delivered to the vagina in the process of ejaculation. The urethra also connects to the bladder to provide an exit for urine.
+ Testes – the site of production of the male gametes (sperm). The singular of testes is testis, but you may also see the term *testicle* (as used in Figure 13.32).

- Scrotum – it encloses and holds the testes outside the body, as they need a slightly lower temperature for normal sperm development.
- Vas deferens – there are two, one for each testicle, and they carry sperm from the testes to the urethra.
- Seminal vesicles – each vas deferens meets a seminal vesicle before coming together to enter the urethra. Seminal vesicles produce a fluid rich in fructose (a monosaccharide) that helps nourish the sperm.
- Prostate – it surrounds the urethra just below the bladder and contributes a fluid that also helps nourish the sperm. Combination of sperm with these two fluids produces semen.

The functions of the relevant components within the male and female reproductive systems

Sexual reproduction provides a mechanism for the survival of the species by producing offspring through the combination of eggs and sperm. However, we know from studying inheritance that sexual reproduction leads to genetic variation, and this is the basis of natural selection and evolution.

The female reproductive system has two functions:
- To produce egg cells. This happens during the menstrual cycle (B2.27).
- To protect and nourish an offspring until birth. This is the function of the uterus and placenta. Part of the embryo grows into the wall of the uterus and develops into the placenta. This has a rich blood supply that is in close contact with that of the mother, allowing for exchange of gases (oxygen and carbon dioxide), supply of nutrients (glucose, amino acids etc.) and removal of waste products such as urea.

The male reproductive system has one function – to produce and deposit sperm (see above).

> **Now test yourself**
> 1. Describe the route taken by sperm from production in the testis to fertilisation of the egg cell.
> 2. Give **two** functions of:
>   a. the cervix
>   b. the male urethra.
>
> TESTED

B2.27 The role of hormones in the reproductive systems

REVISED

Menstrual cycle regulation

The menstrual cycle in females is complex and involves hormones produced by the pituitary, ovaries and uterus. The cycle takes about 28 days, although it is often longer or shorter and can be irregular.

The cycle is regulated by several hormones working together. The cycle starts (day 1) with menstruation, when breakdown of the wall of the uterus leads to bleeding from the vagina (a period). Figure 13.33 on the next page shows the development of a follicle, leading to release of an egg cells (ovulation) and formation of the corpus luteum.
- If fertilisation does not occur, the corpus luteum breaks down and the concentrations of progesterone and oestrogen decrease. This triggers menstruation, on about day 28, and the cycle begins again.
- If fertilisation does occur, the placenta takes over production of progesterone and the lining of the uterus is maintained throughout pregnancy.

There are several negative feedback mechanisms at work:

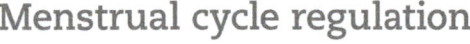

Oestrogen causes a surge in LH → the corpus luteum releases progesterone → progesterone inhibits release of LH and FSH

> **Making links**
> The general function of the endocrine system was covered in B2.14.
>
> B1.28 explained the principles of negative feedback and its importance in homeostasis, but negative feedback is also important in regulation of the menstrual cycle.

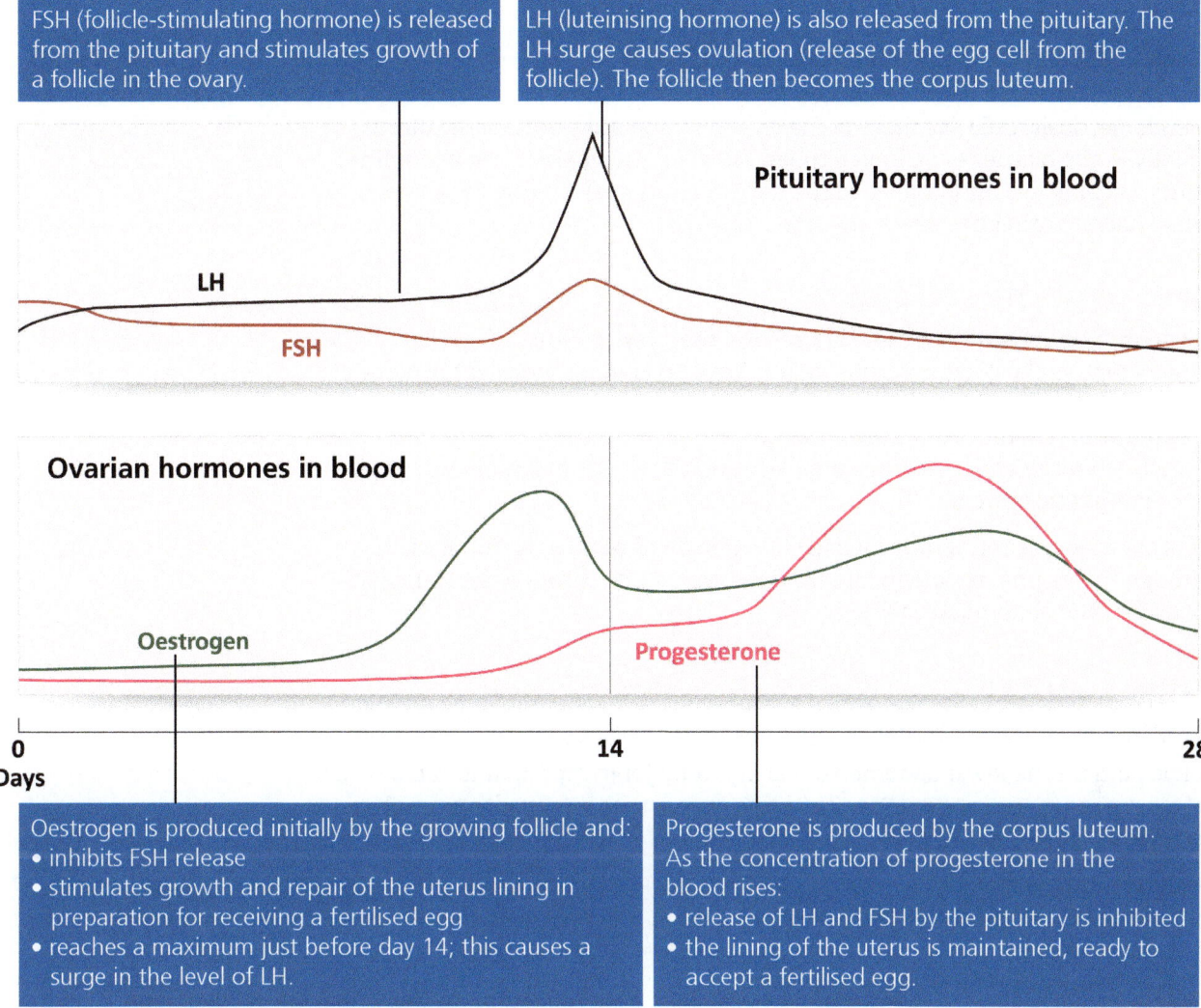

Figure 13.33 The regulation of the menstrual cycle in human females

The growth and development of female/male reproductive characteristics

Oestrogen and testosterone are described as the sex hormones and their actions were covered in B2.14. Males have higher levels of testosterone and females have higher levels of oestrogen, although both hormones are present in both sexes. Puberty is the stage where a child's body develops into an adult body. At puberty:
+ Gonadotropin-releasing hormone (GnRH) (also called luteinising hormone-releasing hormone, LHRH) is released by the hypothalamus and acts on the pituitary.
+ This stimulates the pituitary to release FSH and LH in both males and females.
+ FSH and LH stimulate testes and ovaries to begin secreting the male and female sex hormones.
+ This leads to development of the male and female reproductive organs, as well as secondary sexual characteristics:
  + pubic and underarm hair in both sexes
  + facial hair and increased muscle mass in males
  + widening of the hips and breast development in females.
+ In females, FSH and LH lead to the onset of the menstrual cycle.
+ In males, LH stimulates secretion of testosterone by the testes and FSH makes the testes more responsive to testosterone, leading to sperm production.

> **Revision activity**
>
> Draw the curves for levels of FSH, LH, oestrogen and progesterone as shown in Figure 13.33. Annotate your diagram with:
> + the effects of each hormone as the concentrations rise and then fall
> + how negative feedback helps to explain the shape of the curves.

> **Now test yourself**
>
> 1 Give **one** action of LH in males and **two** actions in females.
> 2 Give the names of **two** structures that secrete progesterone in females.
>
> TESTED

B2.28 The development, impact and management of endometriosis

REVISED

In endometriosis, cells like those of the endometrium grow outside the uterus – usually in the ovaries or Fallopian tubes, but also elsewhere in the abdominal cavity, causing lesions (damage to the tissues or organs) or adhesions (where cells attach to other tissues or organs).

> **Endometrium** A layer of epithelial tissue that lines the uterus.

Causes of the condition

Causes are unknown – but there are several theories:
+ genetics, as the condition runs in families and is more prevalent in some ethnic groups
+ a malfunction of the immune system
+ cells from the endometrium spread through the body in the bloodstream or lymphatic system.

Another theory is retrograde menstruation: instead of flowing out of the body through the vagina, endometrial cells flow backwards through the Fallopian tubes into the abdominal cavity.

Impact on systems within the body and on physical and mental health

Pelvic pain (in the lower abdomen or back) is a major symptom and can be worse during menstruation. Pain can be so severe that it prevents normal activities.

Other symptoms include:
+ nausea (feeling sick)
+ constipation
+ diarrhoea or blood in the urine or faeces
+ very heavy periods.

Diagnosis can take many years.
+ A first step is transvaginal ultrasound – an ultrasound transducer is inserted into the vagina to visualise organs in the pelvic cavity.
+ Accurate diagnosis requires laparoscopy, a surgical procedure that inserts a small camera inside the abdominal cavity to observe lesions or adhesions.

There is increased risk of depression and anxiety disorders. This is partly due to the severe pelvic pain but may be made worse by delays in diagnosis.

How common treatments relieve symptoms or cure the condition

Like many chronic conditions, there is no real cure for endometriosis, so treatments focus on relief of symptoms:
+ pain relief medication, such as ibuprofen and paracetamol
+ hormone-based treatments, including contraceptives; these make periods lighter and shorter, decreasing growth of endometrial tissue and reducing inflammation
+ laparoscopy surgery to remove lesions or adhesions; in more severe cases, all or part of the organs affected can be removed (part of the colon or uterus (hysterectomy)).

B2.29 The process of in vitro fertilisation (IVF) in the treatment of infertility

There are many causes of infertility – some are connected to the male reproductive system and some to the female. The cause of infertility will influence the treatment options.

The main stages of IVF treatment

+ The natural menstrual cycle is suppressed to allow control of the procedure.
+ The ovaries are stimulated to produce more eggs (ovarian hyperstimulation).
+ Progress is monitored using ultrasound scans to check development of maturing follicles.
+ Around 10–30 eggs are collected by inserting a needle through the vagina and into the ovaries.
+ Eggs and sperm are checked and any that are defective are discarded. The sperm and eggs are mixed for a few hours to allow egg fertilisation.
+ Embryos are transferred into the uterus after incubating the fertilised eggs for 2–6 days.

The role of hormones within the main stages of IVF treatment

FSH is used in ovarian hyperstimulation. By suppressing the natural menstrual cycle and hyperstimulating with FSH, more than the usual 1 or 2 eggs will be produced, so enough embryos can be produced to allow successful transfer.

Factors affecting the number of embryos transferred

+ Mother's age – the success rate decreases with the age of the woman having treatment.
+ IVF cycle – one embryo would normally be transferred on the first cycle, but if this is unsuccessful then two embryos would be transferred on the second and subsequent cycles.
+ Quality of embryos – this can be judged before transfer and, if they are not high quality, more than one can be transferred to increase the chances of success.

Infertility can have a negative effect on the mental health of the woman and her partner. However, IVF can also be detrimental to mental health, particularly if it is unsuccessful. Even successful IVF can be stressful because of the effects of the treatment and also the uncertainty in the early stages of pregnancy.

> **Revision activity**
>
> Prepare an information sheet that would be suitable for use with patients considering IVF. This should cover a description of the techniques that will be used, together with a summary of the risks and benefits of IVF.

> **Exam practice**
>
> 1 A 25-year-old woman presents with a history of pelvic pain that has lasted several years and is particularly severe during her periods.
>   a What diagnostic procedures would confirm that she is suffering from endometriosis? [2]
>   b After diagnosis, she is offered pain relief medication, but is told that oral contraceptives might be required to control her condition more effectively. Evaluate the potential impact of each course of treatment. [4]
> 2 A 42-year-old woman has been trying to conceive naturally without success and is beginning IVF. Describe the treatment that she would be given and evaluate the risks and benefits associated with IVF for this person. [9 + 3 for QWC]

Cancer

B2.30 The difference between benign and malignant tumours

REVISED

Cancer refers to a group of diseases where abnormal cells grow and divide uncontrollably. This usually forms a tumour, although some types of cancer, such as leukaemia and other blood cancers, do not involve tumours.

Benign tumours are not cancerous:
+ They are slow growing.
+ They do not invade nearby tissue or spread around the body.

Benign does not mean harmless. A benign tumour may press on key body parts, particularly in the brain, and become life-threatening. In rare cases, benign tumours can become cancerous.

Malignant tumours are cancerous:
+ Some, but not all, are fast growing.
+ They can invade nearby tissue and spread around the body.

> **Tumour** A solid mass of tissue that forms when abnormal cells group together. Tumours may be benign or malignant.

> **Now test yourself** — TESTED
>
> 1 Copy and complete the following:
>   a A tumour is a _____ mass of tissue.
>   b Benign tumours are not _____.
>   c Tumour formation is the result of _____ cell division.
> 2 Are benign tumours harmless? Explain your answer.

B2.31 The development, impact and management of cancer

REVISED

Most cancers do not produce symptoms in the early stages. Doctors use a staging and grading system:
+ Stages are numbered 0–4, where stage 0 means the cancer has just started and not spread and stage 4 means the cancer has spread to at least one other organ; this is known as metastatic cancer. Some types of cancer use a system of letters and numbers to describe the stage.
+ The grade of cancer is based on the appearance of the cells under a microscope. Grade 1 cancer cells resemble normal cells and are not growing rapidly, whereas grade 3 cancer cells look abnormal and grow or spread more aggressively.

Different types of cancer and how common treatments relieve symptoms

Invasive breast cancer
The most common form of breast cancer is invasive breast cancer. Cancer cells develop in the milk ducts and spread to the surrounding breast tissue. One in eight women will be diagnosed with breast cancer, although it can also (more rarely) affect men. Table 13.4 shows common treatments.

Oestrogen can sometimes stimulate breast cancer cells and cause them to grow, so the risk can be increased in women who start menstruating earlier or begin the menopause later (because they are exposed to oestrogen for longer). Pregnancy and breastfeeding interrupt the regular cycle, so they decrease the risk.

> **Making links**
>
> You will notice the term *lymph nodes* used in connection with various cancers – sometimes cancerous cells spread to the lymph nodes. These are parts of the lymphatic system, that play an important part in the body's defence against infection, as covered in the section on immunology (B1.14–B1.22). Lymphocytes get their name because of their association with the lymphatic system, and the immune system can play a part in protecting the body against cancer.

Table 13.4 Treatments for breast cancer

Treatment	Details
Breast-conserving surgery and mastectomy	Lumpectomy is removal of just the tumour; wide local excision also removes a small amount of surrounding breast tissue; partial mastectomy removes up to a quarter of the breast tissue. Mastectomy removes the whole breast and sometimes also lymph nodes in the armpit.
Chemotherapy and/or radiotherapy	This usually follows on from surgery to destroy any remaining cancer cells.
Hormone therapy	Tamoxifen stops oestrogen binding to its receptor in cells and so treats tumours that are stimulated to grow by oestrogen.
Monoclonal antibody therapy	This is a type of targeted therapy. Herceptin® controls growth of cells that have the HER2 receptor (about 20 per cent of breast cancers).
Talking therapies	Talking, counselling and support groups can support the mental health of the patient.

Chemotherapy A form of cancer treatment that uses drugs that are toxic to living cells. Because cancer cells grow more rapidly than most normal cells, they are selectively killed by the drugs.

Radiotherapy This uses high-energy radiation to destroy cancer cells. This can be done using a beam of radiation or by delivery of radioactive materials to the site of the tumour.

Thyroid cancer

There are several types of thyroid cancer; papillary thyroid cancer is the most common. It is usually slow growing but can spread to lymph nodes in the neck. Treatments are given in Table 13.5.

Risk factors include:
+ an under- or over-active thyroid gland
+ exposure to high levels of radiation or radiotherapy
+ a family history of thyroid cancer.

Table 13.5 Treatments for thyroid cancer

Treatment	Details
Thyroidectomy	This is the most common treatment and involves surgical removal of some or all of the thyroid gland. Lymph nodes are also removed if there is a risk the cancer has spread.
Radioactive iodine treatment	This kills cancer cells in the thyroid because the thyroid takes up iodine from the blood.
Talking therapies	These support patients' mental health and help deal with the practical difficulties associated with radioactive iodine treatment.

Non-Hodgkin lymphoma

This is a cancer that develops in the lymphatic system. Lymphocytes start to multiply in an abnormal way. They collect in the lymph nodes and lose their ability to fight infection. Treatments are shown in Table 13.6.

Risk factors include:
+ a weakened immune system
+ autoimmune disease
+ infection with Epstein–Barr virus (EBV) that causes glandular fever
+ infection with *Helicobacter pylori*, a common bacterial infection that causes stomach ulcers.

The appropriate type of treatment depends on the category of disease. High-grade lymphomas grow quickly and aggressively but respond well to treatment and can often be cured. Low-grade lymphomas grow slowly and may not necessarily require immediate medical attention but are harder to cure completely.

Making links

EBV is also thought to be a trigger for the destruction of pancreatic cells that leads to development of type 1 diabetes (B2.16).

Table 13.6 Treatments for non-Hodgkin lymphoma

Treatment	Details
Radiotherapy	This treats early-stage non-Hodgkin lymphoma if the cancer is in only one part of the body.
Chemotherapy	This may be used on its own or in combination with radiotherapy or monoclonal antibody therapy. If the disease does not improve with the initial treatment (known as refractory lymphoma), then a higher dose of chemotherapy is given. However, this will destroy the bone marrow and make it necessary to have a stem cell or bone marrow transplant to replace the damaged bone marrow.
Monoclonal antibody therapy	Rituximab binds to antigens on B lymphocytes and leads to their destruction. Once the treatment is over, a new population of healthy B lymphocytes develops from stem cells in the bone marrow. Monoclonal antibody therapy may last for up to 2 years in combination with chemotherapy.
Talking therapies	These can particularly help support patients with low-grade lymphomas that grow slowly and may not need medical attention but are harder to cure completely.

Acute myeloid leukaemia

Acute myeloid leukaemia (AML) is a cancer of the white blood cells, specifically monocytes and granulocytes. These are types of phagocyte (see B1.20) that differentiate from myeloid stem cells, unlike lymphocytes that differentiate from lymphoid stem cells – hence the term myeloid leukaemia. Treatments are shown in Table 13.7.

Risk factors include:
+ exposure to benzene, found in petrol, cigarette smoke and used in the rubber industry
+ genetic disorders such as Down's syndrome
+ radiotherapy or chemotherapy that can lead to AML many years later.

Table 13.7 Treatments for acute myeloid leukaemia

Treatment	Details
Chemotherapy	This is the main treatment for AML. This will kill as many of the leukaemia cells as possible, which reduces the risk of relapse (the cancer coming back). Intensive chemotherapy and radiotherapy are sometimes used together.
Bone marrow or stem cell transplants	Intensive chemotherapy and radiotherapy destroy the immune system, so a bone marrow or stem cell transplant will also be needed.
Talking therapies	AML progresses quickly and aggressively, usually requiring immediate treatment. Counselling can help support patients through an anxious time.

Germ cell testicular cancer

This is a relatively rare cancer, affecting about 1 per cent of men. It is unusual in that it affects mostly younger men. It is one of the most treatable forms of cancer. Treatments are shown in Table 13.8.

People with testicular cancer are particularly likely to experience high levels of stress.

Check your understanding and progress at www.hoddereducation.co.uk/myrevisionnotes

Table 13.8 Treatments for germ cell testicular cancer

Treatment	Details
Surgery	This involves surgical removal of the affected testicle (orchidectomy). It does not usually affect fertility or the ability to have sex.
Talking therapies	Surgery can lead to issues with self-esteem and body image. Patients recovering from testicular cancer are encouraged to find a counsellor or join a support group.

Causes of the condition

Rapid cell division is not unusual, for example in replacing skin cells as they wear away. Cancer is the result of uncontrolled cell division.

The cell cycle was covered in B1.6 and B1.7. Progress through the cycle is regulated and controlled. Checkpoints ensure there is no damage to the DNA or, if there is, then it is repaired. If the DNA cannot be repaired, the cell undergoes apoptosis – a form of controlled cell death. Mutation in any of the enzymes and proteins involved can lead to tumour formation.

Cell division is controlled by two types of gene:
+ Tumour-suppressor genes slow down the rate of cell division, help to repair DNA or increase the rate of apoptosis in cells with unrepairable DNA. Mutations in these genes can lead to uncontrolled cell division.
+ Proto-oncogenes increase the rate of cell division. Mutations in these genes produce oncogenes that also lead to uncontrolled cell division.

Mutation is a random process, but the rate of mutation can be increased by:
+ damage to DNA from ionising radiation (X-rays or UV light) or chemicals in the environment
+ biological agents, particularly viruses such as HIV and EBV.

Mutation in the genes coding for the enzymes and proteins that check and repair DNA will increase the number of other mutations that go unrepaired.

Besides the risk factors for specific cancers described above, there are general risk factors for cancer:
+ Age – the risk increases with age, as mutations accumulate throughout life.
+ Lifestyle factors – smoking, body mass, diet, level of physical activity, amount of exposure to sunlight and alcohol intake all contribute to the risk of developing cancer.
+ Family history is a factor in some types of cancer, suggesting that there is a genetic factor.

Impact on systems within the body and on physical and mental health

As well as the specific effects of different cancers described above, there are several general effects:
+ Blockages, for example in the blood, lymphatic system or gut, when a tumour presses on surrounding organs. In brain tumours, even if they are benign, this can be life-threatening.
+ Weight loss, which can be due to loss of appetite, nausea and vomiting. Also, cancer cells have a very high demand for energy, so they use a lot of glucose, which leaves less available for other cells in the body.

Exam practice

1. Name **two** classes of gene that can mutate to lead to cancer. [2]

2. A patient presents with a soft lump on their right arm, which is diagnosed as a lipoma. Lipomas are a type of soft-tissue tumour formed from fat cells. They are slow growing and non-cancerous.

   Name the category of tumour that the patient has been diagnosed with. [1]

3. A patient has presented following a series of infections of different kinds and is diagnosed with high-grade non-Hodgkin lymphoma.

   a. Suggest reasons you would give to the patient for being treated as soon as possible. [2]

   b. The patient is recommended to start a course of radiotherapy. They are told that, if this is not effective, there are two options.

   Option 1 is a course of chemotherapy. If that does not bring about an improvement in the disease, then a higher dose will be required, but this will destroy their bone marrow and they will require a bone marrow transplant.

   Option 2 is monoclonal antibody therapy, in combination with lower-dose chemotherapy. This would destroy cancerous B lymphocytes. These would then be replaced naturally by their own bone marrow.

   Evaluate these two options. [6]

Glossary

Accountability To accept that you are responsible for your own actions.

Active site The part of the enzyme where the substrate binds. Its shape is complementary to that of the substrate.

Advanced life support (ALS) Advanced clinical skills for resuscitation. Only professionals that hold, or are in training for, a professional healthcare qualification may be trained in ALS.

Advocacy services Services that provide an advocate for an individual, to help them express their opinions and get their voice heard.

Alveoli Small air-filled sacs at the ends of bronchioles. They have a wall consisting of a single layer of epithelial cells. The singular is alveolus.

Anaemia When the body does not have enough healthy red blood cells.

Antibodies Blood proteins produced in response to, and counteracting, specific antigens.

Anti-discriminatory practice Practice which aims to undermine, reduce or prevent discrimination.

Antigen A substance recognised by the immune system as self or non-self and that stimulates an immune response.

Antimicrobial A substance that kills microorganisms or stops their growth.

Antimicrobial stewardship The effort to measure and improve how antibiotics are prescribed by clinicians and used by patients. Improving antibiotic prescribing and use is critical in continuing to treat infections effectively.

Audit An on-site verification activity, which checks compliance with an agreed standard.

Autoimmune disease Caused by the immune system attacking the body's own cells and tissues, rather than foreign antigens such as those on pathogens.)

Autonomy A person's ability to act in their own interests.

Basic life support (BLS) Uses CPR and/or external defibrillation for resuscitation. Anyone can be trained to use BLS.

Befriending service The organised provision of supportive and reliable friendships, usually through volunteer networks.

Beneficence The act of doing or producing something good.

Biomarkers A broad category of medical signs that can be measured accurately. They can indicate a normal biological process, a pathogenic process (one caused by disease) or a response to medication. Biomarkers range from blood pressure measurements to blood cholesterol tests to chemical reactions at the cellular level.

Caldicott principles Eight principles to ensure people's information is kept confidential and used appropriately.

Calibration Checking that equipment is operating correctly against a required standard and making any adjustments to return it to the standard.

Capacity The ability to decide for yourself what is in your own best interest.

Cardiac arrest When the heart suddenly stops. Blood stops being pumped around the body and the brain becomes starved of oxygen. This causes the person to become unconscious and stop breathing. Death occurs within minutes of the heart stopping.

Cardiopulmonary resuscitation (CPR) Hands-only CPR is giving chest compressions to a person in cardiac arrest to keep them alive until emergency help arrives. CPR with rescue breaths includes respiratory support.

Cartilage A type of connective tissue containing collagen and the elastic protein elastin; it is more flexible than ligaments and tendons but not as hard as bone.

Cell cycle The cycle of division, growth and further division that all dividing cells go through.

Chemotherapy A form of cancer treatment that uses drugs that are toxic to living cells. Because cancer cells grow more rapidly than most normal cells, they are selectively killed by the drugs.

Chromatids Sometimes called sister chromatids. The two identical copies of a chromosome formed as a result of DNA replication. The term *chromatid* is a shorter way of saying 'one of a pair of identical chromosomes'.

Chronic inflammatory diseases Long-term conditions caused when the body's normal inflammatory response, for example to infection or injury becomes excessive.

Civil legal action Used for non-criminal offences, such as breach of contract, personal injury or negligence. Civil law is concerned with the rights and property of individual people or organisations.

Cleaning A process used to physically remove contamination, for example blood or faeces, that does not necessarily destroy microorganisms.

Collaborative approaches Healthcare professionals and agencies, community groups and interest groups such as charities, governmental agencies and individuals all co-operating to improve health.

Co-morbidity The presence of two or more diseases or conditions in one patient.

Competent Having the necessary knowledge, skill or ability to do something.

Condensation reaction A reaction between two small molecules to produce a larger molecule and water. A number of large biological molecules are formed by condensation reactions.

Glossary

Conduct The way in which a person behaves, especially in a particular place or situation, such as at work.

Connective tissue Connects, supports or binds tissues or other organs. It consists mostly of the protein collagen.

Consumables Items used by healthcare providers to treat people that are usually single-use products, for example bandages.

Contamination The unwanted pollution of something by another substance.

Continuing professional development (CPD) A process of continual learning and development to keep skills and knowledge up to date so that employees can work safely and effectively.

Contraindication When a medication or treatment should not be used because it may cause harm, for example if it interacts with food or drink taken, or another medication or treatment being taken.

Controlled conditions Ensuring extraneous variables (those not being studied) are controlled so they do not affect results.

Criminal prosecution Criminal law relates to offences and breaches that have an impact on the whole of society. If an action goes against UK law, this is a criminal offence and criminal legal action is taken.

Cross-contamination When microorganisms such as bacteria are accidentally transferred from one substance or object to another.

Cycle of disadvantage The concept that people who grow up in poverty are more likely to suffer from health problems, social isolation, housing instability and unemployment and are less likely to reach their full potential in life. This disadvantage, in turn, is transmitted to the next generation.

Cytokinesis When the cytoplasm divides to form two daughter cells after nuclear division.

Decontamination A process to remove or destroy contamination. Three processes of decontamination are used: cleaning, disinfection and sterilisation.

Deficiency diseases Conditions that arise due to a long-term lack of a vitamin or mineral in the body.

Depolarisation The reversal of the resting potential; the inside of the cell is now positive.

Deprivation of liberty This is when an individual is not free to go anywhere without permission or close supervision and lacks capacity to consent to this. This is against the law unless done under the rules of the Mental Capacity Act 2005.

Deregistration The act of removing a professional from an official register (of practice).

Diastole The relaxation of the atrium (atrial diastole) or ventricle (ventricular diastole).

Diffusion The movement of a substance from a high concentration to a low concentration.

Disaccharides Made up of two monosaccharides joined by a glycosidic bond.

Disclosure The process in which an individual shares or starts to share information about abuse or neglect.

Disinfection A process used to reduce the number of viable microorganisms (although it may not inactivate certain pathogens).

Disposition A person's usual way of feeling or behaving, for example a person's tendency to be happy and optimistic.

DNA (deoxyribonucleic acid) A double-stranded molecule containing the genetic information responsible for the development and function of an organism.

Duty of care A moral or legal obligation to ensure the safety or wellbeing of others. In this context, employers such as the NHS have a duty of care to their employees.

Effector A gland or muscle that makes changes to return factors to their normal level.

Endemic A disease or condition regularly found in certain populations or local areas.

Endocrine glands These glands release hormones into the blood.

Endometrium A layer of epithelial tissue that lines the uterus.

Epidemic The widespread occurrence of a disease in a community at a particular time.

Equality Ensuring every individual has equal opportunities in life.

Escalation Taking your concern further or to a more senior person.

Ethical values Moral principles that guide behaviour and conduct.

Exocrine glands These glands secrete products onto a surface such as the skin or into ducts such as the pancreatic duct.

Expiration Breathing out.

External defibrillator A medical device used outside of the body to give a person in cardiac arrest a jolt of energy to the heart to re-establish a normal rhythm. Also known as a defib, an AED (automated external defibrillator) or a PAD (public access defibrillator).

Fertilisation Fusion of haploid gametes to produce a diploid zygote with the full number of chromosomes.

First aid Help given immediately after an injury or illness occurs, often at the location where it occurred.

Flagellum (plural, **flagella**) A slender, thread-like structure that is used to move cells, such as sperm cells.

Fluid mosaic model A model of the structure of the cell-surface membrane and how its components are arranged like tiles in a mosaic.

Function The role of a part or system; what it does.

Gametes Gametes (sperm and egg cells in humans) are haploid cells produced by meiosis, a type of cell division that halves the number of chromosomes.

Gaslighting Making an individual question their perception of reality.

Gastrointestinal tract (GI tract) The tube-like structure from mouth to anus that forms a part of the digestive system.

Gender dysphoria Deep sense of distress that may occur when an individual's biological sex does not match their gender identity.

Gene A sequence of bases in DNA that codes for (contains the information to make) a polypeptide (protein).

Gland A group of cells that make chemicals such as hormones or enzymes.

Grievance A concern, problem or complaint someone may have at work.

Half-life The time taken for half of the unstable nuclei in a sample to undergo radioactive decay.

Hazard An event, object, substance, condition or activity that has the potential to cause harm.

Health screening A way of identifying whether apparently healthy people have an increased risk of a particular condition. Part of preventative healthcare.

Hepatitis Inflammation of the liver. It may be caused by drinking alcohol (alcoholic hepatitis) or a virus. There are several types of viral hepatitis, known as A, B, C, D and E.

Holistic Considering the whole person; acknowledging that physical health cannot be separated from other elements of the person (such as psychological wellbeing) and their environment.

Homeostasis The maintenance of an almost constant internal environment despite fluctuations in the external environment.

Hormone A chemical messenger released into the blood by an endocrine gland that acts on a target elsewhere in the body.

Hospice care Care given to individuals with a terminal illness with the aim of improving quality of life and wellbeing, either in a residential care home setting or the service user's own home.

Hospital passport A document that individuals with a learning disability create and carry with them. It explains their healthcare and support needs, learning disability, communication preferences and how to make things easier for them.

Hyperglycaemia When the blood glucose concentration rises above the normal or optimal level.

Hypoglycaemia When the blood glucose concentration falls below the normal or optimal level.

Impartiality Not taking sides and remaining objective.

Infection When pathogens enter a person's body and multiply, causing illness, organ and tissue damage, or disease.

Inflammation A local response to injury and infection.

Injury Damage to the body caused by external force.

Inspiration Breathing in.

Internship The process of working within an organisation, sometimes without pay, to learn and gain experience.

Ionisation The formation of charged particles from neutral molecules or atoms by adding or removing electrons.

Ionising radiation Radioactive particles, X-rays or gamma rays with sufficient energy to cause damage when passing through something, such as cells in the body, due to ionisation.

Isolation Separating infected individuals from others, to prevent the spread of infection.

Joint The area where two or more bones connect.

Legislation A law or set of laws passed by Parliament.

Liability The state of being legally responsible for something.

Ligaments and tendons Both are connective tissues made of collagen. Ligaments join bones together, while tendons attach muscles to bones.

Lymphocytes Small white blood cells. B lymphocytes, or B cells, are involved in the antibody-mediated response. T lymphocytes, or T cells, are involved in the cell-mediated response.

Macronutrients The nutrients the body requires in large quantities for energy: fat, protein and carbohydrate.

Makaton A language programme that uses a combination of symbols, basic signs and speech to enable people to communicate. It is most often used with individuals with learning disabilities.

Menopause When menstruation ceases. This usually occurs in middle adulthood.

Mental capacity The ability to make decisions, by being able to understand information and remember it for long enough to make the decision and then communicate it to others.

Micronutrients The nutrients the body requires in trace (very small) amounts for normal growth and development: vitamins A, B, C, D, E, K and minerals such as calcium, copper, iodine, iron, magnesium and zinc.

Mitosis A process of cell reproduction in which one cell gives rise to two genetically identical daughter cells.

Monosaccharide The most basic carbohydrate. Glucose is a monosaccharide.

Morbidity data Rates of a disease, medical condition or set of symptoms in a population.

Multidisciplinary An approach where health professionals from a range of specialties (disciplines) work together to achieve the best outcomes for service users.

Multidisciplinary team A team made up of people from different professional fields (disciplines) or with different job functions coming together to achieve a common goal for an individual.

Glossary

National Institute for Health and Care Excellence (NICE) An organisation that uses the best available evidence to compile guidelines and quality standards for health and social care provision. These guidelines make recommendations for best practice and what care the public should expect to receive.

Needs assessment A systematic process for deciding how to meet a need, for example how much first-aid provision is required in a workplace.

Negative feedback Returns a factor to its normal level when there is movement away from the normal level.

Nonmaleficence The principle of not causing harm to others.

Nursing associate A healthcare professional that fulfils a nursing role that bridges the gap between healthcare assistants and registered nurses.

Occupational therapist An allied healthcare professional that supports people of all ages to overcome challenges in their daily life, through assessment, goal planning and targeted adjustments to environment and activities.

Omission Failing to do something. Neglect (failing to provide access to care or ignoring medical, emotional or physical care needs) is an act of omission.

Orthotist An allied healthcare professional that provides engineered solutions to people experiencing issues with their neuro, muscular and skeletal systems, for example by designing, making and fitting braces, splints, callipers and so on.

Over-extrapolation To extrapolate (draw conclusions) excessively or well beyond known values.

Oxygen saturation A measure of the percentage amount of oxygen that is bound to the haemoglobin in the blood.

Pandemic A disease outbreak that is prevalent across a whole country or geographical area.

Pathogen A disease-causing microorganism.

Peer review When data/literature is evaluated by other experts in the same field.

Perimenopause The period immediately prior to the occurrence of menopause. May start at the end of early adulthood.

Personal information Any information where the person can be identified, directly or indirectly, including a person's name, address or date of birth. Also called personal data.

Phagocytes Cells that are produced in the bone marrow and circulate in the blood. Some leave the blood and are present in the tissues. They ingest pathogens.

Phagocytosis The process of a phagocyte engulfing and digesting a pathogen or other foreign material.

Phospholipid bilayer A two-layer arrangement of phosphate and lipid molecules that form cell membranes.

Physiological Relating to the functioning of the human body or body system.

Policy A document that sets out what an organisation will do, usually based on laws or regulations.

Polysaccharide A long polymer molecule made up of many monosaccharide units joined by glycosidic bonds.

Pre-existing health conditions Any long-term health conditions that a service user has, is aware of and is being treated for.

Primary research Gathering data that has not been collected before.

Procedure Instructions for how to follow an organisational policy.

Prosthetics An artificial body part, such as an arm, a foot or a tooth, used to replace a part that is missing, either from birth or due to accident or surgery.

Prosthetist An allied healthcare professional that provides engineered solutions to people with limb loss, for example by designing, making and fitting prosthetic legs.

Qualitative data Data that describes qualities or characteristics, or comments on opinion or experience.

Quantitative data Numerical data that expresses how many or how often.

Radicalisation The process by which an individual or a group becomes increasingly extreme in their views in opposition to political, social or religious norms in a society.

Radioactive decay The random process that occurs when an unstable nucleus loses energy by giving out alpha or beta particles or gamma radiation.

Radiotherapy This uses high-energy radiation to destroy cancer cells. This can be done using a beam of radiation or by delivery of radioactive materials to the site of the tumour.

Receptor It detects factors such as temperature or blood glucose concentration.

Referral The action of sending someone for further review, consultation or action, such as a GP referring a patient with a skin condition that is not responding to treatment to a dermatologist.

Reflective practice Thinking about situations and actions in a structured way and drawing points of learning from them.

Regenerative medicine Multidisciplinary science that aims to replace or regenerate human cells, tissues or organs to restore or establish normal functioning.

Regulator/statutory regulator An organisation appointed by the government to control an area of activity, such as healthcare, by means of rules.

Reliability How consistently a method measures something.

Repolarisation The return to the resting potential.

Report line The direction of communication and responsibility within an organisation. Also known as the chain of command.

Check your understanding and progress at www.hoddereducation.co.uk/myrevisionnotes

Reproducibility The extent to which consistent results are obtained when a study or experiment is repeated.

Research validity The extent to which the concept being studied is accurately measured. This requires the design and methods of the study to be well chosen.

Respiratory arrest Respiratory arrest is when a person stops breathing but their heart is still beating. Without rapid intervention, respiratory arrest will quickly lead to cardiac arrest.

Respiratory etiquette Covering the mouth and nose when coughing and sneezing; disposing of used tissues; and washing hands after touching the nose or mouth.

Respite care Planned or emergency temporary care of an individual (usually with complex needs) to provide their usual carers, often family, with a short break.

Resting potential The voltage difference between the inside and outside of a nerve cell. It is usually between −60 mV and −70 mV, i.e. the inside of the cell is more negative than the outside.

Resuscitation To revive someone from unconsciousness. It may be used interchangeably with the term *cardiopulmonary resuscitation* (CPR).

Risk The likelihood of harm occurring and the possible seriousness of that harm.

RNA (ribonucleic acid) A single-stranded molecule that turns genetic information into proteins.

Safeguarding The protection of the health, wellbeing and rights of individuals.

Scholarship A grant or payment made to support a period of learning.

Scope of practice The limit of a professional's knowledge, skills and experience. Comprises the activities they carry out within their professional role.

Screening The process of identifying individuals from the population who may have an increased chance of a disease or condition, so that treatment can begin early.

Secondary research Collating or analysing data that has already been collected.

Sedentary Spending a lot of time seated; a job that requires sitting at a desk all day can be described as a sedentary job.

Self-management Services that encourage, support and empower people to manage their own physical and mental health conditions themselves. Known in the NHS Long Term Plan as 'supported self-management'.

Sharps Equipment and instruments that have the capability of puncturing the skin, for example lancet devices, hypodermic needles and disposable scalpels.

Signposting Recommending or providing the contact details for additional resources, services and support networks.

Social care The provision of services that offer practical support to individuals who require it because of illness or disability.

Social model of disability The idea that people are disabled by barriers within society, rather than an individual impairment or difference. These barriers are seen not just in the physical environment but also in terms of the way that society is organised and operates.

Statutory regulation Regulation required by law.

Statutory training Training that is required for legal compliance. For example, fire safety training is a requirement of the Regulatory Reform (Fire Safety) Order (RRO) 2005.

Stem cells Unspecialised cells that can give rise to other stem cells or differentiate into specialised cells.

Sterilisation A process used to remove all viable microorganisms.

Striated muscle Named for its striped appearance under the microscope, striated muscle is also called skeletal muscle because it is attached to the skeleton and is the main type of muscle involved in movement.

Structure An arrangement of organised elements in a part or system.

Substrate The substance on which an enzyme acts to form the products.

Supply chain The network of all the individuals, organisations and processes involved in the creation, sale and receipt of a product.

Systole The contraction of the atrium (atrial systole) or ventricle (ventricular systole).

Telesurgery Technology that uses robotics and wireless networking to enable surgeons to operate on patients who are not in their immediate geographical location.

Trauma An injury that has the potential to cause disability or death.

Triage Deciding the urgency of a medical case based on signs and symptoms presented.

Tumour A solid mass of tissue that forms when abnormal cells group together. Tumours may be benign or malignant.

Vaccination A treatment given via injection, administered orally (by mouth) or sprayed into the nose. The vaccine triggers the body's immune system to create antibodies against the target disease. Part of preventative healthcare.

Validity How accurately a study or method measures what it intends to measure.

Water potential A measure of the relative tendency of water to move from one place to another by osmosis.

Whistleblowing When an employee passes on a concern of wrongdoing in the workplace that is causing or may cause harm. Or, if an employee has already tried to raise a serious concern about something they have seen but they do not feel it is being dealt with.

Index

6Cs, person-centred care 87–9
abbreviations 60
abuse 120
  action to take 123
  contributing factors 121
  reducing the chances of 124
  types of and signs of 122–3
accountability 12, 64
action potentials 182
active sites 138
active transport 139, 140, 141, 175
acute health conditions 17
acute myeloid leukaemia (AML) 198
adrenal glands 177
advanced life support (ALS) 43–4
advocacy services 83
ageing 104–5
agency job roles 27
alcohol consumption 102
alveoli 171
amino acids 136
anaemia 101
angina 169
antibodies 146
antigens 146
antimicrobial resistance 116
antimicrobial stewardship 117
aorta 164, 165
apps 19–20
arteries 164–5
artificial intelligence (AI) 21, 50
assistive computer technology 20
atherosclerosis 168
atria 164
atrioventricular node (AVN) 166
audit 9, 57
autoimmune disease 162
autonomy 10
Ayliffe handwashing technique 111–12
B cells 147–8
bacteria 144
barriers to healthcare access 19
basic life support (BLS) 43–4
befriending services 83
behaviour, challenging 83
beneficence 11
bereavement 85–7
biomarkers 23
blood 160, 165
blood glucose regulation 178
blood pressure 94, 153
blood vessels 164–5
body mass index (BMI) 100
bones 158–9
breast cancer 196–7
breathing 171
bundle of His 166
Caldicott principles 61
calibration 67–8

cancer 196
  acute myeloid leukaemia 198
  breast 196–7
  causes and risk factors 199
  effects of 199
  testicular 198–9
  thyroid 197–8
capacity 10
capillaries 164–5
carbohydrates 136–7
cardiac arrest 43–4
cardiac cycle 166, 167–8
cardiopulmonary resuscitation 44
cardiovascular system 164–5
  coronary heart disease 167–8
Care Act 2014 41, 71, 119
care needs, changes over the lifespan 75, 105–8
Care Quality Commission (CQC) 63, 73
career pathways 30
cartilage 159
cell cycle 135, 199
cell theory 129
cells 129
  organelles 130–1
  specialised 132–3
chain of infection 109
chemotherapy 197
chromatids 135
chronic health conditions 17
chronic inflammatory diseases 162, 172, 175–6
chronic kidney disease (CKD) 187
chronic obstructive pulmonary disease (COPD) 172
civil legal action 24
classification of diseases and disorders 154
cleaning 66, 110, 114–15
client histories 59
clinical effectiveness 125
codes of conduct 11–12
collaborative approaches 93
communication barriers 80
communication techniques 79–80
community care 22
co-morbidity 82
competence 10
comprehension factors 84
condensation reactions 136, 137
confidentiality 10, 52, 53
conflicts of interest 127–8
connective tissue 159
consent to treatment 10
consumables 68
contamination 66
continuing professional development (CPD) 8
controlled conditions 49
coronary heart disease (CHD) 167–8

co-transport mechanisms 139, 140, 175
COVID-19 31
criminal prosecution 24
Crohn's disease 175–6
cross-contamination 66, 69
cycle of disadvantage 7
cytokinesis 135
data collection 46–8
  recording information 48–9
data protection 55–6, 58, 74
Data Protection Act 2018 51–2
data recording and reporting 48–9
  use of new technology 50–1, 54–5
data sources, strengths and limitations 49
death and dying 85–7
decontamination 114–15
defibrillators 44
deficiency diseases 101
dementia 83–4
depolarisation 182
deprivation of liberty 81
diabetes 179–80
diastole 166, 167
diffusion 139, 171, 175
digestion 174
digestive system 173–5
  Crohn's disease 175–6
disabilities 82
disaccharides 137
disciplinary policies 8
disclosure 123
discrimination 7, 120
disinfection 110, 114, 115
DNA (deoxyribonucleic acid) 130, 142–3
Domestic Abuse Act 2021 120
Duchenne muscular dystrophy 162–3
duty of candour 63
duty of care 41, 63
Eatwell Guide 101
ECG (electrocardiography) 167
eczema 189–90
effectors 152
employment contracts 8
end-of-life care 85–6, 108
endemic diseases 31
endocrine system 177–8
  diabetes 179–80
  role in homeostasis 178–9
endometriosis 194
enzymes 138, 174
epidemics 31
epidemiology 150
equality 7
Equality Act 2010 7, 11, 120
escalation 123
ethical values 10–11
eukaryotic cells 129

Check your understanding and progress at www.hoddereducation.co.uk/myrevisionnotes

evidence-based practice 25–6
exam papers 6
exocrine glands 188–9
expiration 171
external factors 31
facilitated diffusion 140–1, 175
fatty acids 137
fertilisation 191
first aid 41, 42–3
flagella (singular: flagellum) 132
flat organisational structure 26
fluid mosaic model 139–40
funding of services 25
fungi 144
gametes 191
gas exchange 171
gaslighting 122
gastrointestinal tract (GI tract) 173
General Data Protection Regulation 2016 (GDPR) 51
gender dysphoria 18
General Dental Council (GDC) 72, 73
genes 142
glucagon 178
glycerol 137
grief 85, 86
grievance policies 8–9
half-life 155
hand hygiene 111–13
hazardous substances 36, 37
hazards 37
Health and Care Act 2022 119
Health and Care Professions Council (HCPC) 72, 73
Health and Safety Executive (HSE) 37, 74
health and safety incidents 40
Health and Safety legislation 35–7, 41–5
health and safety promotion 38–9
health apps 19–20
health inequalities 92
health promotion 98–9, 151
health screening 18
healthcare providers 15
healthcare sector development 22–3
heart 164, 166–8
heart rate 94, 153
hepatitis 102
higher technical occupations 12–13
holistic approaches 77–8, 103
homeostasis 152, 178–9
    osmoregulation 186
    temperature regulation 189
hormones 177–9
    reproductive 192–3, 195
hospice care 17, 85
hospital passports 83
Human Rights Act 1998 7, 11, 120
hydration 96
hygiene 111–13
hyperglycaemia 180
hypoglycaemia 95, 180
hypothalamus 177, 179
immune response 146–8

incidence 150
independence 84–5
infection prevention and control 109–10
infectious diseases, spread of 145
infertility 195
inflammation 147
Information Commissioner's Office (ICO) 74
information governance 58
informed consent 10
injury, body's response to 148
inspiration 171
insulin 178
    diabetes 179–80
integumentary system 188–9
internships 14
ionising radiation 41, 154
Ionising Radiation Regulations 2017 41
isolation 110
IT systems 54–5
IVF (in vitro fertilisation) 195
job descriptions 29
job roles 27
joints 159
justice 11
kidneys 185–6
    chronic kidney disease 187
learning disabilities 83–4
legislation 7
    data protection 51
    health and science sector 35–7
    and person-centred care 71
    purpose in relation to health sector 41–5
    safeguarding 119–20
liability 48
Liberty Protection Safeguards (LPS) 81
life stages 75
    potential care requirements 106–8
lifestyle choices 92–3, 100–2
ligaments 159
limb-girdle muscular dystrophy 163
lipids 137
lungs 170–1
lymph nodes 196
lymphocytes 147
macronutrients 100
magnification 134
Makaton 79
Making Every Contact Count (MECC) initiative 99
malnutrition 101
manual handling 44–5
    legislation 36
Maslow's hierarchy of needs 78, 79
Medicines and Healthcare Products Regulatory Agency (MHRA) 42
menopause 75
menstrual cycle 192–3
Mental Capacity Act (MCA) 2005 71, 81, 119
Mental Health Act 2007 119
mental health conditions 83–4

micronutrients 100
microorganisms 144
microscopes 134
missions 11
mitochondria (singular: mitochondrion) 130
mitosis 129, 134, 135
monosaccharides 136–7
morbidity 150
morbidity data 47
mortality 150
MRI (magnetic resonance imaging) 149
multidisciplinary teams 18, 28
muscle contraction 160–1
muscles 159–60
muscular dystrophies 162–3
musculoskeletal system 158–61
mutation 199
myotonic dystrophy 163
needs assessment 42
negative feedback 152
nephrons 185
nervous system 181–3
    Parkinson's disease 183–4
neurones 181
NHS 15, 22
    guide to safeguarding 120
NHS core values 76–7
NHS Long Term Plan 92
NICE (National Institute for Health and Care Excellence) 120
non-Hodgkin lymphoma 197–8
nonmaleficence 11
non-profit healthcare providers 15
nonverbal communication 79–80
nuclear medicine 154
nucleotides 142
Nursing and Midwifery Council (NMC) 72, 73
nutrition 96, 100–1
obesity 100, 101
observations 94
oculopharyngeal muscular dystrophy 163
Office for Standards in Education, Children's Services and Skills (Ofsted) 74
organelles 130–1
organisational structures 26–7
osmoregulation 179, 186
ovaries 177, 178
over-extrapolation 49
oxygen saturation 94
pain, signs and symptoms of 95
palliative care 85
pancreas 177, 178
pandemics 31
parasites 144
parathyroids 177
Parkinson's disease 183–4
passive transport 139, 140
pathogens 144–5
    defence against 147
patient safety 125

Index

peer review 49
People and Communities Board (PCB) 77
performance reviews 8
perimenopause 75
person-centred care 93
  6Cs 87–9
  death and dying 85–7
  managing relationships and boundaries 90
  nutrition and hydration 96
  and pre-existing conditions 82
  relevant legislation 71–2, 81
  safeguarding 89
person specifications 29
personal information 51–2, 58
Personalisation Agenda 2012 77
phagocytes and phagocytosis 147
phospholipid bilayer 130, 137, 139–40
physical activity 102, 153
physiological measurements 94, 153
pituitary gland 177, 178
policies 7, 8
  data protection 52
  importance of adhering to 24
polysaccharides 137
positive behaviours 126–7
pre-existing health conditions 18
prevalence 150
Prevent strategy 126
prevention agenda 97
preventive healthcare 17
primary care 16–17
primary research 46, 47
prions 144
private healthcare 15, 22
procedures 7
professional occupations 12–13
professional relationships 90
prokaryotic cells 129
prosthetics 20
proteins 136
protists 144
public health 32–3, 145
qualitative and quantitative data 46–7
quality standards and quality management 9–10
radicalisation 64, 125–6
radioactive decay 155
radiotherapy 197
receptors 152
record keeping 48–9, 57
  reasons for 62–3
  responsibilities 63–4
referral 17, 104

reflex arcs 183
regenerative medicine 23
regulatory bodies 72–4
reliability of data 49
renal system 185–6
  chronic kidney disease 187
repolarisation 182
report line 123
reporting systems 60
reproductive systems 191–2
  endometriosis 194
  role of hormones 192–3
research validity 26
respiratory arrest 43–4
respiratory etiquette 110
respiratory rate 94, 153
respiratory system 170–1
  chronic obstructive pulmonary disease 172
respite care 17
resting potential 182
resuscitation 43–4
revision planning 5
rheumatoid arthritis 162
risk assessment 37–8
RNA (ribonucleic acid) 142–3
robotic surgery 20–1
safeguarding 7, 89, 118
  legislation, policies and procedures 119–20
  reducing chances of abuse 124
  reporting abuse 123
Safeguarding Vulnerable Groups Act 2006 119
scholarships 14
science notation (standard form) 156–7
scope of practice 73
screening 18, 97, 106, 107
secondary care 17
secondary research 47
sedentary lifestyle 102
self-care 84–5
self-management 93
sharing information and data 61–2
sharps disposal 110
SI units 155–6
significant figures 156
signposting 99, 103–4
signs and symptoms 94–5
sinoatrial node (SAN) 166
skeleton 158–9, 160
skin 188–9
  assessment of 94–5
  atopic eczema 189–90
smoking 92, 101, 167, 172

social care services 15, 41
social media use 53–4
social model of disability 82
standard operating procedures (SOPs) 65
statutory training 39
stem cells 131–2
sterilisation 114, 115–16
stock management 68–9
storage of products, materials and equipment 69–70
striated (skeletal) muscle 159–60
substance misuse 102
substrates 138
supply chains 31
surface area to volume ratio 139, 171
synapses 181, 182
systole 166, 167
T cells 147–8
technical occupations 12–13
telesurgery 20–1
temperature 94, 153
temperature control (thermoregulation) 179, 189
tendons 159
tertiary care 17
testes 177, 178
testicular cancer 198–9
thrombosis 168
thyroid 177, 178
thyroid cancer 197
tiered hierarchical organisational structure 27
transmission of pathogens 145
transport mechanisms 140–1
  in small intestine 175
trauma, body's response to 148–9
triage 23
truthfulness 10
tumours 196
units, SI system 155–6
vaccination 18, 97, 107, 148
validity of data 49
veins 164–5
vena cava 164, 165
ventricles 164
villi 174
viruses 144
vulnerable groups 121
waste disposal legislation 36
water potential 179, 186
wearable devices 23
wellbeing, promotion of 92–3
whistleblowing 64, 124
working environments 16